Speech, Language, Learning, and the African American Child

Jean E. v.
San Francisco State University

Gloria Toliver Weddington
San Jose State University

Charles E. DeBose
California State University, Hayward

Allyn and Bacon
Boston • London • Toronto • Sydney • Tokyo • Singapore

Executive Editor: Stephen D. Dragin
Editorial Assistant: Elizabeth McGuire
Editorial-Production Administrator: Joe Sweeney
Editorial-Production Service: Walsh & Associates, Inc.
Composition Buyer: Linda Cox
Manufacturing Buyer: David Suspanic
Cover Administrator: Suzanne Harbison

Internet: www.abacon.com
America Online: keyword: College Online

Library of Congress Cataloging-in-Publication Data

van Keulen, Jean E.
   Speech, language, learning, and the African American child / Jean
E. van Keulen, Gloria T. Weddington, Charles E. DeBose.
     p.   cm.
   Includes bibliographical references and index.
   ISBN 0-205-15268-6
   1. Afro-American children—Language. 2. Afro-American children—
Education—Language arts. 3. Speech and social status—United
States. 4. Black English—United States. I. Weddington, Gloria
T.   . II. DeBose, Charles E.   . III. Title.
PE3102.N42V36   1997
420′.896073—dc21   97-28228
                                                CIP

Printed in the United States of America

10 9 8 7 6 5 4 3 2 1   01 00 99 98 97

To African American Children

*You are empowered, not by becoming something
different, but by being what you are.
Discover your power and partake
in the excitement and
celebration
called
life*

CONTENTS

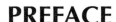

PREFACE

Students in a class on elementary education had just heard a tape-recorded sample of what is commonly known as Black English. Some of them expressed surprise at what they heard: "I've heard that many times," several of them exclaimed, "but I always thought it was just 'bad English.' I didn't realize that it was a language."

The misconception that some African Americans speak "bad" or "incorrect" English—indeed, that there is such a thing as better and worse types of language—is refuted in the first part of this book. The second part focuses on the difference between normal and pathological speech-language in order to support the need for adequate means of assessing speech-language disorders in children of diverse backgrounds. The third part deals with the crucial question of how teachers are to deal with African American language in the classroom.

The overlapping domains of race, language, culture, and ethnicity are introduced in a section entitled, "By Way of Introduction: Race, Culture, Ethnicity, and African American English, which includes a discussion of the way that ethnicity may color the reactions of members of a multicultural society to a variety of language spoken by a stigmatized cultural group. This section begins on page xv.

Chapter 1 surveys the main issues covered and the different fields of academic study that inform the issues at hand.

Chapter 2, "Descriptive versus Prescriptive Grammar," introduces the reader to the important difference between the everyday use of the term grammar and the more precise and technical way that it is used in linguistics, a distinction that is crucial to understanding the validity of attributing to African American English its own system of grammar.

In Chapter 3, "African American Bilingualism," the language situation in Black America is described as a case of societal bilingualism in which African

American English coexists with Standard English in the African American linguistic repertoire.

Chapter 4, "African American English as a Linguistic System," provides a succinct overview of recent work from an Afrocentric perspective that describes African American language as a coherent system containing continuities of patterns that are common to the languages of West Africa.

Chapter 5 focuses on the general communication process and how African American communication styles differ from the dominant American culture. Six psychological themes, oral literature, and expressive patterns of African American communication styles are discussed, as well as the impact of culture on intercultural communication and situational context on code-switching.

The focus of Chapter 6 is the differences between speech-language disorders and African American language. Definitions of speech-language disorders are provided along with causation, and manifestations are presented.

Chapter 7 examines the current practices of assessment of speech and language disorders and presents recommendations for improved assessment of speech and language of African American children. A number of assessment techniques are described and evaluated as well as suggestions for communicating assessment results to parents and teachers.

Chapter 8 examines educational practices in today's schools and problems associated with cultural insensitivity by examiners. Culture and language differences are discussed as related to assessment of African American children and significant court decisions regarding linguistic rights of Black children. Alternative assessment approaches are presented that link assessment and instruction and the multiple intelligence theory that pluralizes the traditional concept of intelligence.

Chapter 9 offers suggestions for treating speech and language disorders in African American children with additional recommendations for teaching mainstream American English to Black children. Teachers are encouraged to use the skills and knowledge about linguistic diversity of the speech-language pathologists in the schools to assist them with developing strategies and lessons that teach mainstream American English in a positive fashion.

Chapter 10 describes the differences between language acquisition and language learning and suggests effective ways to teach mainstream American English to Black children. In addition, a case is made for using foreign language teaching methods when working with African American English speakers.

Chapter 11 highlights and discusses cultural and social variables that interfere with African American students' learning and academic success. In addition, the problem of overrepresentation of African American children in special education classes is discussed with the factors that contribute to this problem. The concept of cultural discontinuity between home and school is explained and how this phenomenon contributes to cultural clashes between teachers and students in the classroom. Psychosocial and cultural variables that contribute to educational inequities and prejudice by teachers are also identified with suggestions for change.

Chapter 12 focuses on African American children's language and literacy in the home and school. This chapter contains information that relates specifically to a recurring debate relative to African American students' language, mainstream American English, and teaching reading. Culture and language variations of African American children are discussed in this chapter, and a literacy framework that is characterized by an interactional process is presented as another approach to the education of culturally diverse students.

Chapter 13 discusses in depth how teachers and parents can empower or disempower African American children. Particular attention is given to ways teachers and parents can enhance pride and empowerment of African American children by developing positive self-esteem and self-discipline. Major emphasis is placed on the importance of love, interaction praise, modeling, encouragement, predictability, and consistency of parents of African American children.

ACKNOWLEDGMENTS

My special thanks and appreciation to my husband, Jacobus van Keulen, and children, Nichole and Obak, for their love, inspiration, and support. JVK

I am grateful for the patience and encouragement from my husband Donald Weddington and daughter Derika. GTW

A few of the many persons who helped and encouraged me in this work, whom I need to acknowledge, include my wife Jacqueline, mother Marie DeBose, my sons, Fred and Charles, Nick Faraclas, Patricia Gardner, Felton Gardner, Marlow Gardner, Jo McNeal, Bill DeBose, Elijah DeBose, Don Bankston, Renee DeBose, Patricia Jones, Cora Aleem, Sam DeBose, and Paul DeBose.

Grateful acknowledgment is also extended to those authors and publishers whose works have been incorporated into our own. Special appreciation is extended to the reviewers for their time and comments:

Owen Boyle, San Jose State University
Alvirda Farmer, San Jose State University
Marion Meyerson, San Jose State University
Stanley Goldberg, San Francisco State University
Thalia Coleman, Appalachian State University
Shirley Thornton, California State University, Sacramento

These individuals read the manuscript and offered vital comments and suggestions.

BY WAY OF INTRODUCTION

Race, Culture, Ethnicity, and African American English

In recent years a large body of academic literature has developed on the language of African Americans that counters traditional misconceptions of it as "bad," "incorrect," or "substandard" English. Largely due to the influence of such linguistic work, attitudes of educators toward African American English (AAE) have begun to change, and school districts have begun to modify their policies toward AAE in ways that are discussed below. In the 1970s, linguists involved in the study of AAE based on tape-recorded data began to use the term Black English (Dillard 1972). Those linguists were, for the most part, not African Americans, and there was a noticeable tendency for their work to focus upon those aspects of African American speech data that differed markedly from European-American dialects of English. Such studies of African American language may be fairly criticized for the fact that they do not contribute to the description of the linguistic competence of native speakers, but rather to the description of their linguistic ethnicity.

Although linguists insist that African American language is systematic and rule-governed, they may have contributed to the perpetuation of negative stereotypes of it by describing "Black English" as a list of features corresponding to the lack or absence of something that is normally present in European-American English. Recent work from an Afrocentric perspective describes African American language as a coherent system containing continuities of patterns that are common to the languages of West Africa.

POLICY OPTIONS

The material presented in the following pages provides the technical basis for recognition of African American language as a legitimate linguistic system, and that, in turn, has implications for the kind of educational policies and classroom practices that are most suitable for American education in general and for AAE speakers in particular. The reader should gain sufficient understanding of the nature of African American language to make an informed decision as to what degree of recognition he or she is willing to extend to it.

The set of policy options available to educators for dealing with African American language in the classroom may be seen as points on a continuum (Figure 1).

SUPPRESSION _____ LIMITED RECOGNITION _____ FULL RECOGNITION

FIGURE 1   Policy options for dealing with African American English.

At one extreme we find the option of *suppression,* that is, the idea that children should be prohibited from speaking African American language, and teachers should gear instruction toward its eradication. At the other extreme, educators may opt for a policy of *full recognition,* one that acknowledges the intrinsic worth of all human language. A policy of full recognition of African American language treats it as a bona fide language, equal in principle to Spanish, Russian, Swahili, and other recognized languages. Somewhere between the two extremes advocates may accept a policy that in some way extends *limited recognition* to African American language.

Few educators can be found who favor total suppression or full and unqualified recognition of African American language. Some educators, however, who would not deliberately pursue a policy of suppression might unknowingly behave in a way that has the same practical consequences. It may involve such innocuous acts as using an inappropriate and scientifically inaccurate term such as "substandard" in reference to salient features of a child's natural language, or calling attention to children's language in a manner that shames or makes fun of them in front of their peers.

Many educators are sufficiently aware of recent scholarship to accept, as an abstract principle, the idea that there is nothing wrong with African American language. Some are reluctant, nevertheless, for practical reasons, to support a policy of full recognition. A good example of such ambivalence is found in a statement by Burling (1973):

> *The policy of full acceptance of the dialect should appeal to our sense of democracy. We may feel that each man should be allowed to speak in his own way and that no child should be handicapped by having to divert his atten-*

tion from other subjects while coping with a new spoken style. But the dangers of this policy are obvious. It is doubtful that even the most splendidly educated young man or woman will find employment if he continues to speak the language of the Black ghetto. (p. 132)

The assumption that monodialectalism limits the employment prospects of speakers of African American language is frequently cited in arguments against full recognition. Such arguments tend to be couched in references to "the real world." Following the above cited passage, Burling goes on to state that "the practical if unjust world demands the standard dialect" (Burling 1973, p. 132).

Most practitioners and scholars who have taken a position on the issue have favored some degree of limited recognition of African American language. The policy of limited recognition differs from the traditional policy of suppression in that the traditional policy aims to instill standard language while eradicating the dialect, whereas the policy of limited recognition seeks to foster *bidialectalism.* That is, advocates of limited recognition consider it desirable to allow dialect speakers to maintain their home and community language while acquiring standard English proficiency and learning to switch from one variety to the other when the occasion demands.

Linguists acting as expert witnesses in the landmark *Martin Luther King Junior Elementary School, et al., v. Ann Arbor School District Board* Black English decision, rendered in 1979 by the United States District Court of Eastern Michigan, contributed to a judicial basis for a policy of limited recognition. The presiding judge in that case found that teachers at Martin Luther King Junior Elementary School in Ann Arbor had failed to teach plaintiff Black children to read and ordered the Ann Arbor School District to provide inservice training to help teachers to teach in a way that takes the children's home and community language, Black English, into account (Baugh 1995; Chambers 1983).

The recognition extended to African American language by Ann Arbor–King is limited in that the decision explicitly states that standard English is the language of "Government, Education, Business and the Arts" while "Black English" is identified as an acceptable code only for use in the plaintiff children's homes and in the African American community. The Ann Arbor–King decision is discussed further in later chapters.

Members of the American Speech and Hearing Association (ASHA) have taken a formal position on the Black English issue, expressing their view that bidialectalism should be the goal of practitioners working with Black English speakers (Committee on the Status of Racial Minorities 1983). The ASHA position is discussed further later in this book. Similar positions have been taken by other professional organizations.

The authors of this book are sympathetic to advocates of the kind of limited recognition of African American language represented by the Ann Arbor decision and the ASHA position paper and are not themselves in full agreement on the question of what should be done about African American language. Rather than advocate any particular policy option, we have decided to help readers decide for themselves by comparing and contrasting the various options and their implications for classroom practice.

The policy of full recognition is in many ways the most consistent and the most democratic. It is often put down, however, as unworkable because it is politically unacceptable to the majority of American citizens. There is considerable merit, nonetheless, in a policy that derives logically from the linguistically sound premise that there is nothing wrong with African American language.

The particular issue of what should be done about African American language is related to the more general question of how American society should accommodate its various racial, cultural, and ethnic groups. To fully understand the formulation and evolution of such policies in the United States, it is necessary to look at two separate spheres of activity: one pertaining to the accommodation of groups by race, the other pertaining to groups of immigrants and their descendants. Before considering those issues, let us establish exactly what we mean by race, in order to distinguish it adequately from the similar and overlapping notions of culture and ethnicity.

Race

The terms "Black English," "African American language," and so on are misleading in that they suggest that speaking Black English is a consequence of belonging to the Black race. Many Americans who belong to the Black race are not culturally African Americans and would not be expected to speak African American language. There is always great variation among members of a cultural group in the extent to which specific traits of that culture occur in particular individuals. Some African Americans speak African American language more than others, and some may not speak it at all. Furthermore, language is acquired through participation in social networks, and there is nothing, in principle, to prevent any person of any race from acquiring any language. In fact, a Caucasian child raised in an African American community may become a speaker of African American language.

Race, in the sense of variation in skin color and certain other genetically transmitted characteristics, is a universal of human experience. The social significance of race varies greatly from one society to another, however, and the majority of humankind is difficult to classify into one of the five traditional racial categories: Negroid, Caucasoid, Mongoloid, Malayan, and Native

American (Bennett 1990). In some societies, the color of one's skin is of no more significance than the size of one's ears. In other societies, race may be one of several criteria used for assigning members to higher or lower, more or less powerful, status.

In the United States, race was formerly used to determine one's place in a system of color caste in that members of the dominant White race enjoyed privileges that were denied to members of the subordinate Black race. Although Black persons presently enjoy equal status with Whites before the law, the remnants of the historical color caste system are manifest in continuing *de facto* segregation in residential patterns, school attendance, and statistical disparities in income, education, employment, and other indicators of the quality of life.

Americans tend to automatically "see" persons as belonging to one race or another, that is, as White or non-White. Many Black Americans look so White, however, that, were their African ancestry not known, they could "pass" for a White person. To be classified Black in American society, a person does not have to look Black, but only to have some degree of Black ancestry. Despite the historical separation of the races in the United States and the existence of laws against interracial marriage, miscegenation has been common and has resulted in numerous persons of mixed racial descent in the Black population.

Many individuals may be seen in the United States who look Black but consider themselves (and are in fact) something else. Many Puerto Ricans, for instance, have dark skin and hair of a texture that is common to Black Americans. So do many Filipinos and persons from the Middle East. They often come from societies, however, in which race does not have the same social significance that it has in the United States, and they often differ greatly from Black Americans in language and culture.

Finally, it should be noted that there are Americans who consider themselves Black, but are of a different culture than African Americans. Certain recent immigrants from African or Caribbean countries or elsewhere in the African Diaspora are Black in race but not African American in culture. Some children of African descent born in the United States are not culturally African American because of the fact that they were raised by non-African American parents. The African American child, therefore, is defined primarily not by genetic race, and not by African ancestry, but by culture.

Culture

In the following discussion we shall use a definition of culture that is based on characteristics of the social situation. Individuals carry into social situations certain expectations based on their previous experiences regarding particular behaviors. For instance, persons they encounter are expected to dress, eat, and act a particular way. Behavior that conforms to such expectations is within the bounds of those individuals' culture.

A simple definition of a *social situation* that may be adequate for present purposes is the following: a time, a place, a set of objects, and set of role relationships that go together, that is, that are congruent. For example, in a scenario, the time might be Wednesday; the place, a room on the sixth floor of the World Trade Center; objects might be present such as a desk, chairs, and file cabinets; and two persons are conversing in the roles of applicant and interviewer. We have just listed some of the essential ingredients of the job interview situation. An individual in that situation wearing a bathrobe would seem out of place. The situation would be rendered incongruent by the inappropriate attire of one of the participants.

Fishman (1972) gives contrasting hypothetical examples of situations, such as those in Figure 2, in which the essential parameters of time, place, and role relationship go together, that is, they are *congruent*. If any of the parameters don't fit, the situation is said to be *incongruent*.

Fishman's examples illustrate the fact that in congruent situations, everything is as expected according to the norms of the culture and tends to go unnoticed, as when a parishioner and priest meet on Sunday morning at church. It is normal and expected and deserves no comment or attention. When a situation is incongruent, however, as when the same parishioner and priest might meet at the race track on a Saturday afternoon, there is something unusual or unexpected about one of the situational parameters, which causes surprise and draws attention.

We acknowledge the existence of unique cultures, not only for the American groups that maintain the customs of a different country after migrating to the United States, but also for various groups of American citizens differ-

ROLE RELATIONSHIP	TIME	PLACE
Boss, Secretary		
CONGRUENT	Monday 11:00 AM	Office
INCONGRUENT	Saturday 11:00 PM	Office
Priest, Parishioner		
CONGRUENT	Sunday 8:00 AM	Church
INCONGRUENT	Saturday 3:00 PM	Race Track

FIGURE 2   Congruent and incongruent situations.

entiated by region, class, race, or religion. Cultural traits frequently spread beyond group boundaries.

An important part of every culture is language. We are expected to talk a certain way and use a particular language or set of languages. We judge one another on the basis of how we speak. African American language and culture have greatly influenced general American culture in the past and continue to do so. There are Americans of various cultural backgrounds who have acquired African American language, and there is no barrier in principle to anyone of any race or culture acquiring African American language. Many African Americans are bicultural and are at ease in situations dominated by European American culture, as well as in situations governed by African American cultural norms. When we discuss African American language in the following chapters, it should be understood at all times that our claims apply specifically to a component of African American culture.

Policy Toward American Minority Groups

Immigrant groups traditionally strove to assimilate to the dominant culture of the United Sates, and those of European descent at least were encouraged to do so. The melting pot came to symbolize the typically positive experiences of European immigrant groups in pursuing and attaining social acceptance and upward mobility. The efforts of non-White groups, especially African Americans, to gain acceptance and prosper economically were frequently stifled by prejudice, discrimination, and hatred. Such groups came to represent the limits of the melting pot ethos: the realization that certain groups do not "melt."

During the Civil Rights Movement of the 1960s and 1970s, the policy debate over the place of African Americans tended to be cast in terms of segregation versus integration, and the melting pot ethos was sometimes appropriated by advocates of the integration option. It is interesting to note that the status of African American language was not an issue in the Civil Rights debate. The race of Black people was the overriding consideration in how they were treated, and it hardly mattered how much or little Blackness was apparent in their speech. African Americans striving for integration were probably as willing to assimilate linguistically as European immigrants had been. Eventually, however, following the lead of groups such as the Nation of Islam, Black Americans opted in increasing numbers for some form of *Black Nationalism* and appropriated symbols of traditional African culture. As linguistic symbols, however, they were more likely to adopt an African language such as Swahili than their native African American language.

As we view the policy debate over African American language in a larger sociopolitical context, it is noteworthy that European immigrants, as part of their assimilation, shifted from a foreign language to foreign-accented English to native-like English. In the case of African Americans, a similar shift occurred from the African languages spoken by many of their earliest ancestors to African-influenced English, that is, African American language. Many, if not most, African Americans remain to the present day only partially assimilated, linguistically and otherwise. Their path to full assimilation appears to be blocked by the lack of opportunities for mobility upward and out of the predominantly Black enclaves where African American language flourishes. The *de facto* segregation, which persists into the 1990s, virtually guarantees the continued transmission of African American language to new generations of children, and educators have to recognize this fact. Anyone who wants to pursue a policy of suppression of African American language should understand that such a policy is not likely to succeed unless African American children attend racially integrated schools and grow up in racially integrated neighborhoods.

In the latter stages of the Civil Rights Movement, the demands of African Americans shifted away from integration and toward *power* and *identity*. Solidarity was expressed through slogans such as "Black Power" and "Black Is Beautiful." Other groups picked up the themes of the Black Movement and called for recognition and empowerment for themselves. Not only ethnic groups such as Chicanos, but also women, gays, and "grays" began to juxtapose the word for their group with the word "power." Out of this development, a new *cultural pluralism* model for the accommodation of American groups emerged to rival the melting pot ethos.

Within the context of competing policies for the accommodation of American cultural groups, the debate over educational policy toward African American language takes on new meaning. The slogan "Black Is Beautiful" implies that all dimensions of African American identity, including African American language, are beautiful. To that extent, there is nothing wrong with it. If there is indeed nothing wrong with it, it seems that a fair and equitable policy would call upon educators to just leave it alone. By advocating a policy of full recognition of African American language, educators might imply the additional message—intentionally or not—that they favor some form of cultural pluralism. Whether one subscribes to cultural pluralism or not, however, the linguistic evidence explored in the following pages strongly supports the full recognition of African American language.

The policy of full recognition is also consistent with the fact that African American language is part of African American culture. In acknowledging the existence of a unique African American culture among certain Americans of African descent (Hale-Benson 1986), we do not claim that African Americans have retained their ancestral African cultures intact. Black Americans have obviously assimilated a great deal of European American culture, beginning with the English language (Levine 1977). Much of what is considered "soul food"—black-eyed peas, cornbread, grits—is not clearly distinguishable from southern food, and the religious and secular music traditions of African

Americans contain a great deal in common with the musical traditions of White Americans.

Clear evidence of African influences can be found in many tangible aspects of present-day African American life, including words such as *okra*, *gumbo*, and *jazz* (Dillard 1972); a rich oral tradition of songs, stories, toasts; characteristic modes of expression such as signifying and playing the dozens (Gates 1988; Goss & Barnes 1989); and the ubiquitous call-and-response pattern of Black performances (Asante 1987). Black culture also has intangible aspects expressed through such elusive conceptualizations as "world view" and "lifestyle" (DuBois 1961). A more extended discussion of African American culture is presented in Chapter 5. Persons who might feel that there is something wrong with African American language and call for its eradication on that basis might be reluctant to subscribe to the premise that there is something wrong with African American culture. Such individuals might be convinced that there is really nothing wrong with African American language by evidence that it is indeed an integral part of African American culture. Making such a point can sometimes be clouded, however, by the way the cultural traits are sometimes perceived as ethnicity.

ETHNICITY

In the early 1980s, an incident occurred in San Francisco, California that serves to illustrate the nature of ethnicity. An African American female reporter was promoted to the position of anchor for the evening news on a local television station and served with distinction until being abruptly terminated. The cause for her termination was widely speculated to be the fact that she appeared in the anchor spot one evening wearing her hair in braids.

In the years directly following the Civil Rights Movement, many Black women adopted a style of tightly braided hair known traditionally as "cornrows," because of the manner in which the braids were aligned, leaving rows of visible scalp between, in the manner of rows of corn in a field. The cornrows hairstyle had become so popular that it had crossed cultural lines and became known as the "Bo Derek look" after the actress who helped to popularize it in a role that she played in the movie "10." In spite of its popularity, however, the television station management apparently found in the act of wearing such braids in the anchor spot grounds for dismissal. What was wrong with the act, we submit, was the inherent ethnicity of the cornrows hairstyle.

The reporter in question is now employed by a local radio station, and her hairstyle is irrelevant to her job performance. One might suspect that she wanted the greater freedom of expression of her ethnicity that the radio medium allowed, because the consequence of her flagrant display of ethnicity on the TV screen was predictable. The cornrows hairstyle was part of a general upsurge of cultural awareness among African Americans that tended to be associated in the popular mind with militant advocacy of political demands that many White persons viewed as extreme. The denial of employment opportunity is just one of a host of predictable reactions to ethnicity.

Many of us have had personal experiences with ethnicity, but if pressed to define it, would have a hard time pinning down exactly what it is. Clearly it has something to do with culture, but what? Are the terms ethnicity and culture synonymous? One way to approach the definition of ethnicity is to examine its relationship to the concepts of *ethnic group*, and *ethnic identity*. Following such an approach, once we have defined ethnic group, we may proceed to enumerate the kinds of traits that, in general terms, contribute to the identity of such a group. We may then use the traits that comprise ethnic identity as a basis for the definition of ethnicity.

Milton Gordon (cited in Bennett 1990) defines an ethnic group in very general terms as a social group distinguished "by race, religion, or national origin" (p. 39). One problem with such a broad definition is the implication that everyone has the same degree of ethnicity. The points we want to make about ethnicity in this section imply that ethnicity is a potentially variable quality. Some persons have more of it than others. Bennett defines ethnic group more specifically as " . . . a group of people within a larger society that is socially distinguished or set apart, by others and/or by itself, primarily on the basis of racial and/or cultural characteristics, such as religion, language, and tradition" (p. 39).

Unlike the more general definition, Bennett's definition emphasizes the notion of being "set apart." This definition satisfies the sense that ethnicity is variable. Others may decide to set apart for special treatment, or special status within a social order, certain persons who manifest the characteristics by which a particular ethnic group is identified. The members of the "set apart" group, according to this definition, have ethnicity, but members of the "others" group do not. Members of the "set apart" group may chose to reject the special status imposed upon them by others and, in so doing, suppress some or all of the traits that establish their ethnic identity.

Bennett's definition enumerates some of the traits that comprise ethnic identity: racial features, religion, and language. Religion and language, of course, are two specific examples of cultural traits. One problem with Bennett's definition of ethnic group is that it does not clearly show how ethnicity differs from culture. If ethnic identity is made up of ethnic traits, how do such traits differ from cultural traits?

It was stated above that culture consists of a set of expectations regarding what is normal behavior within a particular social context. We can think of many instances, however, in which a person who dresses, speaks, or otherwise behaves according to the norms of his or her culture would not be considered to have ethnicity. A man walking down a street in the financial district of San Francisco dressed in conventional business attire would probably not be thought of as ethnic, although such attire is an integral part of his culture. Another person, however, walking in the same area wearing a turban might be seen as ethnic.

To get to the heart of how ethnicity differs from culture, we might imagine the above mentioned turban wearer in a different place, say, a public market in Bombay, India. In that situation, there might be many people similarly outfitted with turbans, and such attire might be normal and expected there. In fact, the situation might be the reverse of what we would imagine in the United States. A person wearing western business attire might be as unusual in some places in India as a person wearing a turban would be in downtown San Francisco. In such places, western dress might be seen as ethnic. In order for an aspect of culture to be considered ethnic, therefore, it apparently must occur in a situation in which it is unusual and unexpected.

When the traits by which a people are identified are viewed from the perspective of others, they are seen as ethnic. Attention is drawn to those very traits that differ markedly from corresponding traits of our own group, be they physical traits such as skin color and hair texture, or cultural traits such as an exotic hairstyle. The cornrows hairstyle thought to have prompted the dismissal of the above-mentioned reporter from her job as a TV anchor meets both of the key criteria of ethnicity: It is a trait of African American culture and it was presented in a situation in which it was unusual and unexpected.

The concept of situational congruity, introduced above, can be applied to the phenomenon of ethnicity. Fishman's examples of incongruent situations—the parishioner and priest at the race track—consist of elements from a single culture. What makes them incongruent is an unusual or unexpected combination of such elements. Although all the elements belong to the right culture, they occur at an unexpected time and place. Ethnicity may be seen as a special case of situational incongruity in which the background elements belong to one culture (X), and the foreground element(s) belong to another culture (Y). In the incident of the cornrows-wearing reporter, the combination of elements from mainstream American culture with elements of African American culture produced an incongruent situation.

African American Language and Ethnicity

In Chapter 3, it is shown that African American language coexists with standard English in the linguistic repertoire of the African American speech community. The occurrence of African American language in such Black cultural events as family gatherings, church meetings, and streetcorner verbal duels is normal and expected. The language of participants is congruent with other situational elements and goes unnoticed. The occurrence of African American language in situations dominated by mainstream American culture, however, is not congruent with other situational elements and fits the definition of ethnicity as the incongruent co-occurrence of elements of different cultures.

Linguistic Features of African American English

There are many commonalties in the English of Black and White Americans, but there are also many points of contrast. Where White Americans would be expected, for example, to say *she's nice*, an African American might say *she nice*. The AAE sentence *she nice* is grammatical in African American language; the reason for this will be made clear in Chapter 2. Labov (1969) wrote an influential paper in which he gave the name "copula deletion" to the tendency for present tense forms of *be* to be absent in African American language where such forms are expected to occur in standard English, e.g., *they at home; we recordin' live*.

The term copula deletion is typical of a marked tendency to label the features of African American language in negative terms. One such feature frequently mentioned in the literature is referred to as "final consonant cluster simplification" (Labov 1972, p. 15). It is used to account for the fact that the final consonant expected in the standard English (SE) pronunciation of words such as *test*, *desk*, *find*, and *told* are frequently not present in African American language. Other Black English (BE) features given negative labels in the literature are "r-lessness," (Labov 1972, p.13) and "l-lessness" (p. 14).

Other features of African American language that have attracted the attention of linguists include the tendency of some African American speakers to pronounce words with the sounds represented by *th* in standard English. A full account of this feature indicates that at the beginning of words, the *voiced interdental fricative* found in words like *this* and *that* tends to be pronounced as /d/. In the middle or at the end of words, the *labiodental* sounds /f/ and /v/ tend to occur in African American speech where the SE interdental *th* sounds would be expected, for example, *bruvver*, "brother"; *mouf*, "mouth."

Two grammatical features of AAE frequently mentioned in the literature are the verb suffixes *-s* and *-ed* (Fasold & Wolfram 1970; Wolfram 1969). It is common in Black speech for a verb to occur with a third person singular subject without the *-s* suffix,—for example, *she make me sick*—and it is common for the *-s* suffix to occur on verbs with non-third person singular subjects, such as *I gets home early*. Verbs frequently occur in BE sentences without the *-ed* suffix where it would be expected in SE, for example, *we pick apples yesterday*.

Other features that have been noted as characteristic of the speech of African Americans includes a feature known variously as "habitual *be*" or "invariant *be*" (Fasold 1969; Labov 1972; Stewart 1966). This feature accounts for the occurrence of *be* in African American language directly following the subject in sentences with "habitual" meaning. The sentence *I be busy*, for example, communicates that the speaker is in the habit of being busy on particular occasions. It does not mean that the speaker is presently busy.

The above-mentioned linguistic features and others do indeed occur in the speech of African Americans, but such a list of features, no matter how complete, does not offer an adequate account of the language of African Americans. In fact, it can render a disservice by describing African American language in negative terms, as the absence of elements that are expected to be present in European-American English. The representation of African American English by lists of features reinforces the tendency to apply a deficit model to African American English and behavior and negate the existence of a distinct African American culture. Such a description, focusing on points of divergence between AAE and the dialects familiar to White researchers, is not an adequate account of the internalized linguistic competence of AAE speakers, but a description of the linguistic ethnicity and culture of Black Americans.

The Ethnic Identity of African Americans

Before we further develop the view of African American language as a part of ethnicity, it will be useful to see how it fits into an overall conception of the ethnic identity of African Americans. We develop such a conception by noting various specific ways in which African Americans tend to differ from Whites, either in their physical appearance or in their cultural behavior. We will consider each such specific point of contrast an ethnic trait and consider the totality of such traits an ideal conception of African American ethnic identity. It is important to stress that the conception is an idealization, or sociotype (Bennett 1990), and individual members of the group differ greatly in the extent to which they manifest any particular trait.

The main physical traits that contribute to the conception of African American ethnic identity are skin color and hair texture. The characteristic dark pigmentation of the Negroid race contrasts with the lack of such pigmentation by Caucasians in a way that causes it to be noticed in settings in which the norms of White culture prevail. Such is also the case with the occurrence of hair of the coarse, or kinky, texture prevalent among persons of African ancestry in White culture. Camera technicians in the movie and television industries are frequently at a loss for effective ways of lighting backgrounds to clearly record the facial features of Black subjects. Barber shops and beauty salons in the United States continue to operate under racially segregated conditions, not so much out of a desire of the operators or patrons to be exclusive or discriminatory, but due to the lack of knowledge of the special characteristics of hair that departs from the relatively straight and fine texture of White hair. Other biological traits that contribute to African American ethnic identity are lip thickness and breadth of the nose.

Many cultural behaviors (as opposed to physical traits) are shared by Black and White Americans, but there are also many ways in which African Americans behave differently from their White compatriots sufficiently to be perceived as African American ethnicity by White people. We have already mentioned several such differences, including linguistic features, and will discuss them further as examples of the claim that there are predictable reactions to ethnicity. Having established that African American language is a component of African American ethnic identity, we may assume that the same kinds of reactions that predictably occur to ethnicity in general may occur in response to African American language in particular.

Predictable Reactions to Ethnicity

Having made the point that African American language is a component of the ethnic identity of African Americans, we may turn directly to the thesis that there are predictable reactions to ethnicity. A list of examples of predictable reactions to ethnicity supported by common experience is presented in Table 1. It is not intended to be exhaustive.

One of the most common reactions to ethnicity is the formation of stereotypes. As members of culture Y accumulate experiences with members of culture X, they begin to associate those traits of culture X to all future encounters with members of that culture. For example, after encountering several Black persons who dance well, a White American might form the general expectation, or stereotype, that all African Americans are good dancers. Another example is Labov's description of the behavior of the copula verb *be* in African American language (1969). He is careful to indicate that some speakers "delete" the copula more frequently than others, and he shows that the variation in the rate of "deletion" by individual speakers is statistically

TABLE 1 Predictable Reactions to Ethnicity

1. Stereotypes
2. Humor
3. Fascination
4. Fear
5. Discomfort
6. Embarrassment
7. Self-hate
8. Cultural appropriation

correlated with a variety of factors besides race, including age and various indicators of socioeconomic status. Although Labov's description is not a stereotype, a less skillful observer might derive a stereotype of Black language from the same linguistic facts. Labov clearly did not intend for the public to gain from his research the generalization that African Americans sentences lack present tense forms of the verb *be*, but the danger certainly exists.

To illustrate the predictability of humor as a reaction to certain types of ethnicity, one only needs to consider how effective ethnic jokes have been in our culture. The success of the popular 1950s radio show "Amos 'n' Andy" exemplifies the predictable humorous reaction a stereotypical imitation of Black language is likely to evoke. The character George "Kingfish" Stevens almost always used the form *is* regardless of the person or the subject—*we is . . . , you is . . . .* Although the use of *is* without standard subject-verb agreement may be observed in real African American language data, it is a variable trait that many speakers seldom or never exhibit. Its exaggerated presence in the language of one of the "Amos 'n' Andy" characters was extremely effective in evoking humorous reactions and reinforcing stereotypes.

Many examples could be given of the way that ethnicity sometimes elicits a reaction of fascination with the ethnic culture. African Americans probably do not mind being stereotyped as good dancers, superb athletes, or gifted musicians as much as they mind negative stereotypes of themselves, and it is such complimentary stereotypes that often evoke reactions of fascination. When historically Black colleges utilize their marching bands and choruses in effective fund-raising efforts, their success may be seen as a predictable fascination with African American music.

A good example of the fear that Black ethnicity sometimes elicits is the effectiveness of the notorious "Willie Horton" commercials utilized during the 1988 Presidential campaign. The stereotype underlying the Willie Horton message is clearly that of the violent street criminal who will commit merciless acts of rape, mugging, and aggravated assault on his victims. Television dramas often portray crime and violence and frequently employ African American male actors to play street hoodlum and violent criminal roles. Such casting decisions are probably influenced partly, consciously or unconsciously, by the fear that tends to be evoked by the perception of certain forms of African American ethnicity.

In an age of increasing concern with political correctness, certain forms of ethnicity might produce a different reaction than would have been expected to occur in our traditional culture. The kind of comedy routines that were hilarious to Americans of all races who listened to "Amos 'n' Andy" might produce a variety of different reactions today. In fact, the television version of the "Amos 'n' Andy" show, after some initial success, was taken off the air in response to protests of the NAACP and others that it was portraying demeaning stereotypes. A university class viewing a documentary of the history of the "Amos 'n' Andy" show reacted in embarrassed silence to excerpts from the show. They might have been amused, but they did not want to incur the risk of laughing at such blatant stereotypes.

A milder reaction to ethnicity than outright embarrassment is discomfort. Consider, for example, how the behavior of participants in certain African American worship services might be perceived by European American visitors. The European American may be accustomed to sitting still on a pew, listening quietly, reverently, and serenely to a preacher who stands behind the pulpit and speaks to a motionless congregation. They might also be used to observing a choir singing while standing straight and moving only their mouths and vocal chords. Such a person might feel somewhat uncomfortable in the emotionally charged atmosphere of the Black worship service, where the preacher is supported by a faithful Amen Corner with steady shouts of *sho nuff, fix it, that's right*, and other indicators that he is preaching well. The choir will sway and rock to the music, unlike the staid choristers to which the European American visitors are accustomed.

There are less obvious predictable reactions to ethnicity, the mention of just two of which will suffice at this time: self-hate and cultural appropriation. As an example of self-hate, consider the use of the term "bad hair" by a curly-haired person in reference to curly hair. Or consider the designation of language replete with *you ises* "bad English" by someone who says *you is*. As an example of cultural appropriation, consider the emergence of rock music through the performance of African American rhythm and blues material by White artists such as Elvis Presley, Pat Boone, and the Beatles. The "Amos 'n' Andy" show might also be seen as cultural appropriation insofar as its White creators Freeman Godsen and Charles Correl relied upon their ability to manipulate dialectal English in such a way as to produce convincing voice representations of comic Black characters.

The academic interest in African American English that has emerged over the years seems to have drawn impetus, in part, from the fascination of mainstream linguists with the ethnicity of African American language. It is understandable how some scholars might have capitalized on the fascination that African American language tends to evoke in order to advance their career. Scholars who engage in the study of cultural phenomena need to be fully aware, however, that the ethnicity of certain topics of academic research may serve as a source of bias in the research product. We are hopefully beyond the time when many scholars were comfortable advocating a "thick lips" theory (Dillard 1972, p. 230) to account for the unique characteristics of African American language. Some reflection on the present state of affairs may be sufficient to confirm how pervasive Eurocentric biases continue to be in the curricula of American schools and colleges.

IMPLICATIONS FOR PRACTITIONERS

Educators responsible for the training of teachers and other practitioners to work with African American children should be cautioned against a "cook book" approach to providing information about the cultural traits of ethnic groups. There is a fine line of distinction between the authentic description of ethnic traits, the idealized portrayal of sociotypes for academic purposes, and the propagation of stereotypes. Well-meaning efforts to disseminate accurate information can result in clumsy attempts to be sensitive in a multicultural setting, which can backfire.

When practitioners look for information on the language of African Americans, with the aim of becoming more sensitive to cultural differences, the available information tends to be presented as lists of features. Although unintended by the authors of the research reports, the practitioners often derive from the information stereotypes such as African Americans pronounce standard English words such as *mouth* with an *f* in the place of the standard English *th*—for example, *teef*, "teeth"; *bof*, "both." Some zealous practitioners armed with such stereotypes may proceed to design lessons to train Black children to pronounce such words "correctly" with *th*.

The points made in this section suggest that if anything is really wrong with African American language, it is that it provokes a variety of predictable reactions. When used in the classroom by a child, few teachers would be so insensitive as to laugh at African American language, but it might make them uncomfortable, and that might be enough for the teachers to take on the mission of teaching the children what they consider "better" language.

SUMMARY

The policy options for dealing with African American language range from a traditional policy of suppression at one extreme to a policy of full recognition at the other extreme. A policy of limited recognition acknowledges the linguistic integrity of African American language, but concedes the lack of public support for a policy of leaving Black Language alone. Such policy options exist in a larger society that traditionally maintained a separate and unequal color caste system, and continues to exhibit *de facto* inequalities in access for African Americans and other persons of different races to economic and educational opportunities.

Race, culture, and ethnicity are similar and overlapping, but ultimately distinct phenomena. The fact that African American language is spoken mainly by members of the Black race is an accident of history. There are non-African Americans who speak African American English, and it is possible in principle for any human being, regardless of race, to acquire any language.

Ethnicity is the perception of traits of one culture by members of a different culture. There are predictable reactions to ethnicity that can help to account for the common perception that something is wrong with African American language. Ethnicity may be defined as an incongruity resulting from the perception of culture X from the perspective of culture Y, or the occurrence of elements of the ethnic identity of group X in situations dominated by the culture of group Y.

REFERENCES

Asante, M. K. (1987). *The Afrocentric Idea*. Philadelphia: Temple University Press.

Bennett, C. I. (1990). *Comprehensive Multicultural Education*. Boston: Allyn & Bacon.

Burling, R. (1973). *English in Black and White*. New York: Holt, Rinehart and Winston.

Baugh, J. (1995). The law, linguistics, and education: Educational reform for African American language minority students. *Linguistic and Education* 7(2): 87–105.

Chambers, J. (1983). *Black English Educational Equity and the Law*. Ann Arbor: Karoma Publishers.

Committee on the Status of Racial Minorities. (1983). Position paper on social dialects. *Asha*, September: 23–24.

Dillard, J. L. (1972). *Black English: Its History and Usage in the United States*. New York: Random House.

DuBois, W. E. B. (1961). *The Souls of Black Folk*. New York: Fawcett World Library. Originally published in 1903.

Fasold, R. W., & Wolfram, W. (1970). Some linguistic features of Negro dialect. In R. W. Fasold & R. W. Shuy (eds.), *Teaching Standard English in the Inner City*. Washington DC: Center for Applied Linguistics.

Fishman, J. A. (1972). *The Sociology of Language: An Interdisciplinary Social Science Approach to Language in Society*. Rowley, MA: Newbury House Publishers.

Gates, H. L. Jr. (1988). *The Signifying Monkey: A Theory of African-American Literary Criticism*. New York: Oxford University Press.

Gordon, M. M. (1966). *Assimilation in American Life*. New York: Oxford University Press.

Goss, L., & Barnes, M. E. (eds.) (1989). *Talk That Talk: An Anthology of African-American Storytelling*. New York: Simon and Schuster/Touchstone.

Hale-Benson, J. E. (1986). *Black Children: Their Roots, Culture, and Learning Styles*. Baltimore: Johns Hopkins University Press.

Labov, W. (1969). Contraction, deletion, and inherent variability of the English copula. *Language* 45:715–762.

Levine, L. W. (1977). *Black Culture and Black Consciousness: Afro-American Folk Thought From Slavery to Freedom*. Oxford: Oxford University Press.

Longstreet, W. (1978). *Aspects of Ethnicity: Understanding Differences in Pluralistic Classrooms*. New York: Teachers College Press.

Stewart, W. (1966). Social dialect. In *Research Planning Conference on Language Development in Disadvantaged Children*. New York: Yeshiva University.

Wolfram, W. (1969). *A Sociolinguistic Description of Detroit Negro Speech*. Washington, DC: Center for Applied Linguistics.

1

HIGHER GROUND

The Knowledge Base of African American Language and Culture Studies

Chapter Overview

Upon reading this chapter you will increase your understanding and appreciation of:

- The need for a high level of awareness among educators of the diverse fields of knowledge that inform the study of African American language and culture
- The nature of human language
- Biases and misconceptions about African American English
- The nature of speech and language disorders
- The need to eliminate cultural biases from established means of assessing normal versus disordered speech-language
- The overrepresentation of African American children in special education classes
- The inadequacy of deficit models of the African American experience
- The inherent danger of viewing the American experience narrowly, and in monocultural terms
- Multicultural education

This book is about African American children who speak African American English (also known as Black English, Black dialect, and Ebonics). The authors address a wide area of knowledge subsumed under the title *Speech, Language, Learning, and the African American Child*. The relevant knowledge base includes the three academic disciplines that are the authors' areas of specialization—education, speech-language pathology, and linguistics—as well as other fields that inform the study of African American language and culture such as sociology, anthropology, history, literature, and ethnic studies.

LINGUISTICS

Readers who lack sufficient training in linguistics may be surprised to discover that African American English (abbreviated AAE) is a familiar variety of language that they had previously mislabeled "bad" or "incorrect" English. Readers who happen to be AAE speakers may be pleasantly surprised to learn that their English is a language in its own right. In asserting that AAE is a language in its own right, we wish to counter the unscientific idea that it is "bad" with linguistic knowledge of its true nature.

We do not wish to argue that AAE is a separate language, and our choice of the label African American English implies as much. There can be no doubting that AAE is a variety of English, and that it shares with other varieties of American English the bulk of its elements and rules. The very idea that AAE consists of elements and rules, as opposed to mistakes and omissions, may be surprising to readers untrained in linguistics and accustomed to negative and pejorative characterizations of AAE. From the discussion of linguistics incorporated into the following chapters, such readers may gain an appreciation for the systematic and rule-governed nature of vernacular language and a willingness to support enlightened policies and practices for dealing with AAE in the classroom.

Readers who presently harbor unscientific notions of good and bad language may elevate their understanding to a new level of sophistication and adopt an attitude that is not judgmental toward language variation. Readers who are already willing to extend some degree of recognition to AAE may, after considering the range of policy options available to educators (Chapter 2), decide for themselves what degree of recognition of AAE is in the best interest of African American students.

LINGUISTIC SYSTEM

While we support the classification of AAE as English, we recognize that it has a distinctiveness to which calling it a *dialect of English* does not do justice.

AAE differs sufficiently in certain ways from other varieties of American English to be considered a different linguistic system. We mean by *linguistic system* the cognitive systems of words, sounds, meaning, and syntactic rules that constitute knowledge of a language: what the linguist Chomsky refers to as *competence* (Chomsky 1965). The notion of competence is developed further in the discussion of descriptive versus prescriptive grammar in Chapter 3. The notion of a linguistic system is developed further in Chapter 5 and serves as a precise technical account of what we mean by the claim that AAE is a language in its own right.

AFRICAN CONTINUITIES

While, as noted above, AAE has a great deal in common with other varieties of English, it also has elements and rules that reflect the continuing influence of African languages that were spoken by the ancestors of present day AAE speakers. Such elements contribute to the distinctiveness of AAE as a linguistic system. African language influences in AAE include syntactic rules for the expression of tense and aspect, as well as the pronunciation, meaning, and grammatical classification of particular words. An AAE sentence like

1. *She tall.*

for instance, in which a predicate adjective directly follows the subject, need not be seen as lacking the English copula verb *is*, since many African languages classify words that would be classified as adjectives in English as stative verbs (DeBose & Faraclas 1993). In such languages, sentences like (1) have the same structure as sentences like (2)

2. *She laugh.*

In the African languages in question, both types of sentences have the structure SUBJECT+VERB. The AAE syntactic patterns represented by sentences (1) and (2) may be seen as the continuation of typical African language structures rather than deviations from standard English patterns. The topic of African continuities in AAE is discussed in detail in Chapter 4.

ALL LANGUAGES ARE EQUAL

Whether we agree with the view that AAE is a different linguistic system, linguistic knowledge can help us to fairly evaluate the distinctive vernacular language that some African American children bring to the classroom. Chomsky's theory of competence emphasizes the universality of human language: the idea that humans are born with the ability to acquire whatever language they are exposed to as young children. All varieties of human language consist of elements and rules and are of equal intrinsic value. That is, no languages are better or worse than others. No matter what race the children are or what their socioeconomic status might be, they are born with the same linguistic capabilities.

In the universalistic sense of linguistic theory, a linguistic system may not be recognized socially and politically as a language. It may be considered a dialect, vernacular, or even worse, as a "corrupt" or "substandard" version of a recognized language. The assertion that a particular variety of language is a language in its own right is usually made to counter an inappropriately negative label that has traditionally been assigned to the variety in question. For present purposes we will say that a communication system qualifies as a language if it consists of words, phrases, and sentences that have established meanings when used in particular ways by members of a community of speakers. We are using the term language, therefore, in a broad and inclusive sense that includes dialects, vernaculars, creoles, and other particular language types (see Chapter 4).

The claim that AAE is a language in its own right is supported by evidence that it has its own grammar and is used in alternation with standard English by bilingual speakers. Although AAE grammar differs from standard English grammar and violates certain prescriptive rules of proper usage, it is consistent with descriptive rules that account for the systematic patterning of African American speech data. The distinction between descriptive and prescriptive grammar is discussed at length in the Chapter 2.

Sociolinguistic concepts introduced in Chapter 3 support the case for African American bilingualism. African American English is described as coexisting with standard English in the African American linguistic repertoire. Elements of the AAE system may be observed alongside elements of the standard English system in code-switching data produced by bilingual African Americans.

SPEECH-LANGUAGE PATHOLOGY

At the same time that we emphasize that AAE is a language in its own right, we also stress the fact that it is not a speech-language disorder. In order to insure that teachers of African American children do not misdiagnose children's normal language as pathological, the teachers should understand and be able to tell the difference between normal language and disordered speech (Chapter 6). By *speech* (as contrasted to language) we mean the more concrete physiological and neurological functions associated with the processing of language *output*. Language itself is located in the mind (Chomsky 1986), and it remains there in a passive state when it is not in use. The process of output begins with the decision of a speaker to say something. Subsequent stages in the output process include the encoding of the message into words and other language forms and its articulation. A full account of speech, in the sense of language output, involves the brain, the nervous system, the lungs, diaphragm, vocal chords, teeth, tongue, and other organs.

Linguists generally disclaim any special knowledge of the physiological functions and processes involved in speech and feel fully capable of studying language without such knowledge (De Saussure 1916). Many linguists have more than a layman's knowledge of articulatory phonetics, the study of the production of human speech sounds, but generally lack expertise in diagnosing and treating disorders that inhibit normal articulation. Speech-language pathologists are interested in normal human language, as well as in understanding the abnormal and pathological conditions that sometimes affect human speech. The basic notion of speech-language pathology is that the study of disordered communication hinges on the understanding and appreciation of the normal processes of human communication. The linguist's knowledge of normal language does not confer any special expertise in the identification and correction of speech-language pathologies, but a rudimentary knowledge of the nature of normal language is required in order to adequately differentiate between normal language and speech disorders.

In many cases the difference between normal language and speech pathology is obvious. Persons who stutter clearly do not lack linguistic competence. They know their language, and it is clear that they know what they want to say. What comes out as stuttering is a disorder of speech fluency and not necessarily a disorder of language itself. In other cases, the distinction between normal language and speech disorders is more subtle. A 10-year-old child in the habit of saying things like *me want to go outside* might be suspected of having a language pathology, but a 3-year-old showing the same usage might be seen as going through a normal process of language development. A child who pronounces words like *this* with an initial *d* sound might be suspected of having defective speech, but it would be premature to make such a diagnosis since such pronunciation variation is normal in some dialects of English. The material presented in Chapters 6 through 9 contributes to the preparation of educators to differentiate between normal language and disordered speech in the particular case of African American children. Without such preparation a teacher might conclude that an African American child is in need of speech therapy when there is in fact nothing wrong with his or her language.

BIASED ASSESSMENT CRITERIA

Speech-language pathologists are accustomed to using assessment methods that take the normal language of standard-English-speaking children as a point of reference for normal and pathological speech. In the last few years, speech-language pathologists knowledgeable of African American English have found that the assessment procedures in which they had been trained frequently led them to conclude that the speech of certain African American children was defective, when it was apparent that the conclusion had resulted from the use of biased criteria (Wyatt 1994, 1995). That is, certain features that suggest pathology when they occur in mainstream American English-speaking children are normal in the speech of certain African American children. Out of such experiences, new unbiased assessment procedures have been developed, which are discussed in detail in Chapter 7. Mainstream American English (MAE) is the acceptable spoken English that conforms to most of the rules of standard English in grammar and phonology, but allows for some errors in both casual and formal conversation as well as regional and social variation.

EDUCATION

Americans have traditionally formulated educational policies and structured classroom practices around the unspoken idea of a learner who embodies the characteristics of European American culture. It is hardly surprising that children of certain racial and ethnic backgrounds tend to score higher than others on standardized tests of achievement, and that African American children in particular tend to fare worse than any other group.

Unsophisticated persons appeal to stereotypes in attempting to account for the low achievement of some African American children. More sophisticated persons have proposed and attempted to defend a variety of explanations including the idea that the tests, and the teaching methods themselves, are culturally biased in favor of European American children (Hiliard 1976). Other scholars have suggested that the educational achievement of African American children, or lack thereof, may be explained in part by the clash between AAE and the standard English expected in academic settings. A detailed discussion of educational testing practices and their effects upon African American children is presented in Chapter 8.

A major focus of this book is on what is happening to African American children in the public schools, and the particular roles that language and culture play. The specific thesis is explored that teachers and other practitioners are prone to misperceive normal characteristics of African American language and culture as pathological conditions requiring remedial and corrective measures.

The clash between African American English and the standard English of academic discourse is a particular instance of cultural discontinuities that permeate the experiences of Black children in classrooms dominated by European cultural values and frequently taught by White teachers. One disastrous consequence of such discontinuities is a tendency for teachers to make inappropriate referrals of bright and capable African American children to special education programs for "slow" or disabled learners. The suspicion that such inaccurate diagnoses and inappropriate referrals occur on a regular basis is supported by statistics showing that African American children, especially boys, are disproportionately referred to speech therapy or special education programs. The overrepresentation of African American children in special education is further discussed in Chapter 11.

AFRICAN AMERICAN EXPERIENCE: PAST AND PRESENT

The idea that there is an African American culture, distinct from general American culture (Hale-Benson 1986), is not without controversy. For years, it was the consensus of American social scientists and historians that the experience of slavery completely destroyed the customs, traditions, and social institutions of the West African societies from which American slaves were taken (Kochman 1981; Levine 1977, p. 4). The result of being forcibly and brutally uprooted from their past lives according to this school of thought, had created a cultural vacuum among the African slaves, a blank slate upon which the experiences of the slave existence would be engraved with no connection to an African past. We disagree with the "blank slate" view of the African American past and offer in the next chapter numerous examples of continuing African influences in the present day experience of African Americans.

DEFICIT MODELS

The negation of a cultural link between African Americans and traditional African societies encouraged the use of deficit models for the analysis of contemporary problems of African Americans. Through such deficit models, the historical assumption that the slaves lost their African cultures is linked with the idea that Black people are presently deficient in certain aspects of European American culture that are considered prerequisites to academic achievement and social mobility. Sometimes the deficit is stated as the lack of a value orientation such as the work ethic. At other times it is attributed to elements of social structure such as the absence of a father or other male figure in the home, or to deprivation of certain "enriching" experiences that middle-class youngsters take for granted such as trips to the museum and stimulating dinner-table conversation (Wiggins 1976). The material presented in the following chapters contains many examples of the distinctiveness of African American culture that contribute to a positive conception of the African American experience that does not involve deficit models.

MULTICULTURAL EDUCATION

One result of the debate and criticism fostered by traditional American educational policies and practices has been a movement to develop alternative approaches to classroom teaching that assume that all children can learn. Such approaches do not assume an ideal learner from mainstream culture and are consciously grounded in the various cultures and ethnicities that American children bring to the classroom. The movement in question is known generally as *multicultural education* (Banks 1989; Bennett 1990), and includes particular inquiries into the educational needs of specific cultural groups such as African Americans.

This book is intended to make a contribution to multicultural education and enhance the reader's ability to make accurate diagnoses and appropriate placement decisions for students whose language performance might be a matter of concern. All three authors have contributed, from their own perspectives, to a growing body of knowledge on the nature of African American English, its history, its social uses, and its implications for educational policy and practice (DeBose 1992; 1994; DeBose & Faraclas 1993; Toliver-Weddington 1971; Wofford 1979).

PEDAGOGICAL IMPLICATIONS

Given the multicultural nature of American society, its legacy of racism, and the dominant role that persons of European ancestry continue to play in all areas of life, including education, a language associated with African Americans is bound to affect educational outcomes in ways that should be consciously understood. Readers may elevate their level of understanding of the nature of language and its role in the African American experience through careful study of the following chapters.

From the higher ground of an enlightened view of African American language and culture, citizens and educators may escape the pitfalls and dangers of applying commonly held misconceptions about vernacular language to the education of African American children. Among other things, they may avoid the danger of misjudging children who speak in a way that is normal within their own communities as affected by disordered or pathological speech.

SUMMARY

The present state of knowledge about African American English is informed by a variety of academic disciplines. The field of linguistics provides theoretical and factual information that can counter public misconceptions about the nature of language, particularly the tendency to label varieties of language inappropriately as "bad" or "substandard" when a more objective analysis would simply label them different. Classifying African American English as a language in its own right, while controversial, is supported by linguistic knowledge.

Knowledge from the field of speech-language pathology can be of great value in deciding what to do about school children who speak AAE. Teachers need to know the difference between normal and disordered speech in order to decide when it is appropriate to refer a child to speech therapy. The overrepresentation of African American children in speech therapy in the nation's schools supports a suspicion that an unacceptably high rate of inappropriate referrals do in fact occur.

The ultimate question of what to do about African American English in American society is informed by knowledge of the nature of American education, the status of standard English in American society, and the function of schools in promoting standard English as a mark of the educated person. Understanding differences in academic achievement among children of diverse racial and ethnic backgrounds is facilitated by theories that focus upon cultural incongruities and the need to consciously and systematically plan the educational experiences of minority children to overcome such incongruities.

The broad knowledge base that fully informs the study of African American language and culture includes, in addition to education, linguistics and speech-language pathology, sociology, anthropology, history, and ethnic studies.

REFERENCES

Banks, J. A. (1989). Multicultural education: Characteristics and goals. In J. A. Banks & C. A. McGee Banks (eds.). *Multicultural Education: Issues and Perspectives* (pp. 2–26). Boston: Allyn & Bacon.

Bennett, C. I. (1990). *Comprehensive Multicultural Education.* Boston: Allyn & Bacon.

Chomsky, N. (1965). *Aspects of the Theory of Syntax.* Cambridge, MA: MIT Press.

Chomsky, N. (1980). *Rules and Representations.* Oxford: Basil Blackwell.

Chomsky, N. (1986). *Knowledge of Language: Its Nature, Origin and Use.* New York: Praeger.

DeBose, C. E. (1992). Code-switching: Black English and Standard English in the African-American linguistic repertoire. *The Journal of Multilingual and Multicultural Development: Special Issue on Code-switching, 13* (1 & 2): 157–167.

DeBose, C. E. (1994). A note on ain't vs. didn't negation in African American vernacular. *Journal of Pidgin and Creole Languages,* 9 (1): 127–130.

DeBose, C. E., & Faraclas, N. (1993). An Africanist approach to the linguistic study of Black English: Getting to the roots of the tense-aspect-modality and copula systems in Afro-American. In S. S. Mufwene (ed.), *Africanisms in Afro-American Language Varieties* (pp. 364–387). Athens: University of Georgia Press.

De Saussure, F. (1916). *Cours de Linguistique Generale.* Geneva: Payot.

Hale-Benson, J. E. (1986). *Black Children: Their Roots, Culture, and Learning Styles.* Baltimore: Johns Hopkins University Press.

Hiliard, A. (1976). *Alternatives to I.Q. Testing. An Approach to the Identification of Gifted Minority Children.* Final Report to the California State Department of Education.

Kochman, T. (1981). *Black and White Styles in Conflict.* Chicago: University of Chicago Press.

Levine, L. W. (1977). *Black Culture and Black Consciousness: Afro-American Folk Thought From Slavery to Freedom.* Oxford: Oxford University Press.

Toliver-Weddington, G. (1971). Introduction: Implications for education. *Journal of Black Studies,* 9: 364–66.

Wofford, J. (1979). Ebonics: A legitimate system of oral communication. *Journal of Black Studies,* 4: 367–382.

Wiggins, M. E. (1976). The cognitive deficit-difference controversy: A Black sociopolitical perspective. In D. S. Harrison & T. Trabasso (eds.), *Black English: A Seminar* (pp. 241–254). Hillsdale, NJ: Lawrence Erlbaum Associates.

Wyatt, T. (1994). *A Variable Rule Approach to the Identification of Language Disorders in African American English (AAE) Child Speech.* Presented at NWAV 23 Conference, Stanford University, October 23.

Wyatt, T. (1995). Language development in African American English child speech. *Linguistics and Education,* 7: 7–22.

2

DESCRIPTIVE VERSUS PRESCRIPTIVE GRAMMAR

Chapter Overview

Upon reading this chapter you will gain understanding of:

- What it means to know a language
- How the term grammar is used in linguistics differently than in everyday usage
- How linguists do grammatical description and analysis
- Specific terms and methods of grammatical description pertaining to vocabulary (lexicon), pronunciation (phonology), word structure (morphology), sentence structure (syntax), and meaning (semantics)
- How language considered incorrect in terms of traditional (prescriptive) rules of grammar can be correct in terms of the system that native speakers automatically follow
- How dialect differences affect the grammatical description of languages

For lay persons, the subject of grammar calls to mind rules that they have been consciously taught to observe, but rules that they approach without confidence. For example, we are taught that it is sometimes correct to use *whom* instead of *who* (Klammer & Schulz 1992). It is such consciously taught do's and don'ts that most people have in mind when they speak of grammar. Such *prescriptive* rules, however, only account for a small part of the linguistic competence of native speakers. The vast majority of the rules that native speakers of a language follow in speaking and writing are not found in traditional grammar books. There is no need to prescribe such rules to native speakers because they always follow them. Some of them can be found in technical linguistic descriptions and are known as *descriptive* rules.

Linguists generally disclaim any interest in prescriptive grammar (Huddleston 1988). They do not see themselves as in the business of prescribing how people should speak or write, but only of describing language as it actually is. Prescriptive grammar rules are taken very seriously by society, however, as criteria for allocating privileges and classifying persons socioeconomically. When we observe violations of prescriptive rules in an individual's speech or writing, we tend to view them as signs of lower class or lack of education. Although we tend to base our standards of correct usage on the native-like language of members of higher social classes, the highest-prestige dialects of spoken English contain features that are at odds with prescribed usage. For reasons that will be made clear below, even educated upper-class English speakers violate prescriptive grammar rules, often unaware that they are doing so, and often feel insecure about their "grammar."

Persons who feel insecure about their knowledge of prescriptive grammar may be pleased to learn that they have "in their heads," so to speak, an extremely complex system of grammatical rules that they follow automatically when they speak or write. Native speakers, although they may have absolutely no conscious knowledge of grammar, tend to speak and write grammatically (Sedley 1990). They can derive a sense of self-confidence from the realization that if something "sounds right" to them it is grammatically correct. We will develop this point further below.

When we claim that African American language has a grammar, it is descriptive grammar, and not prescriptive grammar that we have in mind. In fact, many of the descriptive rules discussed in this section are part of the grammar in the heads of most English speakers including speakers of African American language. Speakers whose grammatical output is not always prescriptively correct may master prescriptive rules by learning how to analyze and make explicit the unconscious and intuitive grammar of their native dialect.

CONTRASTING PROPERTIES OF DESCRIPTIVE AND PRESCRIPTIVE RULES

A key distinction between prescriptive and descriptive rules is that the former make reference to what speakers *should* or *should not* do in order to be considered correct and proper, whereas the latter simply account for what speakers actually do when they speak. Also, as previously noted, prescriptive rules differ from descriptive rules in that the former are consciously taught and enforced, whereas the latter are unconsciously acquired and automatically followed by native speakers. A third important difference between the two types of rules is that native speakers never break descriptive rules. Native speakers may violate prescriptive rules, however, and some do so frequently.

One of the most infamous prescriptive rules of English grammar is violated by sentence (1). It is considered wrong because it contains *ain't*. Many people were consciously taught not to use *ain't* and may have been corrected on more than one occasion. Some people continue to use *ain't* on occasion although they know that it is considered wrong.

1. *Angela ain't at home.*

From the point of view of descriptive grammar, there is nothing wrong with sentence (1). Native speakers actually use *ain't* according to rules that they follow automatically—rules that can be made explicit through linguistic analysis. This writer remembers learning to say jokingly *"ain't* ain't a word 'cause it ain't in the dictionary." As a matter of fact, however, *ain't* is in the dictionary. The *American Heritage Dictionary of the English Language* (Morris, 1976) characterizes *ain't* as "nonstandard" and a "contraction of *am not"* (p. 27). The dictionary goes on to indicate that *ain't* is "extended in use to mean *are not, is not, has not,* and *have not."* The designation "nonstandard" is prescriptive in that it implies that *ain't* should not be used. The dictionary's account of how *ain't* actually is used is descriptive, however.

A more explicit description of *ain't* would show how it fits into, and is an integral part of, an extremely complex system of English sentence negation, which is part of the grammar in the speaker's head. The dictionary's statement that *ain't* may be used "to mean *are not, is not, has not"* is an imprecise way of describing one of several options that English speakers have for making sentences negative. The most basic option is that of placing *not* after certain verb forms as in sentences (2) and (3).

2. *Angela is not going home.*
3. *Angela has not gone home.*

A second option is to substitute a special negated form, known traditionally as a contraction, for the verb after which not would be placed using the basic option. In contrast to sentences (2) and (3), which represent the basic option, sentences (4) and (5) substitute the negated contractions *isn't,* and *hasn't,* respectively, for the basic verbs *is* and *has.*

4. *Angela isn't going home.*
5. *Angela hasn't gone home.*

As a general rule, each English negated contraction may only be used to substitute for a particular verb of which it is a contraction; for example, *can't* substitutes for *can; won't* substitutes for *will;* and so on. The only exceptions are *ain't,* which may substitute for *is, am, are, has,* and *had;* and *aren't,* which may substitute for *am* as well as *are,* in order to avoid using the contraction of *am not,* which happens to be *ain't.*

When native English speakers use *ain't,* therefore, they are engaging in rule-governed behavior. They do not use *ain't* indiscriminately. They would never substitute *ain't* for *can't, won't,* and other negated contractions. Part of knowing how to speak English entails knowing how to use *ain't.* It is part of the grammar that English speakers have in their heads, their linguistic competence.

The rule that people should not use *ain't* is a prescriptive rule. It is consciously taught and enforced, but native speakers may break it, and some do so frequently. The rule against using *ain't* is a small part of English speakers' knowledge of how to negate sentences. The general rule for negating English sentences using *not,* and the special options for substituting negated contractions (including *ain't*) for the verbs after which *not* would otherwise be placed, are descriptive rules. Native speakers follow them automatically and unconsciously and never break them.

NATIVE SPEAKER INTUITIONS AND GRAMMATICALITY

Although native speakers never violate the descriptive rules of their language, those who lack special training in grammatical analysis are usually incapable of explaining those rules. Native speakers have highly reliable intuitions, however, of what constitutes native-like tokens of their language, that is, of what "sounds right" to them. Consider, for example, how native English speakers automatically alternate between using *much* with certain nouns and *many* with others. Most native speakers would agree that examples (6) and (7) below sound fine. The same speakers would reject (8) and (9), however, as sounding wrong. Asterisks (*) such as those before examples (8) and (9) are used in linguistics to indicate unacceptability to native speakers.

6. *I cooked too much rice.*
7. *I cooked too many apples.*
8. * *I cooked too many corn.*
9. * *I cooked too much noodles.*

Although most native speakers are unable to explain what is wrong with sentences like (8) and (9), the correct usage of *much* versus *many* is accounted for in descriptive grammars of English by subclassifying nouns as "count nouns" which refer to countable entities such as apples and noodles; and "mass nouns," which stand for things like rice and corn, which are not countable. As a rule, English speakers use *many* with count nouns and use *much* with mass nouns. Native English speakers automatically use *much* and *many* correctly, although most of them are incapable of explaining why they do it and do not know a count noun from a mass noun.

In linguistic argumentation the judgments of native speakers are taken as evidence of *grammaticality*. Sentences that sound right to native speakers are considered *grammatical*, and those that sound wrong are considered *ungrammatical*. Using the facts represented by particular grammatical or ungrammatical examples, we try to arrive at general statements that accurately explain the unconscious and intuitive knowledge that native speakers have of their language.

One of the most common prescriptive rules of American English is that you should not use double negatives, as in sentence (10).

10. *We didn't tell nobody.*

Many English speakers actually produce sentences with double negatives, and such sentences may sound fine to them. In that sense, they are grammatical. It is possible, therefore, for a sentence that is considered "incorrect" from a prescriptive point of view to be "correct," that is grammatical, from a descriptive point of view. Sentences that break prescriptive rules might sound wrong to those who are well educated and have been taught that they are wrong. It should be clear, however, that the kind of "wrong" involved in breaking prescriptive rules is a lesser magnitude of "wrong" than what is represented as an ungrammatical string (e.g., 11)

11. * *we nobody tell didn't.*

Linguists explain the grammaticality of sentence (10), in part, by showing how it is systematically related to a positive sentence such as (12).

12. *We told somebody.*

Sentence (10) is an instance of the second of the above-discussed options for English sentence negation, namely that of substituting a negated contraction of the verb after which *not* would be placed according to the basic option. (Although the related positive sentence [12] does not contain a verb after which not can be placed, native English speakers know intuitively to use a form of the auxiliary verb *do*, i.e., *did*, in such cases.)

People hardly realize how complex the native speaker's knowledge of the English language is until they try to make it explicit. In fact, to fully describe sentence (10) as a negated version of (12), people need to account for the occurrence of *nobody* in (10) where *somebody* occurs in (12). English seems to restrict the indefinite pronoun *somebody* to positive sentences, when it occurs in the predicate after the main verb, as in (12). When such sentences are negated, English speakers may substitute *nobody*, as in (10), although it results in a violation of the rule against using double negatives. They may also substitute the word *anybody*, of course, and be prescriptively correct, as well as grammatical.

The ability of native English speakers to produce and recognize grammatical utterances supports the theory that they have unconscious and intuitive knowledge of a vast and complex system of descriptive rules. Although native speakers may violate prescriptive grammar rules such as the prohibition of *ain't* and double negatives, native speakers never violate descriptive grammar rules. Descriptive rules, as the specifications of what constitutes native-like language, are always grammatical by definition. Production of an ungrammatical string of words of a language is evidence that the speaker does not know the language.

To reinforce the fact that most speakers are not conscious of descriptive rules, let us consider some ungrammatical strings that represent violations of particular descriptive rules.

13. * *Alice will giving you the information.*
14. * *They have spent money their.*
15. * *The hikers arrived the summit.*

Examples (13) to (15) do not sound right to most native speakers. In that sense they are ungrammatical, that is, they violate descriptive rules. The examples do not sound right because they are inconsistent with a native speaker's intuitive and unconscious knowledge of particular descriptive rules. A naive native speaker could correct (13) by substituting *give* for *giving*, but would be hard put to explain why the correction is necessary. Those who have been trained in descriptive grammar could specify that what is wrong with (13) is that a *modal auxiliary* such as *will* must be followed by the stem form of a verb. The stem form of the main verb of (13) is *give* not *giving*.

To account for what is wrong with (14), a speaker untrained in grammatical analysis might say that *money* and *their* are in the reverse order of what they should be. A trained linguist would recognize it as a violation of the general principle that *determiners* such as *their* precede the nouns that they modify. A naive native speaker might respond to the intuition that (15) is wrong by correcting it, adding a preposition such as *at* between *arrived* and *the*, but would probably miss the generalization that an intransitive verb such as *arrived* cannot take an object. The intransitive verb analysis can be supported by substituting a transitive verb such as *reached* for *arrived* in (15) and noting that the result, example (16), is grammatical.

16. *The hikers reached the summit.*

The descriptive rules violated by examples (13) to (15) may be summarized as follows:

1. A modal auxiliary (e.g., *will, can, should*) must be followed by the stem form of a verb.
2. A noun phrase may consist of a determiner (e.g., *the, each, their*) followed by a head noun.
3. An intransitive verb such as *arrive* cannot take an object.

Such are the kinds of unconscious, intuitive rules that we have in mind when we speak of descriptive grammar. Although untrained native speakers are not conscious of them, they indicate that they know such rules intuitively by speaking in a manner that is consistent with them, by recognizing that ungrammatical strings do not sound right and by their ability to correct violations of such rules in the language of nonnative speakers.

GRAMMAR AS A DESCRIPTION OF A LANGUAGE

When linguists use the term grammar in technical discussions, it is understood that it is descriptive, not prescriptive, grammar that they have in mind. In linguistics, the term grammar simply denotes a description of a language. In the present context, a grammar is a description of the linguistic competence of a speaker of the language in question. No linguist has yet come close to producing a complete description of what native speakers know about English, or any other language, nor is one likely to do so in the near future.

In order to produce a complete descriptive grammar, it would be necessary to describe not only the entire set of words that speakers employ, including the pronunciation and meaning of each word, but also the restrictions on how words may occur in grammatical sentences. The explicit description of just one part of a language, the *lexicon*, the part of the grammar in your head that is like a dictionary, is a monumental task in itself (Burling 1992).

Consider what is involved in the complete description of a single word, say, *man*. The most straightforward part of the description of this word is its pronunciation, or *phonology*. It can be described in part as a sequence of three sounds, or *phonemes*, represented conventionally by the sequence of letters "m," "a," and "n."

If the entire task were to describe the pronunciation of all of the words of a language, that would be challenging enough, but at least it seems possible. Each word can be described as a sequence of phonemes selected from a small and known set. English has approximately 39 phonemes that are familiar to linguists, and we know what they are (allowing for dialect differences discussed below).

Since the task also includes describing the meaning of each word in the language, it would help if the meaning of the word could be broken up into minimal parts similar to the way that the pronunciation of words is divided into phonemes. As a matter of fact, linguists have found a useful way of analyzing the semantic composition of words in the idea of *semantic features*. Using such an approach, the meaning of the word *man* can be shown to be composed of such features as ANIMATE, HUMAN, ADULT, and MALE. Such an analysis shows how the meaning of *man* has some of the same features as the words *woman, girl*, and *boy*. Each of the words *woman* and *boy* differ in meaning from *man* by just one feature: the former is FEMALE not MALE, and the latter is not ADULT, but CHILD.

While it seems possible to adequately describe the meanings of certain words in terms of semantic features, it is difficult to achieve a satisfactory analysis of the semantic composition of the vast majority of the words of English. Many words in the English lexicon are not easily described in terms of semantic features (Burling 1992). How, for example, is the meaning of *window* analyzed into semantic features?

Linguists have yet to develop a comprehensive set of semantic features adequate for the general analysis of the meanings of the words of a language, and that is one reason why no one has produced a complete descriptive grammar of English or any other language. A more general reason is that language is extremely complex. Linguists, who spend their professional lives studying language, understand this better than most people. Realizing that the definitive description of a language is not technically feasible, in the short run, linguists develop and work with theories that stipulate in general terms how languages are structured and organized. One such theory is the idea that native speakers of English have a grammar of the English language in their heads. Their linguistic competence is organized into several different components.

The lexicon is in many ways the most central component of a grammar. As noted above, a complete description of the lexicon cannot be done without reference to other components. Not only is each word in the lexicon given a phonological and a semantic description, as discussed above. Each word is also assigned to a syntactic category such as "noun" or "adjective," which determines how it occurs in grammatical sentences. In order for a sentence to be grammatical, the individual words must be arranged in a way that is consistent with the rules of English *syntax*, or sentence structure.

Other components of descriptive grammar that English speakers intuitively follow belong to the level of *morphology*. Certain words may be subdivided into two or more meaningful parts known as *morphemes*. The adjective *unbreakable*, for example, consists of three morphemes—the prefix *un-*, the stem *break*, and the suffix *-able*—that may be added to most English forms to derive an adjective.

Most English speakers are unable to consciously account for the grammatical structure of a sentence in very much detail. The fact that they can produce and understand sentences, however, and recognize grammatical and ungrammatical strings of words, supports the theory that they have unconscious and intuitive knowledge of a language in their heads.

DIALECTAL DIFFERENCES

The attempt to classify specific rules of a language as descriptive or prescriptive is complicated by the existence of dialect differences. Although all English speakers have a grammar in their heads that they use to encode and decode utterances, the grammar in your head, while similar to mine in many ways, is not the same as the grammar in my head. What sounds fine to me might not sound right to you, and vice versa. For instance, speakers of American English tend to disagree on the grammaticality of sentences like (17) and (18). They sound right to some speakers, but wrong to others.

17. *My car needs fixed.*
18. *William might can fix it.*

Some speakers insist that in order for (17) to be correct, it should have the sequence *to be* inserted between *needs* and *fixed*. Other speakers insist that (17) sounds fine as is. Sentence (18) also sounds right to some native speakers and wrong to others for whom either *might* or *can* must be removed in order for it to be grammatical. Their grammar does not accept the sequence **might can*. If native speakers disagree on whether a given sentence is grammatical, it may be due to dialectal differences.

For many Americans, a dialect is something that someone else speaks. Bostonians, Texans, New Yorkers, and Oklahomans are more likely to be thought of as speakers of dialects than are people from places like Ohio and California. In this section we want to make two key points about dialects:

- Everyone speaks a dialect.
- All dialects are equal (although some are more equal than others).

To say that everyone speaks a dialect is simply to acknowledge that when a language is spoken in several different geographical areas and social strata, dialect differences will develop. The most conspicuous of such differences are in the lexicon. Some speakers may employ a different word than others for the same meaning. Some Americans, for example, use the word *soda* to denote a "soft drink," while other Americans use the word *pop*. Some speakers use *expressway* where speakers of other dialects use a different word such as *freeway* or *turnpike*.

More subtle differences may be noted in other aspects of a language, such as the pronunciation of words. The word *syrup* is pronounced by most Americans in one of three ways. One variant has a vowel similar to that of *sear* in the first syllable. Another has a vowel like that of *sir* in the first syllable; the third has only one syllable that rhymes with *burp*. Other pronunciation differences affect whole classes of words containing the same sound, and there is variation in how the sound is pronounced in different dialects. The words *how, now, brown, cow*, and many others have a common vowel sound that some people pronounce as a diphthong, or two-phase vowel. For some speakers, the onset of the diphthong is like the *a* in *father*, and the termination is like the *oo* in *shoot*. Other speakers pronounce that sound as a diphthong that terminates with *oo*, but has an onset like the *a* in *cat*, or like the *u* in *cup*.

Some speakers of American English pronounce certain sets of words alike, while other speakers pronounce them differently. Many Californians pronounce the verb *caught* identically with the noun *cot*, whereas other speakers pronounce those words distinctly. Many of the same persons who pronounce *caught* and *cot* the same also pronounce *horse* the same as *hoarse*.

When we say that everyone speaks a dialect, then, we simply mean that where a language has different words for the same thing, different pronunciations of the same word, and so on, everyone uses one or another of the available options. Everyone says either *pop* or *soda* and everyone pronounces *horse* the same as *hoarse* or differently. To say that all dialects are equal is to affirm that when such differences exist, one choice is just as good as the other. The dialect that says *pop* is no better and no worse than the one that says *soda*. The fact that *soda* has one more syllable than *pop* and one more sound is of no consequence whatsoever.

Although feelings exist among speakers of English that certain dialects are better than others, there is no scientific basis for such feelings. To the contrary, the statement that all dialects are equal is strongly and unanimously confirmed by scientific studies of human language. The parenthetical expression that "some are more equal than others" is an acknowledgment of the existence of attitudes among speakers of English that afford greater prestige to certain dialectal variants than others. Take, for instance, the variant pronunciations of *creek*. Most Americans feel that the pronunciation that rhymes with *week* is better than the variant that rhymes with *sick*. There is really no scientific basis for maintaining that the former pronunciation is better than the latter. The belief is widespread among Americans, however, and to that extent the former is "more equal."

It was pointed out above that the distinction between descriptive and prescriptive grammar is complicated by dialect differences. To illustrate this, let us suppose that a teacher had two students who pronounced *creek* differently—one with each of the above-mentioned pronunciations—and insisted that both should produce the higher prestige pronunciation. The resulting rule that you should pronounce *creek* a certain way might be considered a prescriptive rule insofar as it contains the word "should." It is a rule that one of the students follows automatically, however, and never violates. For her it is actually descriptive of how she speaks, and telling her that she *should* speak that way is like telling the sun to rise every morning—as if it were not going to do so anyhow. For the other student, however, who normally says *crick*, the requirement is truly a prescriptive rule, consciously taught and enforced by the teacher. The student may learn to produce the prescribed pronunciation in the teacher's presence in order to receive good marks, but once outside the teacher's earshot is likely to revert to the natural dialectal pronunciation.

The variations in the English system of sentence negation discussed above correspond to dialectal differences in the area of syntax. If all dialects are truly equal, dialects that frequently break prescriptive rules against the use of *ain't* and double negatives are equal to those that use such stigmatized forms rarely. In a classroom setting, however, teachers are likely to require that all students conform to the norms of the dialects that tend to automatically conform to the prescriptive rules. Another syntactic rule that speakers of many varieties of American English tend to follow automatically is the use of the verb suffix -*s* with third person singular subjects. In some varieties of English, however, sentences like (19) and (20) are grammatical.

19. *Mary have three sisters.*
20. *We takes the bus to school.*

The use of -*s* in agreement with third person singular subjects is clearly a prescriptive rule for speakers of such dialects, although it is a descriptive rule for speakers of dialects that automatically follow it. Practitioners influenced by traditional attitudes might feel strongly that such dialectal patterns should be corrected because of their low prestige. Before acting on such feelings, however, they should keep in mind that all dialects are equal. Dialects that negate sentences with *ain't* are just as good as those that only use *ain't* as a special option to a basic system that uses *not*. Patterns of native-like language, whatever the socioeconomic status of the speaker, are grammatical, even though they may violate traditional norms of correct usage.

PRESCRIPTIVE RULES FREQUENTLY VIOLATED BY SPEAKERS OF HIGH-PRESTIGE DIALECTS

Most of the prescriptive rules discussed so far are rules that are violated more frequently by poor and uneducated persons and by speakers of particular varieties such as African American language. It should be clear, however, that all varieties of spoken American English contain features that are contrary to prescribed usage (Klammer & Schulz 1992). One is the occurrence of what are known as "dangling prepositions," as in sentence (21).

21. *She is the one I was telling you about.*

Most speakers, whatever their social class, would accept (21) as grammatical, although there is a long-standing prescriptive rule that you should not end a sentence with a preposition. To make sentence (21) comply with that rule, however, it would be necessary to change it in a manner that might sound worse that the so-called wrong version (21):

22. *She is the one about whom I was telling you.*

Although the prescriptively corrected sentence might sound worse, there is some value in being able to know when a sentence that sounds right to you is considered incorrect and being able to produce the so-called correct version. In the case of dangling prepositions, the key to being able to recognize and correct them is clearly the ability to recognize prepositions. In order to develop the ability to recognize prepositions, it is necessary to study descriptive grammar. Although our ultimate goal is to improve our ability to comply with prescriptive grammar rules, we need to study descriptive grammar along the way to simply make sense of certain prescriptive rules.

Another prescriptive rule frequently violated by speakers of most dialects of American English may be referred to for convenience as the "he and I" rule. This rule requires that subject pronouns always be used in compound subjects where two noun phrases are conjoined. Sentences (23) and (24) are both grammatical, but the latter is not prescriptively correct due to the occurrence of the object pronoun *her* in the subject *Her and Alice*.

23. *Robert and I were appointed to the committee.*
24. *Her and Alice went to the committee meeting.*

Many English speakers attain partial understanding of this rule and they understand it as requiring that you should always use subject pronouns such as *I*, *she*, and *he*, instead of the corresponding object forms *me*, *her*, and so on in the kind of compound noun phrases in question. With such partial understanding, such speakers might be tempted to "correct" a sentence like (25) or (26), although there is nothing wrong with it descriptively or prescriptively.

25. *The President appointed me and Robert to the committee.*
26. *A table near the exit was reserved for her and Alice.*

English speakers actually produce on a regular basis such *hypercorrect* sentences as (27) and (28) by applying a prescriptive rule in an instance where it does not properly apply.

27. *The President appointed Robert and I to the committee.*
28. *A table near the exit was reserved for she and Alice.*

Although the compound noun phrase Robert and I is prescriptively correct in (23), since it functions as the subject, it is not correct in (27), where it functions as the object of the verb *appointed*. Since it functions as the object, the object pronoun *me* that occurs in (25) is correct. Just as the ability to recognize prepositions is key to the ability to spot and correct a dangling preposition, the ability to correct and avoid hypercorrection of the "he and I" rule depends upon the speaker's being able to tell when a compound noun phrase is functioning as a subject or an object.

Pedagogical Implications

One implication of the material presented in this chapter that some practitioners may find disturbing is that the traditional practice of correcting students' language to conform to prescriptive rules be reevaluated. What is disturbing is the feeling that a teacher might be abdicating his or her responsibility to prepare speakers of low prestige dialects for the expectations of the "real world." We do not advocate any such abdication of responsibility. We do suggest that the reader reflect upon what are *effective* ways of teaching speakers of all dialects to produce language that conforms to prescribed usage when they so desire.

SUMMARY

In linguistics, the term grammar simply denotes a description of a language. It has none of the prescriptive connotations associated with the everyday usage of the term grammar. Prescriptive grammar rules prescribe how one should speak or write in order to be considered correct. Descriptive grammar rules describe how a language is actually spoken by native speakers. Another important difference between prescriptive and descriptive grammar is that the former consists of rules that are consciously taught, whereas the latter are unconsciously acquired by native speakers in early childhood. Native speakers are capable of violating prescriptive grammar rules, and some of them do so frequently. Native speakers automatically follow descriptive rules, however, and never violate them.

A descriptive grammar is a representation of the knowledge that speakers use to produce and recognize grammatical sentences. Everybody speaks a dialect, and all dialects are equal, although some are more prestigious than others. Because of dialect differences, what is grammatical for one native speaker may be ungrammatical for another.

Violations of certain prescriptive rules occur more frequently in dialects spoken by persons of low socioeconomic status. Some prescriptive rules are frequently violated by speakers of high-prestige dialects, and one consequence of teaching prescriptive rules is the linguistic insecurity felt by speakers who are aware that their language is sometimes incorrect according to prescriptive grammar, but unable to eliminate such errors from their usage.

REFERENCES

Burling, R. (1992). *Patterns of Language: Structure, Variation, Change.* San Diego: Academic Press.

Huddleston, R. (1988). *English Grammar: An Outline.* Cambridge University Press.

Klammer, T. P., & Schulz, M. R. (1992). *Analyzing English Grammar.* Boston: Allyn & Bacon.

Morris, W.(Ed). (1976). *The American Heritage Dictionary of the English Language.* Boston: Houghton Mifflin Company.

Sedley, D. (1990). *Anatomy of English: An Introduction to the Structure of Standard American English.* New York: St. Martin's Press.

3

AFRICAN AMERICAN BILINGUALISM

Chapter Overview

Upon reading this chapter you will gain understanding of:

- How we vary our language according to the nature of the situation in which it is used
- How the determination of what is correct in language depends to some extent on our sense of what is appropriate for the situation in question
- How the description and analysis of language is affected by stylistic variation
- How African American English coexists with mainstream American English in the African American linguistic repertoire
- The role of language in African American culture
- Technical concepts and terminology for the description of bilingualism, bidialectalism, and other societal patterns of language use

In this chapter we introduce material that validates frequent references in the literature to the *duality* of the African American experience, focusing on the realm of language use. What DuBois aptly summarizes as a ". . . . twoness— an American, a Negro; two souls, two thoughts, two unreconciled strivings; two warring ideals in one dark body . . ." (1961, p. 17) has a linguistic dimension that is often clouded by the controversy over the status of African American language and its implications for educational policy. Policy makers need to be aware, however, that a strong case can be made for treating African Americans as a bilingual and bicultural community.

In a multicultural society such as the United States, the question of what constitutes appropriate behavior is complicated by the fact that many of us live in two or more cultures simultaneously. It is commonly acknowledged that many members of certain groups—for example, Mexican Americans—are bicultural as well and bilingual. It is less commonly acknowledged, but just as true, that many African Americans are bicultural and bilingual. Some scholars are more comfortable with the term *bidialectal* as a descriptor of the dual linguistic competence of African Americans. Since we are using the term language in a way that includes dialects, the term *bilingualism* is synonymous with *bidialectalism* in our usage.

The bicultural individual must cope with the constant need to behave in different, sometimes conflicting ways, depending upon which cultural norms are in force at a given time. When African American children are at home or at church, it may be normal and appropriate to speak African American language. When the children participate in the general American culture, however, they may find that use of their home/church language is not always considered appropriate.

In discussing the assessment of the language capabilities of African American children later in this book, the importance of using the norms of the children's own community as a standard of reference is emphasized. The material presented in this chapter provides a detailed account of the norms of language use in the African American community in terms of the situations in which African American language is appropriate. In the following chapters, we will account for some of the specific lexical, syntactic, phonological, and morphological features that signal the presence of African American language.

THE SITUATIONAL NATURE OF LANGUAGE USE

In Chapter 2 we introduced one way of moving beyond traditional notions of correct usage in dealing with African American language. Although AAE contains violations of prescriptive grammar, it is grammatical in that it is consistent with the descriptive grammar of African American language. In this chapter we will look at an aspect of the question of correctness that is derived from the realization that what is correct, more often than not, cannot be stated in categorical terms. It often depends on the situation (Fishman 1972). What might be wrong in one situation might be perfectly correct in another situation.

In the last chapter we saw how grammaticality can be a useful addition to our terminology for evaluating symbols of language. In this chapter we will focus upon the dimension of appropriateness. A given instance of language might be correct in the sense that it is grammatical and yet be considered an inappropriate choice. In order to develop this idea, we will broaden the theoretical perspective of our discussion from a specific emphasis on language itself to include the social context of language.

As we explore the implications of the situational nature of language use for the issues raised in this book, we want to be careful not to just adopt the term "inappropriate" as a euphemism for "bad" or "incorrect." We also want to explore the point of view that language that is normally considered "bad" might be appropriate and acceptable for particular situations. It might be more appropriate, for example, for a football coach speaking to his team in the locker room at halftime to urge his charges to "get out there and kick some asses," than it would be for him to use a milder expression such as "kick some behinds."

In addition to *ass* and *behind*, English has a variety of words for the part of your anatomy known euphemistically as your *bottom—fanny, butt, rump*, and *derriere*, to name a few. This is one of many examples of how we maintain sets of synonyms that have the same literal meaning but differ in their social connotations. Such *situational synonyms*, as we might call them, seem to fulfill a similar purpose to that of diverse items of clothing in our wardrobe. We have something appropriate for every situation.

Consider the various words we use for the condition denoted by the word *drunk*. If your next door neighbor, an average person, is in such a state, the term *drunk* might be an appropriate choice for reporting that person's condition. A police officer would probably choose a different term, however, in writing a report of your neighbor's behavior while *under the influence*. If you were privileged to attend a posh function at the White House, and the First Lady were seen in an *inebriated* condition, you would be careful to choose the right word to describe her in subsequent gossip. Neither *drunk* nor *intoxicated* appears to be adequate for such a situation, and perhaps someone of such high standing could never get beyond being *tipsy*.

SOCIOLINGUISTICS

Much of the regularity and patterning in language and a good deal of what native speakers know about their language is of a nature that cannot be adequately explained by a model of descriptive grammar such as was presented in Chapter 2—a model that consists solely of structural elements such as words, phrases, and sounds. When an American wife says to her husband, for example:

Will you take out the garbage?

A structural analysis of the sentence uttered does not correctly account for the intended meaning. The sentence is in the form of a question that, by its internal structure, demands an answer of "yes" or "no." In American culture, however, such a question is intended to be taken as a command when spoken by a wife to a husband. The subfield of linguistics known as *sociolinguistics* developed in response to the need for a way of analyzing language as part of a larger social context.

Sociolinguistics is usually defined as the study of language in its social context. Fishman (1972) defines sociolinguistics, or, as he prefers to call it, *the sociology of language*, as the study of who says what to whom, when, and why. Insights into the nature of sociolinguistics may be derived from the study of *sociolinguistic phenomena*, such as the above-mentioned situational synonyms, which illustrate in various ways how our use of language takes cues from the social context. Other sociolinguistic phenomena explored in this chapter are *status-marked forms of address, stylistic variation, diglossia*, and *code-switching*.

THE CULTURAL CONTEXT OF SOCIAL SITUATIONS

In general terms, the social context of language is culture. For the issues raised in this book, it will be useful to think of African American language as situated in African American culture. In Chapter 1 we briefly sketched a model of the social situation based on the notion of congruity of time, place, and role relationships. One particular type of situational congruity, discussed in the following section, is the fact that certain words selected by speakers should be appropriate for the particular person to whom they are speaking.

Status-Marked Forms of Address

English has certain sets of words among which speakers may chose that imply something about the relative status of the person addressed to the speaker. In England, the special forms *Your Highness*, and *Your Majesty* are reserved for use in addressing royalty. There is no comparable status to British royalty in American society, but we do have special forms of address reserved for certain persons of exalted status. The term *your honor*, for example, is reserved specifically for addressing the judge in a courtroom situation. The choice of a term such as *sweetheart* or *baby* as a form of address implies a special status such as spouse or lover. Some individuals use such forms of address loosely and unadvisedly, however, when it would be more appropriate to call the individual being addressed *ma'am, sir*, or something more formal.

Studies of the use of forms of address in corporate America indicate that reciprocal use of first names is common among business executives, and that reciprocal use of title plus last name is also common. Asymmetrical exchanges also take place among corporate executives when there are age differences or differences of occupational rank. An older person might refer to a younger peer by his or her first name, while the younger person would use the more formal title plus last name (Ervin-Tripp, 1972).

Without going into the question of the appropriateness of African American language for the job interview situation, there are clearly important issues of language choice of which job applicants need to be mindful. One has to do with the choice of forms of language to be used by the applicant and the interviewer in addressing one another. Is it appropriate for either to address the other by his or her first name, or should they use the more formal title plus last name in this situation? Should the applicant refer to the interviewer as "sir" or "ma'am"? Or is it preferable to avoid such deferential forms of address?

It is interesting to note that the terms *sir* and *ma'am* were required of Black people addressing White people in the system of racial etiquette that prevailed in the Southern United States under the color caste system. Black people were not allowed to respond with a simple "yes" or "no" to questions or directions from members of the highest caste. It was always necessary to respond "yas-suh" or "nossuh" to a male addressee, and "yasm" or "no'm" to a female of the dominant group. In the context of such a painful history, it might be difficult for an African American applicant to employ similar forms of address toward a European American interviewer in a job situation, although similar behavior in a racially neutral context might be appropriate.

Another way that language was used to reinforce the asymmetrical role relationships between Black people and White people in the caste system was through the use of the terms *boy* and *girl* by Whites in reference to Black adults in communities throughout the Old South. If the African American addressees were so elderly that the practice of addressing them as youngsters seemed ridiculous, they were addressed by White people as "Aunt" or "Uncle."

Dr. Alvin Poussaint reminds us that such practices have survived the caste system to some extent as he reports a painful personal experience in which a policeman confronted him on a public street and asked him:

"What's your name, boy?"

Although Dr. Poussaint responded,

"Dr. Poussaint. I'm a physician . . ."

the policeman went on, undaunted to ask:

"What's your first name, boy? . . ." (Ervin-Tripp 1972: 218)

Such differential treatment of African Americans by police officers continues to be a common occurrence in contemporary America.

The characteristic use of status-marked forms of address to reinforce the asymmetrical status and role relationships between Black people and White people in the American color caste system poignantly illustrates one particular aspect of the situational nature of language use. It also reminds us that because of its historical role in the oppression of African Americans, words normally considered innocuous, when used by White Americans to address African Americans, may communicate more than is intended.

The discussion of status-marked forms of address in the context of the issues raised in this book would be incomplete without reference to the infamous term *nigger*. When used by White people to address or refer to African Americans, the term is an insult, a fighting word of the worst kind. It may be puzzling for someone who is aware of the insulting and demeaning connotations of the term to observe African Americans using the term *nigger* in reference to themselves, or as an endearing form of address to a friend or family member. It is not so puzzling when we consider the situational nature of language use. It is inappropriate for a White person to use the term *nigger*, but some African Americans are comfortable with the term in situations where no White people are present, and its meaning is roughly equivalent to that of *guy*, or *fellow*; for example, *he's a tall, husky nigger = he's a tall husky guy*. To more fully analyze the use of the term *nigger* in African American culture, it will help first to introduce the phenomenon of stylistic variation.

Stylistic Variation

In this section we look at a type of variation in language that contrasts with the dialectal variation discussed in Chapter 2. Unlike dialects, which are spoken by different persons of differing regions or social backgrounds, different *styles*, or *registers* of a language are used by the same individuals on different occasions. Language styles may be characterized by varying degrees of formality, or symbolize a relationship between speaker and addressee characterized by some particular quality such as *intimacy, familiarity, distance, solidarity* or *camaraderie*. A football coach describing the quality of his team's recent victory to a fellow coach might select a style that conveys a spirit of camaraderie in which the expression *We kicked their asses!* would be appropriate. Such a colloquial style would be inappropriate if the two were discussing the victory with a reporter on a television program. In that situation, the same information could be expressed appropriately as *We dominated them totally!*

According to Joos (1961), English has exactly five styles: a *formal* style, a *consultative* style, a *casual* style, an *intimate* style, and a *frozen* style. In the formal style, all of the prescriptive grammar rules discussed in the previous chapter, including the use of *whom* instead of *who* and the avoidance of dangling prepositions, would be expected to be followed. Although language is considered incorrect to the extent that it violates such rules, it may be appropriate to suspend some of the rules of correct usage in certain situations, and certain styles. Most Americans learn at some point in their schooling that it is incorrect to say *It is me*. We are told that the subject pronoun *I* should be used instead of *me* in such sentences because it refers to the same person as the subject pronoun *it*. Whatever the justification might be for insisting that it is correct to say *It is I*, most Americans continue to say *It's me* when called upon to identify themselves as a caller at the door or on the phone. Such situations are frequently between a caller and listener who are on familiar terms, whereas the expression *It is I* is formal to the point of sounding stiff and unnatural.

A good example of the consultative style might be the language that we consider appropriate for the job interview situation. One way in which the consultative style differs from the formal style is in the selection of the various options for sentence negation discussed in Chapter 2. The basic option of placing *not* after a particular verb is the most formal. In the consultative style, the use of the contractions *isn't, aren't, didn't*, and so on, are also acceptable, but the use of *ain't* and double negatives are not. The consultative style is relaxed but businesslike. It is the style we associate with radio and TV broadcasts. Blatant violations of prescriptive grammar rules tend to be avoided, although speakers often lack full understanding of the rules and produce hypercorrect forms such as *You and I* in places where *you and me* are prescriptively correct, for example, *between you and I*.

As we reflect upon the expectations for correct language in a job interview situation, it is apparent that African American is not the only variety of American English that does not naturally conform to those expectations. The use of "like I said" to introduce a summary statement is common among speakers of high-prestige dialects of English, but might be recognized by some job interviewers as a deficiency in the ability to speak properly. In view of that fact, one has to wonder why it is that speakers of African American language are so often singled out as needing special instruction in order to ensure adequate performance in job interviews.

An example of a situation in which the casual style is appropriate might be an annual employees' picnic for a particular work unit. The participants are not necessarily intimately related and may have no dealings with one another whatsoever outside of the work situation. Participants who occupy professional or managerial positions in the organization may be accustomed to employing a consultative style, interspersed with the jargon of their particular occupation, in their communication with each other on the job. In the casual style, rules of correct grammar would be relaxed even more than in the consultative style, and certain slang expressions could safely be uttered by persons who would avoid them at work. Pronunciation of certain words may change in casual English. The words *for* and *your* sometimes change to *fer* and *yer*; words such as *something* and *nothing* are frequently reduced to *sumpm* and

nuttin; and certain word endings such as the *ing* suffix tend to be relaxed—
workin', hitt'n'.

The intimate style would be reserved to use among persons who are close enough socially to feel confident sharing details about themselves that could be embarrassing or damaging if disseminated more widely. Within such relationships it is most likely that a taboo word such as *nigger* might be uttered.

Slang

The subject of the situational nature of language use clearly includes the topic of slang. In the context of the present focus on African American language it needs to be emphasized that African American language is not slang. To the contrary, it is a language in the sense that has a lexicon, a phonological component, semantics, syntax, morphology, and so on. A small part of the lexicon of any language may consist of recently created words, or of existing words to which new meanings have been given that are known only to selected persons within special networks. Two slang terms that have gained currency among African Americans are *bad*, with the special meaning "fantastic," and *ride*, with the meaning "automobile." Many speakers of African American language seldom use slang, although they normally speak with characteristic African American grammatical patterns. Sentence (1)

1. *They daddy have a really nice car.*

is grammatically African American English, although it contains no slang. Sentence (2)

2. *They daddy have a bad ride.*

has the same grammatical structure as (1), as well as the same meaning, although it contains slang words.

The tendency to confuse African American language with slang may be explained by the fact that African American culture, and African American language in particular, has contributed a great deal of what is unique about American culture. Several of the most original contributions of American culture to world culture in the field of music are African American in origin, including spirituals and jazz. With the spread of the jazz idiom, many of the special terms that developed in the in-group language of jazz musicians became everyday slang expressions, first among Black Americans, then among Americans in general. The terms *cat* ("male person"), *chick* ("female person"), *cool* ("nice"), *hip* ("wise"), *groovy* ("positively valued"), and *cop* ("to obtain, or procure") are just a few of the rich lexicon of slang terms that have originated in Black culture. Such slang is not what we have in mind, however, when we speak of African American language.

Diglossia

The concept of *diglossia* (Ferguson 1959) offers a model of the dual nature of language in certain speech communities that accounts (with some notable exceptions) for the functional distribution of African American English and Standard English in a way that specifies their appropriateness for different situations of use, as well as for grammatical and lexical differences between the two codes. African American English may not differ as greatly from standard English as the vernacular (L) varieties in Ferguson's sample cases of diglossia differ from the standard or classical (H) varieties with which they coexist (e.g., Haitian Creole [L] differs greatly from standard [H] French), but it has a similar functional distribution to such cases.

Table 3-1, adapted from Ferguson (1959), illustrates the typical functional distribution of H and L in a diglossic language situation.

In applying the diglossia model to the language situation in Black America, we consider African American language the L variety and standard English the H variety. The main exception to the functions specified for H in Table 3.1 would be in the variety that would be used for a sermon in an African American church. While some congregations might expect the minister to preach in standard English, some African Americans appear com-

TABLE 3-1   **Functional Distribution of H and L Varieties of Language with Diglossia**

Function	Variety
Formal speech	H
Public lecture	H
News broadcast	H
Soap opera	L
Newspaper editorial	H
Caption on a political cartoon	L
Conversation with family and friends	L
Sermon in church or mosque	H
Poetry	H
Folk literature	L

fortable with worship services in which the sermon is preached in African American English, or at least in which the minister frequently switches to the L variety in order to reach a new level of spiritual fervor or underscore the seriousness or sincerity of the message.

The question of the appropriate choice for Black preachers between Standard and African American English is a live issue among African American seminarians. According to Dr. Louis-Charles Harvey, President of Payne Theological Seminary:

> . . . a [Black] preacher must learn to communicate to those assembled. There are times you can use idioms from [African American English] and be accepted. But a steady diet of [such language] and idioms would not be accepted at this time in most African American churches (personal communication).

While the appropriateness of African American language in the pulpit remains controversial, its role in other aspects of African American worship is clearly established. The traditional Negro spirituals are typically in African American language and contain in their lyrics such memorable lines as

Steal away to Jesus,
I ain't got long to stay here

and

I ain't gon' study war no more.

The frequent occurrence of *ain't*, double negatives, and other violations of prescriptive grammar rules does not detract from the beauty and power of Negro spirituals. If anything, the language seems to contribute positively to such qualities. Contemporary African American gospel music also frequently employs language forms that might be considered inappropriate in other settings.

In addition to spirituals and gospel lyrics, Black language is frequently employed in African American literature. Notable examples of poetry in African American language include "When Malindy Sings," "The Party," and other dialect poems by the famous bilingual poet Paul Lawrence Dunbar. Langston Hughes produced numerous prose and poetry works in African American language. Hughes' poem "Mother to Son" is a noteworthy instance of the effective use of Black language in a literary work, as is his entire collection of "Simple" stories. Teachers may find in African American literature a rich and effective means of maximizing the relevance of language arts instruction to the everyday lives of Black children.

AFRICAN AMERICAN ORAL LITERATURE

The discussion of African American literature would be incomplete without reference to a rich oral tradition the roots of which scholars have traced to ancient Africa (Gates 1988). One of the most famous and frequently quoted works of the Black oral tradition is "The Signifying Monkey," an extended narrative of the genre known as *toasting* (Abrahams 1964). "The Signifying Monkey" and other folk poems have been handed down from generation to generation of Black Americans through oral performances on street corners, in back alleys, in taverns, and other secular, or male, gathering places. The monkey embodies the typical qualities of the trickster hero and employs a traditional Black expressive style known as *signifying*.

Signifying—and other characteristic Black modes of verbal expression known by such terms as *marking, woofing, sounding, shucking,* and *jiving*—attest to the importance of verbal art in African American culture. Mitchell-Kernan (1972) analyzes signifying in depth. She notes that one sense in which the term signifying is used is in reference to either of several traditional forms of verbal dueling: *capping* and *playing the dozens*. The former consists of two or more adversaries who attempt to exceed each other in spontaneous performances of witty, creative, hilarious, and outrageous put-downs of each other. The latter is like the former but consists specifically of insults about the female parent of the other.

Labov (1972) analyzes the discourse structure of playing the dozens as he observed it among participants in his study of the language of teenagers in Harlem, New York. Labov noticed that playing the dozens could take the form of casual, playful, and not very creative responses to spontaneous put-downs such as the simple interjection:

Yo mamma!

offered in response to an equally uncreative put-down such as

M------f-----, you ain't got the sense you was born with!

At its best, however, playing the dozens involves two highly skilled adversaries who hold an audience of onlookers captivated with the humor and eloquence of their banter. The following examples cited by Labov (1972), and attributed to Abrahams (1962), are typical of what this author experienced in street-corner sessions as a youth (offensive words have been deleted from the original versions).

I ----ed your mother on top of the piano
When she came out she was singing the Star Spangled Banner.

Iron is iron, and steel don't rust,
But your mamma got a ----- like a Greyhound Bus.

In the all-male gatherings where the dozens are traditionally played, the frequent use of taboo words that would be grossly offensive in many other situations is appropriate.

Mitchell-Kernan analyzes another dimension of the concept of signifying that lacks the element of "game playing" found in such rituals as playing the dozens. In this regard, signifying

> . . . refers to a way of encoding messages or meanings in natural conversations which involves, in most cases, an element of indirection. (1972: 165)

As one example of such "indirection," Mitchell-Kernan relates a conversation that took place in the home of an informant, Barbara, who invited her to come back by on Saturday, at which time she was going to "cook some chit'lins." Barbara then interjected jokingly, still ostensible talking to Mitchell-Kernan:

> "Or are you one of those Negroes who don't eat chit'lins?" (p. 166)

It turned out that the message was actually intended for a third participant, Mary, who interjected indignantly in response to the comment about some Negroes not eating chitterlings:

> ". . . That's all I hear lately—soul food, soul food. If you say you don't eat it you get accused of being saditty . . ." (p. 166)

Mary continues to interject that while she had eaten such soul food as "Black-eyed peas and neck-bones" during the depression, she couldn't "get too excited" about it. She goes on to explain her present eating preferences:

> "I eat prime rib and T-bone because I like to, not because I'm trying to be White . . ."

Mary then leaves, and Barbara makes the key observation:

> "Well, I wasn't signifying at her but like I always say, if the shoe fits, wear it." (p. 167)

Mary's behavior, and Barbara's analysis of it, both validate Mitchell-Kernan's claim that signifying involves an element of indirect communication.

Mary got the message that she was considered the kind of assimilated Black individual often compared to an Oreo cookie—Black on the outside and White on the inside—even though the message was ostensibly not directed to her.

THE LANGUAGE SITUATION IN BLACK AMERICA: CLASS-STRATIFICATION OR CODE-SWITCHING

The term *language situation* is used in sociolinguistics in reference to the overall pattern of language use in a particular speech community. As we have discussed, a bilingual or diglossic model adequately accounts for the language use of African Americans. It is commonly asserted in the literature, however, that the language situation in Black America is one of *class stratification*; that is, African American English is spoken by poor and uneducated Black people and Standard English is spoken by middle class African Americans.

Mitchell-Kernan's description of the conversation between Barbara, Mary, and herself appears to support the class stratification model in that the three Black women speak to each other in Standard English. In another conversation reported in the same article, however, Mitchell-Kernan shows that she is bilingual. The reported conversation takes place between Mitchell-Kernan and a male informant encountered in a public park, who opens the conversation by complimenting her, in African American Language:

"Mamma you sho is fine." (1972: 170)

Mitchell-Kernan displays her competence in African American language in her reply:

"That ain' no way to talk to your mother." (p. 170)

and in her subsequent behavior in this conversation.

DeBose (1992) presents evidence of code-switching in spontaneous conversations of African American adults recorded in Oakland, California in 1987. One of the informants is a middle-class female, "P," who frequently switches to African American language. P's code-switching was recorded in two different sessions in her home, with the researchers, her husband, and her daughter present.

From listening to the first few minutes of the recording, one might get the impression that P is a monolingual standard English (SE) speaker. As the sessions progress, however, she makes several notable switches to AAE. Code-switches to AAE are set in regular type.

In the following excerpt from the beginning of the first tape P speaks SE exclusively to the researcher N. The classification of her first utterance as SE is supported by the SE pronunciation of *can't*, which contrasts with the ethnically marked *cain't*.

P: I just can't stay in the bed late. I can't do it!

One of several code-switches occurs later in the tape when P narrates an incident in which she "fusses" at her daughter L, who is late coming home from a music rehearsal and admits having spent time at a local shopping mall "looking around." P switches to AAE mainly to describe her conversation with L in direct quotation.

> . . . I said *'L ! Bring yo ass (laughter)!* . . . I said *'Where have you been all day! Where have you been!'*
> *'We just went up to the Mall. We was, we just walkin' around. We just lookin' at the Mall.* I said *'Lookin' at the Mall? Thugs and hoods hang out at the Mall! I ain't raise no thug and hood, here!* You know. So then she *'Well, we didn't, we wasn't, we just lookin around and we got us sumpm to eat and stuff'.*
>   Oh I fussed and I cussed. I said *'You on punishment now for six months. You cain't look at no T.V. You cain't do nothin!* . . .

In the second session, P frequently speaks AAE interspersed with SE as she returns home to join her husband and the researchers after taking her youngest daughter K to a Saturday computer class. Her use of AAE in the following excerpts suggests that she now defines the situation as one in which the choice of AAE is appropriate.

> Okay, let's go. (unin.) Let's run up here real quick cause (unin.) *They gon be on time. They ain't gon be on time.*
>   *I'm'on run L up here for this computer class* . . . *They suppose to start the Dad's club. I think it's starting now so I'm'o run up here and* see what they're doin,' it's about fifteen after, *they suppose to have from ten to twelve* . . . *They gon try to start some Saturday activities at the school* . . .

DeBose (1992, p. 165) states in the conclusion that

The evidence considered in this paper is striking counter evidence to the claim that [AAE] is spoken mainly by poor and uneducated persons . . .

Evidence of code-switching by Black Americans supports the claim that the African American speech community is bilingual. Not only are two different language, AAE and SE, maintained in the community's linguistic repertoire, they are often spoken by the same bilingual individuals. The class stratification model is refuted by evidence that African Americans of all socioeconomic levels speak African American language.

The bilingual nature of the African American linguistic repertoire is also supported by evidence discussed in the next chapter to the effect that AAE is a language in its own right.

SUMMARY

Language that is normally considered "bad" might be appropriate and acceptable for particular situations, and language that is correct, in the sense that it is grammatical, might be considered an inappropriate choice. A good deal of what native speakers know about their language is of a nature that cannot be adequately explained by a model of descriptive grammar of the internal structure of language.

Insights into the nature of sociolinguistics may be derived from the study of sociolinguistic phenomena—such as situational synonyms, status-marked forms of address, stylistic variation, diglossia, and code-switching—that illustrate how our use of language takes cues from the social context. In general terms, the social context of language is culture. African American language is situated in African American culture.

Member of particular cultures can tell what the situation is at any given time, and act accordingly. A social situation may be defined as a time, a place, a set of objects, and set of role relationships that go together. In congruent situations, all of the elements are normal and expected and tend to go unnoticed. In incongruent situations there is something unusual or unexpected, which causes surprise and draws attention.

Evidence of code-switching by Black Americans supports the claim that the African American speech community is bilingual. Two different languages, AAE and SE, are maintained in the linguistic repertoire of the African American speech community and are often spoken by the same bilingual individuals.

There are many situations for which African American language is the appropriate choice including the home, the church, sacred and secular music, and oral and written literature. African Americans have an exceptionally rich oral tradition of folk stories, songs, poetry, verbal games, and a variety of named genres of verbal expression, such as signifying and playing the dozens. Although slang expressions originating in African American culture have contributed richly to American culture, African American language is not slang. Slang expressions only comprise a small part of the lexicon of African American language.

African American language may be inappropriate for the job interview situation. However, if both White and Black children speak dialects that differ from the expected language of the job interview, there is no justification for singling out African American children to be taught Standard English.

REFERENCES

Abrahams, R. (1962). Playing the dozens. *Journal of American Folklore*, 75:209–18.

Abrahams, R. (1964). *Deep Down in the Jungle: Negro Narrative Folklore from the Streets of Philadelphia*. Chicago: Aldine Publishing Company.

DeBose, C. E. (1992). Code-Switching: Black English and Standard English in the African-American Linguistic Repertoire. In Carol M. Eastman (ed.), *The Journal of Multilingual and Multicultural Development: Special Issue on Codeswitching, 13* (1 & 2): 157–167.

DuBois, W. E. B. (1961). *The Souls of Black Folk.*Greenwich, CN: Fawcett Publications (originally published in 1903).

Ervin-Tripp, S. (1972). *On Sociolinguistic Rules: Alternation and Co-occurrence*. In J. J. Gumperz & D. Hymes (eds.). *Direction in Sociolinguistics: The Ethnography of Communication* (pp. 213–50). New York: Holt, Rinehart and Winston.

Ferguson, C. A. (1959). Diglossia. *Word*, 15: 325–40.

Fishman, J. A. (1972). *The Sociology of Language: an Interdisciplinary Social Science Approach to Language in Society*. Rowley MA: Newbury House Publishers.

Gates, H. L. Jr. (1988). *The Signifying Monkey: A Theory of African-American Literary Criticism*. New York: Oxford University Press.

Gumperz, J. J., & Hymes, D. (eds). (1972). *Direction in Sociolinguistics: The Ethnography of Communication*. New York: Holt, Rinehart and Winston.

Joos, M. (1961). *The Five Clocks*. New York: Harcourt, Brace and World,

Kochman, T. (1981). *Black and White Styles in Conflict*. Chicago: University of Chicago Press.

Labov, W. (1972). *Language in the Inner City: Studies in the Black English Vernacular*. Chapter 8: Rules for Ritual Insults (pp. 297–353). Philadelphia: University of Pennsylvania Press.

Mitchell-Kernan, C. (1972). *Signifying and Marking: Two Afro-American Speech Acts*. J. J. Gumperz & D. Hymes, (eds.), *Directions in Sociolinguistics: The Ethnography of Communication* (pp. 161–79). New York: Holt, Rinehart and Winston.

4

AFRICAN AMERICAN ENGLISH AS A LINGUISTIC SYSTEM

Chapter Overview

Upon reading this chapter you will gain understanding of:

- The linguistic nature of African American language
- The nature of dialects, vernaculars, pidgins, creoles, and other particular types of linguistic systems
- How African American language differs from other dialects of American English in its lexicon phonology and grammar
- The relationship of African American language to African and Caribbean creole languages
- Arguments for and against a policy of full recognition of African American language

What is this thing that we have been calling African American English and that is commonly referred to as Black English? Is it a language? A dialect? A vernacular? A creole? Is it some, all, or none of the above? Whatever term best characterizes African American English as a *linguistic system* (Stewart 1970), what should it be called? In this chapter, we will attempt to answer such questions on the basis of the present state of linguistic knowledge. Our primary aim is to develop the case that AAE is indeed a language. Such an affirmation, we will show, is not only appropriate, but also a crucially important component of a new paradigm of English language arts instruction in which the traditional notions of "good" and "bad" English have no role or function.

Linguists unanimously reject the idea that African American English is "bad" and support the view that it is systematic and rule-governed. Some linguists may be uncomfortable for political reasons, in view of the ambiguity of the term language, to endorse the affirmation that AAE is a language. Most linguists acknowledge the existence of a unique dialect of American English spoken by African Americans, although they differ on a number of issues concerning its linguistic nature, and its relationship to the English of White Americans. The most heated and persistent debate has focused on two related questions: Whether AAE is fundamentally the same as dialects spoken by White Americans and different in superficial ways, or vice versa; and whether AAE evolved from the same historical source as dialects spoken by Whites, or from a different source, such as a creole (Dillard 1972).

As noted in Chapter 3, many linguists tend to characterize the distinctive qualities of African American language in terms that suggest the absence of elements that are present in varieties spoken by White Americans, and deny the existence of a unique linguistic system for African Americans. We reject that view of African American language and support a *bisystemic* model of African American language variation. That model assumes that African American language coexists with standard English in the African American linguistic repertoire, and that many speakers are bilingual. Although all linguists agree that AAE is systematic and rule-governed, some argue that it is the same system as standard English except for the features listed in their descriptions of Black English. It is interesting to note that the assertion that African American English is a language in its own right has greater force when supported by evidence that it is a *different* system than standard English. The assertion that African American language is a language can also be strengthened or weakened by our decision to call it by one or another of the various names that have been suggested for it.

WHAT SHOULD THE LANGUAGE OF AFRICAN AMERICANS BE CALLED?

Contributors to the emerging field of African American language studies have employed a variety of terms for African American language. Earlier studies, conducted at a time when African Americans were commonly referred to as Negroes, employed such terms as Negro Dialect, or Nonstandard Negro English. As Black Americans began to reject the label "Negro" and express a preference for "Black" as the appropriate label for their group identity, however, terms such as "Black English" and "Vernacular Black English" became increasingly commonplace. The term "Ebonics" was coined in 1979 by a group of African American scholars, dissatisfied with the Eurocentric connotations of the term Black English (Covington, 1976).

The term "nonstandard Negro English" is obsolete due to the obsolescence of the term "Negro." Moreover, use of the modifier "Non-standard" shows insensitivity in defining African American language in negative terms. The term Black English is consistent with the established practice for labeling regional dialects of English, for example, Texas English, British English, and so on. If African American language is considered a social dialect of American English, the term "Black English" is appropriate. The subordination of African American language to English implied by the term "Black English" may be avoided by terms such as "Ebonics" which make no reference to the English language.

In considering the question of what to call African American language, we must not neglect the perspective of ordinary people. To ordinary African Americans, the language that they speak is simply English. It is impossible to predict what will happen in the future as the findings of recent scholarship on African American language become known to the masses of its speakers, and they begin to deal with the realization that it is not "bad" English, as they had been taught, but a language in its own right. When the issue is taken up by the African American community, whatever they decide as a group to call their language, whether Ebonics, Black English, African American English, or none of the above, that is what it will be called.

The issue of what African American language should be called is part and parcel of the more general concern for sensitivity in the naming and labeling of the various cultural groups of a pluralistic society and the cultural traits of those groups. We cannot tell the reader which of the prevailing terms for African American language to use, although each of us has his or her preferences. As a general practice, however, the reader is advised to avoid any particular label whenever possible and to be aware of the relative appropriateness of various terms for various situations. The only terms that we categorically reject as totally inappropriate are those that imply that African American language is "bad," "incorrect," or "substandard."

IS AFRICAN AMERICAN LANGUAGE A DIFFERENT SYSTEM FROM STANDARD ENGLISH?

Afrocentric scholars recognize African American language as a language in its own right, which is best and most adequately described in terms of its own internal structure or grammar (i.e, lexicon, semantics, phonology, morphology, and syntax) without reference to standard English. From such a grammar, one may judge for oneself the extent to which African American language is similar to or different from other varieties of English.

An honest evaluation of the facts leaves no doubt that African American language is a variety of English, and that it has many elements and subsystems that are the same as, or very similar to, varieties of English spoken by Whites. It is clearly not the same as European American English, however, and the main point of contention should be whether the differences are sufficient or of such a nature as to support its classification as a different linguistic system.

In support of our position, we show below that African American language has a number of differences from standard English that Eurocentric accounts have tended to understate. A case in point involves the lexicon. Many of the features of "Black English" described by some linguists as phonological simplifications or deletions may also be accounted for using the notion of lexical alternation (Vaughn-Cooke, 1986). After discussing some examples of lexical alternation, we show that African American language has a different system of sentence negation than the standard English system which we briefly alluded to in Chapter 1. As in all cases of grammatical description, there is no intention of attributing the usage in question to any particular individual speakers. The only claim is that the forms in question are in widespread use. Some individuals may use them frequently, or occasionally, in alternation with standard English forms. Other individuals may never use them.

THE UNIQUENESS OF THE AFRICAN AMERICAN ENGLISH LEXICON

Eurocentric accounts of African American language often understate the uniqueness of its lexicon by arguing that many lexical items that are similar to their English equivalents are the same, but subject to phonological variations. Many African American words are very similar to standard English in sound, grammar, and meaning, and many of those differ phonologically in ways that may be expressed through phonological rules. For example, a set of African American words such as /fo/ "four," /flo/ "floor," /do/ "door," /mo/ "more," and so on may be derived from their standard English equivalents by deleting final /r/. Eurocentric analyses account for such lexical correspondences by attributing to "Black English" such phonological features as r-lessness and final consonant cluster simplification.

The phonological features analysis may be adequate for certain cases in which a simple phonological difference separates the African American form from its standard English equivalent. In the case of words such as *test*, *desk*, *find*, *told*, it makes sense to argue that African American language has the same lexical items as standard English, even though speakers pronounce them differently. Such a concession, however, does not negate the claim that African American language has a different lexicon, in totality. After all, certain different languages such as Spanish and Portuguese have many common words. African American language has quite a few lexical items that are different from their standard English etymon. Some such words are the same in sound, but differ in some of their meanings. A case in point is the adjective *yellow*. As used in African American language *yellow* not only denotes the color "yellow," as in other dialects, it also has a special meaning among African Americans when it is used in reference to a light-skinned person. The term *high-yellow* is also used with reference to a light-skinned person. Another example of an African American lexical item that has special meanings beyond its common English meaning is the term *po*, which not only means "destitute," but also "skinny" or "emaciated." A third example of this type is the adjective *fine*, which means "attractive" or "good-looking" in African American language as well as its standard meaning.

The lists of features approach also leaves unaccounted for African American words that differ in pronunciation from their standard English equivalents in unsystematic and unpredictable ways. The African American language word *sho* "sure" is pronounced in a way that is not accounted for fully by the deletion of *r* from standard English *sure*. The African American language word for "hungry" has a distinctive pronunciation *hongry*, but African American language does not have a general rule by which words containing the vowel of *sung* are transformed in pronunciation to match the vowel of *song*. African American language also has its own characteristic pronunciation of *sister*, with an initial vowel similar to the vowel of *took*. Many bilingual speakers of African American language and standard English maintain both forms of such words in their lexicon and select one that they feel is appropriate for any given situation.

Another way of presenting the uniqueness of the African American lexicon, despite its similarity to standard English, is to display sets of words such as personal pronouns, some of which are the same as, or very similar to, their standard English equivalents, but others of which are markedly African American. The African American language personal pronouns (Table 4-1) differ from those of standard English, not only in having a distinct second person plural form y'*all*, but also in having special variants *I'm* and *it's* of the first and third person singular forms I and it.

TABLE 4-1 The Subject Pronouns of African American English

	singular	plural
first	I I'm	we
second	you	y'all
third	he she	they
	it it's	

The use of apostrophes in the spelling of these forms (*I'm*, *y'all*, and *it's*) is for consistency with conventional practice, and in recognition of African American historical derivation from standard English contractions of *I+am* and *it+is* respectively. The reader should understand clearly, however, that in the African American system they are classified as pronouns, each consisting of a single morpheme.

The classification of *I'm* as a pronoun is supported by anecdotal evidence of casual observers as well as by formal linguistic analysis. The soul singer James Brown, for example, in a television interview quoted his father, whom he described as "an uneducated man," as saying to Brown when he was a child

I'm is yo daddy. You is not my daddy.

The classification of *I'm* and *it's* as pronouns is supported by recent formal analyses of African American grammar (DeBose & Faraclas 1993) in which predicates are classified as *stative* or *nonstative*. The special pronoun variants are described as co-occurring with stative predicates such as predicate adjective phrases (e.g., sentences 1 and 2).

1. *I'm tired.*
2. *It's cold.*

The basic forms I and it co-occur with nonstative predicates or verbs (e.g. sentences 3, 4)

3. *I got tired.*
4. *It got cold.*

Another form of evidence in support of the classification of I'm and it's as monomorphemic pronouns is the occurrence of such forms in certain archaic varieties of African American language in ways that are clearly not contractions of a pronoun + a form of the verb be. In the dialect of English spoken in Samana, Dominican Republic, for example, I'm frequently occurs before been and got, as in the following excerpt from a conversation recorded by DeBose in Samana in 1979 (DeBose, 1983; 1988).

. . . I'm been Miami, I'm been Spain . . . I'm got some brothers . . .

One particular set of words in the African American lexicon that has no direct counterpart in the standard English system are *catenatives*, so called because they function to link a subject to a prototypical complement such as a verb phrase or predicate adjective. As predicates, catenatives are classified

TABLE 4-2   African American Catenatives

catenative	meaning	stativity
gon'	future time	+
be	habitual/irrealis	−
done	completive	+/−

according to their stativity (+) or (−) as shown in Table 4-2. The stativity classification of a catenative plays a major role in determining how it may occur in catenative constructions.

The stative classification of *gon'* correctly predicts its co-occurrence with the special subject pronoun *I'm* (sentence 5), and the nonstative classification of be (sentence 6) correctly predicts its occurrence with the basic pronoun *I*.

5. *I'm gon' be at home.*
6. *I be at home.*

The catenative *gon'* takes a nonstative complement (be in sentence 5, cook in sentence 7), whereas the catenative *be* takes a stative complement (*at home* in sentences 5, 6, *cookin'* in sentence 8):

7. *I'm gon' cook dinner.*
8. *I be cookin' dinner.*

The catenative *done* is classified for stativity as +/− in recognition of the fact that it patterns like stative predicates when it follows the catenative be as in sentence 9, but, unlike other stative predicates, tends to co-occur with the basic pronoun I rather than the special variant *I'm* (sentence 10).

9. *I be done got tired.*
10. **I'm done got tired.*

As noted above, standard English does not have a lexical category comparable to the African American catenative. Nor does it have a grammatical equivalent to the stative/nonstative contrast so fundamental to the grammar of African American language. Eurocentric accounts of AAE are content to observe that the forms *gon'*, *be*, and *done* are phonologically similar to standard English forms. They hardly entertain the possibility that those forms might be different in subtler and more abstract ways such as we have just illustrated.

Sentence Negation in African American Language

As a final illustration of how different African American language is from standard English as a linguistic system let us briefly sketch the basic elements of the African American language system of sentence negation. Remember that in Chapter 2 we characterized the standard English sentence negation system in terms of a basic option of placing not after the first auxiliary, a secondary option of substituting a special negated contraction for the auxiliary after which not would otherwise be placed, and a third option of selecting ain't instead of certain negated contractions.

The African American system has a basic option for negating sentences that is completely different from the standard English system. Depending on the type of predicate, either *ain't*, or *don't* is placed before the predicate (Bailey 1965; DeBose & Faraclas 1993; Dillard 1972). To apply this rule correctly, predicates are classified as stative, nonstative type a, and nonstative type b, as illustrated by sentences 11 to16 in Table 4-3.

Sentences 17 to 23 represent the negated versions of sentences 11 to 16 by means of the basic African American language option, which selects *don't* with "nonstative 6" predicate types and *ain't* with others.

17. *She ain't mean.*
18. *They ain't my cousins.*
20. *He ain't at school.*
21. *He ain't went to school. or He ain't go to school.*
22. *We don't go to school.*
23. *We don't be at school.*

In addition to the basic option for negating sentences in the manner just illustrated, African American language speakers have other options for negating sentences that avoid the use of the stigmatized form *ain't*. One such

TABLE 4-3   Types of Predicates

	Stative	Nonstative/A	Nonstative/B
11. *She mean.*	+		
12. *They my cousins.*	+		
13. *He at school.*	+		
14. *We went to school.*		+	
15. *We go to school.*			+
16. *We be at school.*			+

option is to select *not* instead of *ain't* for the negation of sentences with stative predicates (sentences 24 to 26, for example):

24. *She not mean.*
25. *They not my cousins.*
26. *He not at school.*

To avoid using *ain't* for the negation of a type A nonstative sentence, African American language speakers may select the option of using *haven't* or *didn't* (DeBose 1994) as in sentences 27 and 28:

27. *He haven't went to school.*
28. *He didn't go to school.*

The *ain't*-avoiding sentence negation options available to AAE speakers sometimes result in sentences that are the same as standard English on the surface. In many instances, however, they result in sentences that retain the outward appearance of African American language.

The evidence just considered concerning the uniqueness of the African American lexicon and its unique system of sentence negation support the affirmation that African American language is a language by showing that although it is English, it is not the same linguistic system as that of Standard English.

WHAT TYPE OF LINGUISTIC SYSTEM IS AFRICAN AMERICAN LANGUAGE?

The term language is often used in an excessively narrow sense that sets high prestige varieties of language with unquestioned social recognition apart from those with lower prestige and lesser degrees of social recognition. In that narrow sense, the term language excludes dialects, vernaculars, creoles, pidgins, and other particular types of languages of marginal social status. Because of the many ambiguities surrounding the term language, we will resort, when necessary, to the more technical term linguistic system.

In asserting that what African Americans speak is a language, we are in agreement with the unnamed social commentator who defines a language as "a dialect that has its own army and navy." Such a definition recognizes the essentially sociopolitical nature of many typological classifications for language varieties. In the following pages we will explore the criteria developed by linguists for classifying a linguistic system in one way or another, that is, as a dialect, vernacular, standard, pidgin, or creole.

The most commonly assigned classification to African American language is that of a dialect. A dialect is technically a language variety that lacks autonomy (Stewart 1970). That is, it is considered to be one of several different ways in which a particular language is spoken and does not have a separate identity. The decision as to whether a given variety should be classified as a language or a dialect is complicated by the fact that the attitudes of speakers are more important than any objective assessment of how similar or different a given variety might be from the language of which it is supposed to be a dialect.

Some varieties of Norwegian and Danish are so similar that their speakers can understand one another without switching languages. Despite their mutual intelligibility, however, Norwegian and Danish are considered different languages by their speakers, and so they are classified thus. Some dialects of Chinese, however, differ so much that their speakers cannot easily understand one another, yet they are not considered different languages, but dialects of a single language. In both cases, the final decision as to whether it is a case of different languages or different dialects is based more on sociopolitical considerations than on objective degrees of similarity or difference between the varieties in question.

The fact that African Americans consider their language English supports the classification of African American language as a dialect of American English. That does not preclude the possibility that it might in the future be classified as an autonomous language. Perhaps African Americans will develop a new collective consciousness of their language around a consensus that it is *not* English, either through the unplanned spread of scientific knowledge and accurate information about African American language or through a systematic campaign to change its status. However it would come about, such a change in the speakers' attitudes toward African American language would require a change in its technical linguistic classification from dialect to autonomous language.

The technical classification of African American language as a dialect does not conflict with the statement that it is a language in the broad inclusive sense. Nor does the frequent classification of African American language as vernacular, creole, or post-creole (DeCamp 1971) in technical linguistic literature. In technical usage, a *vernacular* is a language that lacks standardization in the sense of prescribed norms of correct usage, and a body of written literature (Stewart 1970). African American language is normally used only in spoken form. The main exception to this is the frequent use of African American language in literary works for dialog, folk narrative, and quotations. The present classification of African American language as a vernacular language does not preclude its possible future classification as a standard language following the acceptance of authoritative grammars and dictionaries and the publication of literary works entirely in African American language.

A *creole* may be defined in simple terms as a mixed language (Hymes 1971). It derives its lexicon primarily from a particular existing language but contains words and grammatical patterns from various languages. Technically, a creole is defined as a pidgin that has acquired a community of native speakers. A *pidgin*, in turn, is defined as an emergency code consisting of a small vocabulary sufficient for communication in a limited set of circumstances such as warfare and trade (Hymes 1971).

Pidgins frequently develop in frontier areas and war zones where speakers of two or more different languages are forced to communicate in a language that most of them barely know. In such situations, gestures and body language are often relied upon to make up for the limited set of words and syntactic patterns available to the group. A pidgin is similar to what we commonly refer to as broken language—broken English, broken French, and so on (Ferguson & DeBose 1977). African American language is not presently a pidgin or a creole, and it is inappropriate to refer to it as broken English.

THE ORIGIN OF AFRICAN AMERICAN ENGLISH

Research on the origin of African American language has generated debate among linguists over the pros and cons of what has come to be known as the *creolist* hypothesis. Simply put, the creolist hypothesis claims that pidgin English was used by many of the ancestors of present day African Americans, and that creole English was acquired by many of the children of African captives born into slavery on American plantations (Dillard 1972). The evidence for the prior creolization of African American language is largely circumstantial and includes the fact that Africans enslaved by Europeans depended upon their limited knowledge of the European languages not only for communication with their captors, but also for communication with other Africans.

The West African areas from which many of the ancestors of African Americans came are extremely multilingual. In Nigeria alone, for example, over 200 different languages are spoken. The millions of Africans brought to America as slaves undoubtedly included speakers of many different African languages such as Yoruba, Hausa, Twi, Ibo, Efik, Fulani, Ewe, Wolof, Mende, and Mandinka, to name a few. The likelihood was considerable that any given group of African captives would include many who could not understand each other's languages. To further complicate matters, the European slave traders established a practice of deliberately separating captives from the same ethnic and linguistic groups from one another in order to lessen their ability to plot insurrection.

Conditions were ideal among the captive Africans for pidgin English to develop as a means of emergency communication and become established as the primary means of communication among Africans in the new plantation societies. It was inevitable that as children were born in captivity, their African ancestral languages would be lost and replaced by English, or possibly, an English creole. The creolist hypothesis is supported by striking similarities between African American language and acknowledged English creoles such as Gullah, spoken on the sea islands of South Carolina and Georgia, Jamaican Patois, Guyanese Creole, and Taki Taki of Surinam (Alleyne 1980). The same similarities that can be observed between African American language and certain creoles, however, are also seen in comparisons of Black Language to many of the languages of West Africa.

Dillard (1972) supports his version of the creolist hypothesis mainly with written evidence of pidgin and creole features in the language attributed to African Americans in travelers' accounts of visits to North America in earlier times, and in language attributed to fictional characters by early American authors. Additional evidence in support of the creolist hypothesis is reported in recent studies of the archaic English dialect spoken in Samana, Dominican Republic by descendants of Free Africans who migrated to Hispaniola in the early 1800s (DeBose 1983; 1996).

Although there is considerable evidence in support of the creolist hypothesis, there is also abundant evidence in support of a third way of interpreting the origin of African American language using the notion of African continuities. The African continuities analysis is not in conflict with the creolist hypothesis, and it has the desirable quality that it can be used for teaching African American children about their language in a way that emphasizes its African roots.

African Continuities in African American Language

Recent work from an Afrocentric perspective describes African American language as a coherent system containing continuities of patterns that are common to the languages of West Africa. Afrocentric scholars avoid the devaluing of African American language implicit in the practice of describing it as the absence of elements present in standard English by emphasizing the presence of features that have been retained from African languages. For example, instead of attributing the absence of standard English *th* sounds to African American language, Afrocentric scholars emphasize the fact that speakers of other languages, when exposed to English, frequently replace the *th* sounds with similar phonemes in their native languages (Williams 1991).

The interdental fricative sounds spelled *th* in English are rare among the languages of the world. French speakers frequently substitute /z/ for the English voiced interdental fricative producing pronunciations such as *zis*, and *zat*. The phoneme /z/ is a voiced dentoalveolar fricative, similar enough to the English voiced interdental fricative for which it substitutes to be comprehensible to English speakers. The phoneme /d/, in the African American forms *dis*, and *dat* is a voiced dentoalveolar stop that, unlike the voiced interdental fricative of *this* and *that*, is in the phonemic inventories of many West African languages. It was normal for African captives to use the similar sounds of their native languages in the place of the unfamiliar English sounds. The use of those sounds in African American language may be seen as the continuation of phonemes from African languages rather than the absence of the English interdental fricatives represented by the letter th.

The notion of African continuities can account for any of the features of African American language that have been previously described as the absence of something present in standard English. Instead of alluding to "final consonant cluster simplification," for instance, to account for such African American forms as *tes* "test," and *tole* "told," Afrocentric scholars describe such forms as representing continuities of typical West African phonotactic patterns that permit sequences such as CONSONANT-VOWEL (abbreviated CV), and CVC, but not the CVCC pattern underlying such standard English forms as *test* and *told*.

It is interesting to note that in order to describe African American language in terms of African continuities we are forced to resort to more rigorous methods of linguistic description than listing features and attaching labels to them. When speaking to an audience of non-linguists it has been convenient to use their familiarity with standard English as a point of departure. Typical African American language pronunciations such as *flo* "floor" have been described as instances of the "r-lessness" feature. To avoid the negative characterization of African American language inherent in the feature label, the Afrocentric scholar cannot simply substitute a more complimentary label for the feature, but must look again to the typical phonotactic patterns of West African languages for evidence that /r/ does not tend to occur in those languages after vowels or at the end of words as it does in English words such as fourth and floor.

The various morphological and syntactic features listed separately in Eurocentric descriptions of African American language may be seen as continuities of a system found in West African languages and creoles in which differences of aspect (Comrie 1976) take precedence over differences of tense (Comrie 1985). In English the reverse is true. In English, every predicate is marked present or past tense by the form of the first member of the verb phrase. In the African and creole languages in question, however, the classification of events is primarily on the basis of whether or not the action or state is completed. That is, where English speakers are obligated to grammatically mark the occurrence of an event as past or present tense, many African languages and creoles are set up to classify events in terms of *completive* or *noncompletive* aspect based on whether the predicate is classified stative or nonstative (Mufwene 1983; Turner 1949). The description of the African American language tense-mood-aspect system developed in DeBose and Faraclas (1993) makes a fundamental distinction between completive and non-completive aspect and between stative and nonstative predicates. As such, it strongly supports the creolist hypothesis and the hypothesis of African continuities.

Pedagogical Implications

The rich and growing body of knowledge on African American language presents an opportunity and a challenge to educators who are committed to maximizing the relevance of lesson content to the various experiences and cultural perspectives that children bring into the classroom. The availability of detailed grammatical descriptions of African American language provides the basis for teaching the concepts of grammar in a way that is validated by the internalized linguistic competence of speakers of all varieties of American English.

The question of the origin of African American language involves content from a variety of disciplines including history and geography, as well as linguistics. Such material may be used to develop replicable models for the infusion of multicultural content into the elementary and secondary curricula.

SUMMARY

Two issues have dominated academic research on African American language: the question of whether it is the same or a different system than standard English; and the question of whether it originated in the same way, or in a different way than other varieties of American English.

Scholars disagree on whether African American language should be called "Black English," "Ebonics," or something else. To the ordinary African American, however, the language that he or she speaks is simply English. It may be prudent to avoid, whenever possible, any particular label for African American language.

Although linguists insist that African American language is systematic and rule-governed, they may have contributed to the perpetuation of negative stereotypes of African American language by describing it as a list of features corresponding to the lack or absence of something that is normally present in Mainstream American English, that is, as Standard English Minus. Recent work from an Afrocentric perspective describes African American language as a coherent system containing continuities of patterns that are common to the languages of West Africa.

REFERENCES

Alleyne, M. C. (1980). *Comparative Afro-American: An historical-comparative study of English-based Afro-American dialects of the New World.* Ann Arbor: Karoma.

Bailey, B. L. (1965). Toward a new perspective in Negro dialectology. *American Speech* 40:171–77.

Comrie, B. (1976). *Aspect: An introduction to the study of verbal aspect and related problems.* Cambridge: University Press.

Comrie, B. (1985). *Tense.* Cambridge: University Press.

Covington, A. (1976). Black people and Black English: Attitudes and deeducation in a biased macroculture. In D. S. Harrison & T. Trabasso (eds.), *Black English: A Seminar* (pp. 255–264). Hillsdale, New Jersey: Lawrence Erlbaum Associates.

DeBose, C. (1983). Samana English: A dialect that time forgot. *Proceedings of the Ninth Annual Meeting of the Berkeley Linguistics Society,* pp. 4–53.

DeBose, C. (1988). *Be in Samana English, Society for Caribbean Linguistics, Occasional Paper No. 21,* St. Augustine, Trinidad.

DeBose, C. (1994). A Note on Ain't vs. Didn't Negation in African-American Vernacular. *Journal of Pidgin and Creole Languages* 9:1, 127–30.

DeBose, C. E. (1996). *Creole English in Samana.* Frances Ingemann (ed.), *1994 Mid-American Linguistics Conference Papers,* II, 341–50.

DeBose, C. E., & Faraclas, N. (1993). An Africanist approach to the linguistic study of Black English: Getting to the roots of the tense-aspect-modality and copula systems in Afro-American. In S. S. Mufwene (ed.), *Africanisms in Afro-American Language Varieties* (pp. 364–387). Athens: University of Georgia Press.

DeCamp, D. (1971). Towards a generative analysis of a post creole continuum. Dell Homes (ed.), *Pidginization and Creolization of Languages* (pp. 349–70). London: Cambridge University Press.

Dillard, J. L. (1972). *Black English: Its History and Usage in the United States.* New York: Random House.

Ferguson, C. A. &. DeBose, C.E. (1977). Simplified registers, broken language and pidginization. In Albert Valdman (ed.), *Pidgin and Creole Linguistics* (pp. 99–125). Bloomington: Indiana University Press.

Green, L. (1993). *Topics in African American English: The Verb System Analysis.* Unpublished doctoral dissertation. University of Massachusetts, Amherst.

Green, L. (1995). Study of Verb Classes in African American English. *Linguistics and Education* 7(1): 65–81.

Hymes, D. (ed). (1971). *Pidginization and Creolization of Language.* Cambridge: University Press.

Morgan, M. (1993). The Africanness of counter language among Afro-Americans. S. Mufwene (ed.), *Africanisms in Afro-American Language Varieties* (pp. 423–35). Athens: The University of Georgia Press.

Mufwene, S S. (1983). *Some Observations on the Verb in Black English Vernacular.* Austin: African and Afro-American Studies and Research Center, University of Texas.

Mufwene, S. S. (1996). African-American English, Caribbean English Creoles, and North American English: Perspectives on their geneses. Frances Ingemann (ed.), *1994 Mid-American Linguistics Conference Papers,* II, 305–30.

Stewart, W. A. (1970). A sociolinguistic typology for describing national multilingualism. Joshua Fishman (ed.), *Readings in the Sociology of Language* . The Hague: Mouton.

Turner, L. D. (1949). *Africanisms in the Gullah Dialect*. Chicago: University of Chicago Press.

Vaughn-Cooke, F. B. (1986). Lexical diffusion: Evidence from a decreolizing variety of Black English. In M. Montgomery & G. Bailey (eds.), *Language Variety in the South* (pp. 111–130). Tuscaloosa: University of Alabama Press.

Williams, S. W. (1991). Classroom use of African American Language: Educational tool or social weapon? In Christine E. Sleeter (ed.), *Empowerment Through Multicultural Education*. Albany: State University of New York Press.

5

AFRICAN AMERICAN COMMUNICATION STYLES

Chapter Overview

Upon reading this chapter you will gain understanding of:

- The general communication process
- Six psychological themes in language, oral literature and expressive patterns of African Americans
- Meanings and values of Black and White culture and communication
- Intercultural communication
- Communication competence within the Black community
- African American communication styles
- Code-switching and situational context

In previous chapters the point was made that African Americans have a distinctive cultural tradition influenced by patterns and behaviors of African American origin. In this chapter we develop the point that culture plays a major role in the communication process among individuals from different cultural and language backgrounds. This phenomenon is particularly true and noticeable among African Americans and European Americans living in the United States. When African Americans and European Americans interact, they bring to the communication process different filters through which their messages are sent, received, interpreted, and understood. The speakers and listeners from both cultural and language backgrounds bring to the communication process their past experiences, perceptions of the listener or speaker, their emotional involvement with the message, and their understanding of the verbal content. They also bring their world views, interpretation of the other's behaviors, and the reasons they are interpreting the interaction as they do.

Communication differences between European Americans and African Americans are seldom discussed; yet, Blacks and Whites often say to each other, "I didn't understand what you said," or, "I didn't understand what you meant," or, "I misunderstood, I thought you said. . . ." These statements are often the result of what we commonly call communication breakdown or miscommunication.

Unless there are reasons to think otherwise, many European Americans assume that the messages and meanings they assign when communicating with African Americans are understood and interpreted in the same way. Thought is seldom given to the fact that most African Americans translate the messages they receive into their own words and create their own version of what they thought was said. During the *translation* process, three "Vs" of communication are involved: verbal, vocal, and visual elements—the central ingredients of the communication process (Alessandra & Hunsaker 1993).

THE GENERAL COMMUNICATION PROCESS

According to Kochman (1981), the chief cultural differences are often ignored when interracial communication styles fail between Blacks and Whites. In most cases, both groups assume they are operating according to identical speech and cultural conventions and that these conventions are the ones established by the socially dominant White group as standard. This assumption reflects the general sentiment of most White and Black Americans; however, most Whites fail to recognize that Blacks' communication norms and conventions differ considerably from their own. These differences are due in major part to cultural affiliation—culture and communication are not separable. Communication is meaningful because of the culture that frames it and culture is expressed through communication (Hecht, Collier, & Ribeau 1993).

Communication is a two-way process and includes five basic elements: two people (a speaker and a listener), two processes (sending and receiving), and a message (Alessandra & Hunsaker 1993). Figure 5-1 illustrates this process.

It should be noted that language, in the sense of the linguistic code through which verbal communication takes place, is just one component of the process. The problem faced in any communication is how to get the ideas from one person's head to another. This problem is further compounded when the speaker's communication style, culture, and language are different from the listener's. These differences provide considerable opportunity for

SPEAKER > ENCODING > MESSAGE > DECODING > LISTENER

FIGURE 5.1   Communication Process

misunderstandings. As shown in Figure 5-1, speakers start the communication process with what they want to say—the message.

To send a message, the speaker translates the message into words and actions; that is, words are selected to convey the meaning and a variety of gestures, facial expressions are used to help transmit the message. The message being communicated is then carried by the three "V" elements—verbal, vocal, and visual cues. The vocal element includes the tone and intensity of the voice and other vocal qualities that are often referred to as the "music" we play with our voice. The visual element incorporates everything that the speaker does to convey meaning to the message and what the listener can see. Of the three "V" elements of communication, the visual element is the most powerful and memorable. Dynamic visual, nonverbal communication gets and holds the listener's attention. It is through strong visual, nonverbal elements that effective communication begins—getting the listener's attention first then holding it by using powerful vocal and verbal elements to transmit the message.

Once the message is transmitted using the three "Vs," the listener "receives" the message through a series of filters: (1) past experiences (2) perceptions of the speaker (3) degree of emotional involvement with the message (4) level of understanding of the verbal content (5) level of attention and (6) opinion about the speaker's communication style, voice quality, rate, and accent. In other words, the listener busily translates the message received into his or her own words and creates his or her own opinions about the speaker and what the speaker said.

During the communication process, problems typically arise in three major areas: sending the message, the environment in which the message is sent, and receiving the intended message. For example, communication can be derailed by sending inappropriate visual messages that contradict the vocal messages. A specific example of a speaker's inappropriate visual message that contradicts the vocal message is a suppressed smile while verbalizing words of grief and sorrow to the listener. Typically, when this happens, the speaker is referred to as sending a "mixed" message. Mixed messages usually leave the listener confused and untrusting of the messenger. Since the visual element of communication is the most powerful first impression and people tend to respond visually before words are spoken, the listener in the example given will most likely remember the visual behavior (suppressed smile) and not the message—words used to express sorrow and grief. Nonverbal (visual) communication can add to or detract from the meaning of words communicated. Therefore, it is important that the speaker's visual and vocal elements work in harmony to send messages. This is particularly true in intercultural communication where cultural values, attitudes, and behaviors influence interpretation and understanding.

The environment definitely influences the communication process. Situation context influences how speakers talk, their choice of words, and the type of visual elements used. For example, communication style of African Americans in the workplace is usually different from that used at home with family, school, church, and street corner. The same is true for African American students—their communication styles are considerably different in the home with their parents than with their teachers in school. Likewise, their communication styles are different with their peers socially than with adults socially. The environment or setting, place and time are elements that greatly influence the communication process and styles across different cultures.

Environments can be a problem for effective communication between individuals from different cultures because environments influence a speaker's choice of words and visual and verbal expressions. Environments influence communication style and the appropriateness of the styles used by children and adults.

The other problematic area of communication is reception. How does the listener receive and translate the message? Numerous factors can influence the listener's reception of the message. Some of the factors which affect the ability of the listener to receive the message intended are the individual's emotional state, perception of the words, meaning and value, judgments about the speaker, cultural differences, value differences, and language differences.

PSYCHOLOGICAL THEMES

Although social scientists, barring a few exceptions, have promoted the view that African culture was all but destroyed by slavery, White (1984) views the holistic, humanistic ethos described by Nobles (1972) and Mbiti (1970) as having a definite correspondence between the African ethos and the African American world view in terms of African psychology, emotional vitality, interdependence, collective survival, the oral tradition, perception of time, harmonious blending, and the role of the elderly.

The careful examination of African Americans' communication styles reveal that there is a correspondence between the African ethos and the African American's oral tradition. African American culture and communication reflect the recognition of an African past, today's social reality, and the complexities of life in America where environments are replete with institutional racism and discrimination (van Dijk 1987). According to Collier (1992), ethnicity and culture are the frames through which to view and understand African American communication. As noted earlier, ethnic culture connotes "the social or communicative system shared by a group with similar heritage." These groups are constituted by membership in a system with common patterns of interaction and perception and a historically transmitted system of symbols, meanings, and norms (Collier 1992; Geertz 1973; Schneider 1976).

Ethnic culture is said to be an individual, social, or societal construct (Middleton & Edwards 1990). On an individual level, ethnic culture is a characteristic of a personal world view that is at least partially shared in common with other group members. On a social level, ethnic culture is enacted and maintained in conversation among group members (Giles & Johnson 1987). In this regard, ethnic culture is described as a patterned social network with shared history, tradition, practices, power dynamics, communication norms, rituals, and institutions. Ethnic culture is described as a system of interdependent patterns of conduct and interpretations, communication patterns of actions and meaning that are deeply felt, commonly intelligible, and widely accessible in creating, defining, and communicating identity or personhood (Carbaugh 1988).

Six themes have been identified as recurring psychological themes in the language, oral literature, and expressive patterns of African Americans. These themes provide a psychological and historical perspective that serves as the foundation for communication styles and unique expressions of African Americans in different sociocultural contexts. These themes, symbolizing the affective, cognitive, and cultural flavor of the African American psychological perspective (White & Parham 1990) are: emotional vitality, realness, resilience, interrelatedness, the value of direct experience, and distrust and deception.

Emotional Vitality

Emotional vitality represents the sense of aliveness, animation, and openness to feelings expressed in the language, communication style, oral literature, song, dance, body language, folk poetry, and expressive thought of African Americans (Redmond 1971). Jeffers (1971) describes Black dance and oral literature of Black folks as vivacious, exuberant, sensuous, and wholesomely uninhibited—"a statement that life should abound and flourish with the vigorous intensity of the Funky Chicken. . . . rather than the sedateness of the waltz or fox trot" (p. 57). Similarly, Holt (1975) describes the Black oral tradition as the act of speaking as a performance on the stage of life. Capturing and holding the attention of the listener is an art form where the Black speaker is expected to make words come alive, to use ear-filling phrases that stir the imagination with heavy reliance on tonal rhymes, symbolism, figures of speech, and personification. The vitality expressed in communication patterns by Black people is viewed as life-affirming and the feelings related to the affirmations of life are freely shared with others through vibrant Black speakers, preachers, singers, and performers who tell it like it is (White & Parham 1990).

Realness—Tellin' It Like It Is

Much of Black poetry, the blues, and gospel music tell it like it is. The messages are usually related to real-life experiences, learning to survive, paying one's dues, disappointments, tragedy, or setbacks. Although the listener might assume that the blues and gospel lyrics represent resignation and despair, in the Black ethos, tragedy, defeat, and disappointment are not equated with psychological destruction (White & Parham 1990, p. 57. Instead, the goal by Blacks in the face of tragedy is to keep on keepin' on, to keep the faith and maintain a cool steadiness.

Resilience and Revitalization

Although blues and gospel artists incorporate oppression, hardship, and struggle encountered by Blacks in their work in their music, this does not reflect the total spectrum of their work. From a Black psychological perspective, an emotional balance of renewed experiences, joy, and laughter help troubles to pass and happiness to emerge. The consciousness of pain, sorrow, and hurt expressed in blues and gospel music is not accompanied by feelings of guilt, shame, and self-rejection. Instead, Black blues and gospel singers are fully aware of the excitement and euphoria created by the lyrics, rhythm, and sounds of their music. In spite of real pain or loss, grief, or defeat, the blues and gospel lyrics are powerful and capable of communicating moving messages that can pique the spirit and bring about happiness and joy to African Americans. These communication experiences through music revitalize the spirit and transcends feelings of joy (White & Parham 1990, p. 59).

The words used to communicate by blues singers, folk poets, comedians, and preachers are powerful, uplifting, healing, inspiring, and revitalizing. Their messages come in large measure from their ability and adeptness to reach out and touch others through words and style that both speaker and listener can bear witness to.

Interrelatedness, Connectedness, and Interdependence

These concepts are viewed by Nobles (1976) as the "unifying philosophic concepts in the African American experience base." Nobles maintains that these concepts are prominent themes in Black language with respect to the interactive dynamics between speaker and listener, the power of words to control, cognitive style, timing, and communicative competence. He also indicates that the language of "soul folks," wherever it occurs, is characterized by the interrelatedness of speaker and listener. For example, White and Parham (1990) quote Holt (1975), who says that "the act of speaking is a dramatic presentation of one's personhood to those who share a background of similar acculturation" (p. 64). The listener acts as an echo chamber, repeating, cosigning, validating, and affirming the message of the speaker with "amens," "right-ons," "yes sirs" and "teach-ons." Spillers (1971), in White and Parham (1990), illustrates an interactive exchange between a Black preacher and the congregation that went like this:

Preacher: The same Christ, the same man.

Congregation: Same man.

Preacher: Who sits high and looks low, who rounded the world in the middle of his hands?

Congregation: Middle of his hands.

Preacher: The same man who fed 5,000 and still had some left over.

Congregation: Yes sir! Had some left.

Preacher: The same man who raised the dead and who walked the waters and calmed the seas.

Congregation: Let's hold him up church.

Preacher: This same man is looking out for you and me. (p. 64)

In this example, the Black preacher establishes a form of situational control by defining a reality using vivid imagery drawn from a body of collective experiences that the congregation understands and can relate to in their lives. The preacher also controls the situation linguistically with words that touch the psychoaffective rhythms that cause joy, laughter, sadness, strength, and optimism. Another example of interrelatedness that draws on a picture of reality that Black listeners could affirm comes from Dr. Martin Luther King, Jr. He used metaphors to describe the reality of Black people's dissatisfaction with the slow pace of the civil rights legislation in August, 1963 when he said, "Justice rolls down like water and righteousness like a mighty stream" (White & Parham 1990, p. 65).

The extensive use of metaphor in Black speech reflects a cognitive style where likeness, correspondence, similarity, and analogous relationships between ideas, events, and concepts are shown by using picturesque imagery that appeals conjointly to the intellect and emotions. Black people use colorful poetic sketches that arouse feelings and visual symbols to draw pictures of what is happening. Examples of visual imagery communicated by Black youths are illustrated in the following statements:

- Gettin over like a fat rat in a cheese factory
- That aint nothing man, ice it
- Higher than nine kites on a breezy day
- Man that dude was really stroking
- Just as cool as she wanted to be
- I don't know what page you on (White & Parham 1990, p.66)

According to Spillers (1971), the metaphor in Black language is a teaching device. African Americans depend on the common background between themselves and their listeners to establish an impact and associate meanings to the words. Visual imagery is used as a substitute to expand and clarify meanings from an African American cultural perspective. Black children learn to use this linguistic style, which is saturated with Black folk expressions, metaphors, visual imagery, and figures of speech. Their ability to communicate with peers in this expressive style is an expectation within the culture. Conflict arises when they cannot easily translate isolated words and literal meaning of the conventional European American language style into their normal speech patterns, and when teachers will not permit them to use their expressive patterns in the classroom.

In 1969, Rap Brown describes conflict arising from his verbal competence in Black expressive styles and the expectations of his teachers with respect to learning traditional English poetry. Rap ran down his verbal wizardry by telling another brother:

> *Man you must not know who I am,*
> *I am sweet peeter jeeter, the womb beater.*
> *The baby maker the cradle shaker.*
> *The deer slayer the buck binder the woman finder,*
> *Known from the gold coast to the rocky shores of Maine,*
> *Rap is my name and love is my game. (White & Parham 1990, p. 67)*

In the example shown, Rap Brown said, "and the teacher expected me to set up in class and study poetry after I could run down stuff like that, if anybody needed to study poetry, she needed to study mine." This example evidences one type of conflict that arises between Black students and teachers—the students feel competent and proud of their linguistic rhythms that are synchronized by a reciprocal command of timing and pace. Conflicts arise because European American teachers do not understand Black students' communication style, the significance of the style to African American language and ethnic culture, and the goal of the communication style, that is, to be in time with the beat, pulse, tempo, and rhythm of the speech flow. Likewise, the same communication style and principles apply to Black adolescents' rap music, playing the dozens, signifying, and sounding.

In the Black community, a large number of linguistic terms are used to designate different forms of social-linguistic interaction. In Table 5-1 a list of fifty-four social-linguistic terms have been compiled by Smith (1974, p. 70).

TABLE 5-1   Terms Used to Designate Social-Linguistic Interaction

1. Bad Mouth, Mouthin'	28. Mau Mau, Mauing
2. Base, Basin'	29. Mumblin'
3. Blow, Blow on	30. Pimp Talk
4. Call and Response	31. Protection Talk
5. Cappin	32. Pull Coat
6. Cop a Plea	33. Rappin'
7. Cop on	34. Rhapsodize
8. Cover snatch, Snatchin'	35. Runnin' It Down
9. Dozens, Dirty Dozens	36. Scat Singin'
10. Drop a Dime	37. Screamin'
11. Fat Up	38. Showboatin'
12. Fat Mouth, Mouthin'	39. Shuckin' and Jivin'
13. Frontin' Off	40. Signify, Signifyin'
14. Gate Mouth, Mouthin'	41. Soundin
15. Gibb, Gibbin' (Jibb)	42. Spilo Wibbin'
16. Gripp, Grippin'	43. Stuff Playin'
17. Group, Grouped	44. Sweet Mouthin'
18. High Siding	45. Talkin' Proper
19. Horrah, Horrahin'	46. Talkin' Shit (Talking Trash)
20. Jaw Jackin'	47. Talkin' in Tongue
21. Jeffin'	48. Tautin'
22. Jivin'	49. Testify - Testifyin'
23. Jonin'	50. Toast, Toastin'
24. Larcen, Larcenin'	51. Tom Tom, Tommin'
25. Lolly Gaggin'	52. Whop Whoppin' Game
26. Lug Droppin'	53. Woffin', Woofing
27. Mack, Mackin'	54. Woof (Wolf) Ticket

Source: Adapted from E. Smith, "Evolution and Continuing Presence of the Oral Tradition in Black America," unpublished doctoral dissertation, University of California–Irvine, 1974. Reprinted by permission.

Communicative competence within the Black community means a high level of receptive and expressive ability to break down the message, stay on top of a situation verbally, tune into what others are saying (running down), and when it is appropriate, use a particular social-linguistic category (White & Parham 1990). The oral tradition is viewed as an integral part of Black identity and the emotional, psychological, and cultural tone of the Black ethos is expressed by means of the spoken word.

Value of Direct Experience

The actual experiences of living in the Black ethos provide experiences of natural facts, eternal truth, wisdom, and precepts of survival that influence Black oral expression and communication style. The lessons learned from experiences of life are carried forward from one generation to the next by the oral tradition. Black children are taught the precepts of life through a vast oral literature from older Black adults. Parables, folk verses, folk tales, biblical verses, songs, and proverbs are valued cultural lessons that have passed on from generation to generation. Some of the sayings that Black parents and grandparents have passed on to their children are as follows:

> The truth will come out.
>
> Don't sign no checks with your mouth that your a_ _ can't cash.
>
> Hard head make a soft behind.
>
> You better be yourself or you gonna be by yourself.
>
> One monkey don't stop no show.
>
> Only a fool plays the golden rule in a crowd that don't play fair.
>
> If you lay down with dogs you gonna come up with fleas.
>
> What goes around, comes around.
>
> You better learn how to work before work works you.
>
> You don't git to be old being no fool. (White & Parham 1990, p. 71–72)

Each generation has passed on the oral literature and each generation of Black people has reshaped and expanded the meanings to encompass the events of their time and place. The older people in the Black community are respected for their accumulated wisdom during their experiences and lifetime. They are respected as storehouses of oral tradition and the keepers of the heritage. African Americans consider elders as having seen the "comings and goings of life" and when death comes, it is viewed as a testament to the fact that a life has lived and the end of the earthly journey has been completed. Understanding and interpreting the Black world view, as it is communicated by Black oral expressive styles, come about as a result of experiencing and living the Black ethos.

Distrust and Deception

In general, the experiences of slavery, institutional racism, and ongoing economic oppression in America have caused African Americans to distrust European Americans. As a result of distrust, the use of a common language with culturally different semantics enables Black people to conceal what they mean from White people while still maintaining a high level of clarity in their communications. Words, phrases, and statements that are thought to mean one thing when interpreted from a European American frame of reference can mean something entirely different when translated through an African American ethnotropic filter (White & Parham 1990). For example, because familiar gospel songs were sung by the slaves in the presence of their masters, they had to contain hidden meanings that could be interpreted differently. When the slaves sang, "Steal Away to Jesus," "On My Journey Now," and "Dis Train Is Bound for Glory," they meant, "I'm getting ready to steal away from here, to start on my journey on a secret train [underground railroad] bound north to freedom." (p. 80)

Multiple meanings can be hidden in the messages communicated by African Americans in songs and words. Linguistic deception continues to be used as a way of controlling undesirable psychological imagery and devaluative labels used to describe African Americans. Therefore, Black people have translated the undesirable words Whites use into meanings that are desirable. For example, in Black cultural semantics, "bad" means good—someone to look up to, a hero. Black children sometimes confuse teachers when they turn undesirable labels around to mean something positive and admirable. An example is the use of such labels as "clumsy lips" by some teachers to suggest that Black children who consistently use African American language have a speech defect. Black children, on the other hand, may refer to someone with "clumsy lips" as a Black brother who has power with words—can "run it down" or "talk that talk" (White & Parham 1990, p. 81).

MEANINGS AND VALUES OF BLACK AND WHITE COMMUNICATION STYLES AND CULTURES

In this section, attention is focused on meanings and values that Black and White students attach to their own and to each other's behavior and fundamental aspects of Black and White culture and communication in the classroom. America's classrooms, with large enrollments of Black and White students as well as other racially, culturally, and linguistically different students, provide numerous opportunities to observe different patterns of behavior and communication styles that are meaningful, valued, and reflect social and cultural significance.

One area where there is considerable difference and often misinterpretation between White and Black students is *modes of behavior*. For example, when Black and White students engage in a public debate on an issue, the modes of behavior that are considered appropriate for each group are considerably different with respect to their stance and level of spiritual intensity (Kochman 1981). The Black student's mode is typically high-keyed: animated, interpersonal, and confrontational; whereas the White student's mode is relatively low-keyed: dispassionate, impersonal and non-challenging. The first mode is characteristic of involvement; it is heated, loud, and generates affect; the second mode is characteristic of detachment and is cool, quiet, and without affect (Kochman 1981).

Black and White students classify behavior modes differently based on context and cultural framework. For example, Black students give different meaning to the words "argument" and "discussion" than White students. There are formal, functional and situational differences. Black students distinguish argument used to debate from argument used to ventilate anger and hostility. Formally, both modes consist of effect and dynamic opposition; however, the resemblance is only superficial. Arguments used for debates are considered modes of persuasion in relation to the debaters' material. The presence of persuasion indicates that the Black students are sincere and serious about what they are saying. In arguments for persuasion, Black students assume a challenging stance with respect to their opponents, but the students are not antagonistic. Instead, they view themselves as contenders cooperatively engaged in a process that hopefully will validate their opposing ideas.

Argument that is a ventilation of anger and hostility is more intense than in persuasive argument. The opponents are viewed as antagonists, givers and receivers of abuse, and not contenders engaged in a struggle to produce a valid thought or idea. Because Black students define and use "argument" functionally differently in Black culture, they are aware of the formal elements that distinguish the two and the situations in which one meaning is applied instead of the other.

White students, on the other hand, fail to make these distinctions because argument for them functions only to ventilate anger and hostility. It does not function as a process of persuasion. For persuasion, White students are taught to use discussion that is without affect and dynamic opposition (Kochman 1981). Consequently, White students feel that Black students are not engaging in persuasion when affect and dynamic opposition are present. The mere presence of opposition, regardless of focus or intensity, is seen as the preliminary to an argument with ventilated anger and hostility. Because the White students fail to make the same distinction as Black students about their behaviors and meanings of words, they misinterpret the Black students' intentions and do not believe they are acting in good faith.

Because of the cultural differences toward argument as a process of persuasion in the White culture, White students typically regard the Black students' argumentative mode as dysfunctional because of their view that reason and emotion work against each other. Conversational behaviors and styles of African Americans express ethnic identity. Studies have been published on the conversational style of African American ethnic culture that reflects the cultural mode of conversing that is expressed in language, relationships, and verbal and nonverbal messages (Cazenave 1983; Clark 1985; Cromwell & Cromwell 1978; Gray-Little 1982; Ransford & Miller 1983; Robinson 1983; Smith 1983). For example, African American and European American communication style differences are affected by such variables as in-group/out-group status, gender, socioeconomic status as well as contextual and regional factors. Body movement (kinetic behavior) is influenced by both race and gender, with body lean and eye gaze differences more pronounced for females than males (Smith 1983). African American females look at the conversational partner less and lean toward each other more than White females (Smith 1983).

Research studies have also focused on African American language style and core symbols of communication style. The remainder of this chapter will focus on these concepts and results from studies conducted in these areas.

LANGUAGE STYLE

African Americans, like other cultural groups, define themselves in part through language and identify themselves through language use. African Americans are a pluralistic communication community in which regional and social class differences are apparent (Jenkins 1982). African Americans' linguistic behavior is not necessarily homogeneous. Physical isolation, sociocultural orientation, age-group affiliations, and gender variations in older members affect social networking and the linguistic style of African Americans.

African American English, like other language forms, is governed by rules with specific historical derivations and is passed on through socialization. It is now recognized as a legitimate language form with a unique and logical syntax, semantic system, and phonology that varies depending upon which African language influenced it and in which region it was developed (Jenkins 1982; Smitherman 1977; Stewart 1970). The distinctiveness of African American speech style marks the speaker as a member of the group for in-group acceptance, promotes identity, and is reinforced by group members.

This creates a double bind for African American children growing up in neighborhoods where mainstream American English is fiercely ostracized by the Black teen culture, yet rewarded by the mainstream American culture. Since mainstream American English is the preferred language, other forms are considered as nonstandard and relegated to lower prestige status. This rejection of African American English as a legitimate linguistic style has harmed the development of child speakers (Seymour & Seymour 1979).

Recent studies of European American perceptions of "sounding Black" indicate that negative evaluations do not pervade all judgments. Johnson and Buttny (1982) found that contrary to predictions, European listeners did not respond more negatively on all dimensions to speakers who "sounded Black" than to speakers who "sounded White." The effects depended on the content of the speech. When the content was narrative or experimental, there were no differences attributable to speech style. However, when the topic was abstract and intellectual, "sounding Black" produced lower ratings from European Americans. Their findings indicate that European Americans do not have uniformly negative global predisposition toward African American speech, but selectively bias their evaluations to be consistent with cultural stereotypes.

Code-switching is another communication style that encompasses the selective use of African American English and mainstream American English depending on the situation. Three types of code-switchers have been identified by Seymour and Seymour (1979). The first group consists of African Americans who are less formerly educated and have difficulty using mainstream American English. This group has difficulty when mainstream American English usage is situationally expected. The second group is formally educated and fluent in mainstream American English, but members of this group have difficulty expressing themselves in African American English. This group has difficulty when African American English is preferred. The final group is educated and able to use both language systems. This third group is a prototype of pluralistic language use and should be encouraged in educational settings.

Code-switching also appears in cultures other than those residing in the United States. While it is not uncommon for effective communicators to adapt their style to fit the situation regardless of their ethnicity, the power dynamics of the American society and the history of African American oppression permeate this type of switching with a political meaning. African Americans change their communication style to fit the racial and gender composition of the dyad (Hecht, Collier, & Ribeau 1993).

African Americans adjust their communication style to the situation. For example, African Americans talk with each other to relax, to develop or maintain friendships out of mutual interest. The communication style in these situations will likely include the use of slang, lots of laughter, in-group gestures,

African American English, and assumed intimacy; whereas, in Black–White conversations there is restraint and an awareness of grammar usage.

Code-switching choices are usually automatically triggered based on situational factors and influences. Some systematic situational factors that influence switching from one communication style to another include: (1) the frequency of contact with conversant, (2) the familiarity of the contact, (3) the perception of the other as a member or non-member of Black street culture, (4) the presence of females, (5) the topic being discussed, and (6) the intensity of emotion concerning the topic. These types of situational factors will influence the style choices and switches from deep slang and full stylistic manner to toned-down versions of Black street speech or to increased amounts of mainstream American English prescriptive forms.

CORE SYMBOLS OF COMMUNICATION STYLES

Communication is more than just the use of language. Language is used to create messages that involve topics, meanings, and verbal/nonverbal styles of expression (Hecht, Collier, & Ribeau 1993). Communication style expresses the core symbols of the ethnic culture and identity. African American communication style incorporates core symbols that represent stylistic tendencies in African American culture.

Rose's (1982/1983) work on African American psychology and literature found that there are five basic symbols or values in African American culture:

- Sharing one's life with family and close relationships
- Uniqueness or individual style
- Affective humanism or positive attitudes
- Disunital orientation (viewing things as both good and evil rather than either/or (p. 95)
- Assertiveness (style literature suggests this symbol)

African American communication styles are seen as expressing these symbols or values and, conversely, shaping and recreating them.

Sharing

The symbol of sharing is characterized in a number of different aspects of African American communication style. This is exemplified by the call-response pattern in which a speakers' statements are affirmed through messages such as "amen," "right on," "yes sir," or partial sentence feedback as illustrated earlier between the preacher and the congregation. Sharing is played out in a variety of communicative forms, for example, touch, distance, relationship intimacy, rituals, distance. Sharing is viewed as a highly unifying concept in African American culture.

Touching

African Americans touch members of their group more than they touch European Americans—this is particularly true of lower socioeconomic status African Americans. Interracial dyads touch less than interracial dyads among both European Americans and African Americans (Willis, Reeves, & Buchanan 1976).

Distance

Distance preferences are also a part of the core symbol of sharing. Close distances signal connectedness and bonding. Halberstadt (1986) found across a variety of studies that African Americans establish closer distances than European Americans when communicating. These close communication distances begin in early childhood when African American children establish closer distances in play (Hecht, Collier, & Ribeau 1993).

Relationship Intimacy

Many African American communication symbols and nonverbal behaviors of touch and distance signal involvement, connection, and intimacy that result in closer, more intimate friendships than European Americans (Hammer & Gudykunst 1987) and in general across the topics of religion, school and work, interest and hobbies, and physical condition (Hecht & Ribeau 1984). European Americans seem to develop more intimacy regarding love, dating, sex, emotions, and feelings (Hammer & Gudykunst 1987).

African Americans do not usually carry this core symbol of relationship intimacy into out-group relationships with European Americans. As a result African Americans may appear to be indifferent or uninvolved in their interactions with European acquaintances and strangers (Asante & Noor-Aldeen 1984; Ickes 1984). In these situations, European Americans are more likely to experience such interracial interactions as somewhat difficult, burdensome, and awkward. As a result, they tend to feel a particular responsibility and concern for making the interaction work. They talk more, look at the others, and smile more, which reflects a form of overaccommodation on the part of European Americans (Giles & Coupland 1991).

Eye contact patterns are communication symbols that are used differently between African Americans and European Americans. When European Americans speak they tend to look at their partner less than they do while listening (Hecht, Collier, & Ribeau 1993). Whereas, for African Americans this pattern is reversed with listeners looking less and the speakers looking more (LaFrance & Mayo 1976). This communication style difference may contribute to misinterpretation of communication style and intent between European American and African American speakers. Since European Americans do not look at each other frequently when communicating, their communication style with African Americans may be interpreted as boredom or lack of interest. Similarly, when African Americans are communicating with European Americans, their frequent eye contact may be interpreted as intensity, hostility, or power (Hecht, Collier, & Ribeau 1993). In either case, misunderstanding communication styles often leads to misinterpreted communication and cross-cultural communication clashes between in-group and out-group communicators.

Rituals

Communication rituals are part of African American culture and communication style. Communication rituals are used to affirm allegiance to the group and cultural identity. Communication rituals are demonstrated in forms of shared communication activities that demonstrate a commitment to the group. A number of communication rituals are common and observable in African American culture: for example, call-response, various types of jiving, boasting and toasting, and playing the dozens. These rituals are played out in the home, church, street corner, playgrounds, and schools. Social context is important and can enhance or diminish communication rituals.

Jiving

Jiving is a communication style developed by African Americans based upon improvisation and accentuation of behaviors that are believed to be highly acceptable. These behaviors are used with European and African American audiences with varying forms of recognition and positive reward (Cogdell & Wilson 1980). Six types of jiving have been identified by Cogdell and Wilson for different purposes and in different ways.

The first type of jive perpetuates the European American myth that all Blacks have rhythm, can sing and dance and act uncouth. This type of jive is usually acted out by Black entertainers via songs, jokes, dance, and acting. The second type of jive involves the use of slang, informal African American English, and figures of speech that reflect African American English codes. The third type of jive is comprised of foolish talk as a means of getting and holding a reputation for not being serious. Foolish talk is also used sometimes to ease tension that under normal circumstances could erupt into expressions of anger or overt hostility. The fourth type of jive comes from the "hipster." The hipster is usually a highly resourceful, creative, intelligent African American male who can talk circles around the average person. The fifth type of jive involves overt teasing. Pleasure is derived from playing tricks on other African Americans in order to evoke laughter and to make the victim feel foolish. The intent is not to do harm and the tricks are not malicious. The sixth type of jive is known as the swing. This type of jive is usually found in professional work environments where African Americans have a need to congregate and party together to relieve stress experienced in settings dominated by European Americans (Hecht, Collier, & Ribeau 1993).

Another communication ritual is the folkloric speech event known as "playing the dozens" (Garner 1983). This is an aggressive contest often using obscene language in which the goal is to ridicule and demean the opponent's family members, notably the mother. Garner (1983) states: "The game is an important rhetorical device which promotes community stability and cooperation by regulating social and personal conflicts. This expressive game influences, controls, guides or directs human actions in ways consistent with community norms" (p. 47).

Boasting
Boasting is a ritualized speech act which reflects the oral nature of African American communication. Garner (1983) indicates that boasting occurs as a source of play and entertainment and functions to enable the speaker to gain recognition within a group. African American boasting often contains humorous exaggeration. Boasting is also used in conflicts to help bring harmony and cohesiveness to the group. Boasting is usually accompanied by an African American audience and verbal and physical reactions of the audience such as shouts, laughter, applause, and catcalls. The audience members often serve as the referee and judge the performers. A boasting performance cannot succeed without an audience that is psychologically prepared and able to participate in the event (Edwards & Seinkewicz 1990).

Uniqueness

African American communication styles and symbols are important and unique to acknowledging and endorsing the group. One unique characteristic of African American communication is the demonstration of individuality while embracing commonality of the group in interactions with others (Rose 1982/1983). The ritualized forms of communication behaviors provide opportunities where the two competing forces can be combined. For example, hand slapping has become a stylized, communal activity in which individuals have developed their own unique style of "gimme five" (Cooke 1980).

The dual function of sharing and uniqueness is also observable in ritualized boasting. For example, boasting serves to promote group harmony and cohesiveness while calling attention to individual performance.

The values of uniqueness and sharing are learned in early childhood by African American children. The values are communicated to them verbally and nonverbally. They are taught to do their best and not to compare themselves to others (Rose 1982/1983) and to "be real" and not "phony." These values are expressed through individual stylized nonverbal presentations (Cooke 1980; Kochman 1981) and the stylized walk that is used by African American males to attract attention and admiration.

Assertiveness

Assertiveness is reflected in a variety of communicative behaviors and cultural rituals. Playing the dozens and woofing are examples of assertive communication. Woofing involves a type of threat that is not intended as imminent action (Kochman 1981). During these types of activities, communication may include a loud, strong voice, threats, slang, and street talk. The communication level may vary in intensity depending on the type of activity from calm arguing for persuasion to more intense forms of anger (Kochman 1981).

African Americans and European Americans differ in their interpretations of these actions (Kochman 1981). Many of the assertive and aggressive forms of African American communication (shouting, threatening) are viewed by European Americans as signals for physical confrontation when none is intended. These types of communication style differences contribute to misunderstandings that often result in negative consequences for African Americans—particularly males.

SUMMARY

Communication is a complex, multidimensional process and African American communication is no exception. African Americans have many communication styles and codes that are used in particular contexts. Communication style and code varies according to situational context (formal/informal), the audience (in-group/out-group), age, and gender. African Americans' communication style differences often contribute to European Americans' confusion and misinterpretation of messages communicated and received. These differences are attributable to cross-cultural communication clashes between African Americans and European Americans. Cross-cultural communication clashes can be observed in conversations between African American students and European Americans in public, in school classrooms between teachers and students, and in the workplace.

Communication styles and ritualized forms are embedded in African tradition, historical experiences, and psychological themes. The psychological themes that have been identified in African American language and expressive patterns are: (1) emotional vitality, (2) realness, (3) resilience, (4) interre-latedness, (5) the value of direct experience, and (6) distrust and deception (White & Parham 1990).

In African American culture, oral tradition and communication perfor-mance are highly valued. Communication style expresses the core symbols of the ethnic culture when enacted in ritualized forms and promotes allegiance to the group. African American children learn early the value of communi-cation to their cultural and ethnic identity. The four basic values in African American culture are: (1) sharing one's life with family and close relationships, (2) uniqueness or individual style, (3) affective humanism or positive attitude, and (4) disunital orientation, which means viewing things as both good and evil rather than either/or.

The communication process across cultures involves more than speaking and listening. The speakers and listeners bring their experiences, perceptions, and emotional involvement to the communication process. These variables influence interpretation and understanding of messages communicated and received. Communication is an expression of culture and ethnicity. Culture and communication are inseparable; culture is expressed through communication.

PRACTICAL APPLICATION

To enhance students' knowledge and understanding of the concepts and communication style differences presented in this chapter, some exercises are recommended.

Exercise 1. Have the students choose a partner (preferably from a differ-ent ethnic/cultural group). Once the students are paired, each dyad of students should tell the partner a 3-minute story about an event that caused them to feel isolated and/or ignored. The speaking partner should concentrate on the details of the story and the feelings he or she believes are associated with it. When listening, the partner should carefully try to remember the important details of the speaker's story. After 3 minutes, the roles switch—the listener will speak and the speaker will listen. At the conclusion of the storytelling and lis-tening, each student will tell the partner what was heard (the message) and the interpretation (perception/understanding) of the speaker's feelings (body lan-guage) as associated with the message. The playback of the messages from each student will be evaluated for accuracy of the interpretation (perception/understanding) and of the speaker's feelings (body language).

Although this exercise may seem simple, it often reveals the degree of inaccuracy that transpires in communication within and across cultures. It also demonstrates how individuals from different cultures perceive and interpret speaker's messages, feelings, and/or emotional state when communicating. Openly share and discuss what happened among the students.

Exercise 2. Have the students visit an African American church, play, community or festival to observe differences in African American communication styles from a contextual perspective. The students should note distinct communication differences observed among children, adults, males, and females for later discussion in class. Notice the common and different communication styles observed by students and how situational context influences communication style.

Exercise 3. Assign readings from articles referenced in this chapter for discussion in class and enhanced awareness.

REFERENCES

Alessandra, T., & Hunsaker, P. (1993). *Communicating at Work.* New York: Simon & Schuster.

Asante, M. K., & Noor-Aldeen, H. S. (1984). Social interaction of Black and White college students. *Journal of Black Studies,* 14:507–516.

Carbaugh, D. (1988). Comments on "culture" in communication inquiry. *Communication Reports,* 1:38–41.

Cazenave, N. A. (1983). Black male–Black female relationships: The perceptions of 155 middle-class Black men. *Family Relations,* 32:341–350.

Clark, M. L. (1985). Social stereotypes and self-concept in Black and White college students. *Journal of Social Psychology,* 125:753–760.

Cogdell, R., & Wilson, S. (1980). *Black Communication in White Society.* Saratoga, CA: Century-Twenty-One Publishers.

Collier, M. J. (1992). *Ethnic Friendships: Enacted Identities and Competencies.* Manuscript submitted for publication.

Cooke, B. G. (1980). Nonverbal communication among Afro-Americans: An initial clarification in R. L. Jones (ed.), *Black Psychology* (2nd ed.). New York: Harper & Row.

Cromwell, V. L., & Cromwell, R. E. (1978). Perceived dominance in decision making and conflict resolution among Anglo, Black and Chicano couples. *Journal of Marriage and the Family,* 40:759.

Edwards, V., & Seinkewicz, T. J. (1990). Oral Cultures Past and Present. Cambridge: Basil Blackwell.

Garner, T. E. (1983). Playing the dozens: Folklore as strategies for living. *Quarterly Journal of Speech,* 69:47–57.

Geertz, C. (1973). *The Interpretation of Cultures.* New York: Basic Books.

Giles, H., & Coupland, N. (1991). *Language: Contexts and Consequences.* Pacific Grove, CA: Brooks/Cole.

Giles, H., & Johnson, P. (1987). Ethnolinguistic identity theory: A social psychological approach to language maintenance. *International Journal of the Sociology of Language,* 68:69–99.

Gray-Little, B. (1982). Marital quality and power processes among Black couples. *Journal of Marriage and the Family,* 44:633–646.

Halbertstadt, A. G., (1986). Family socialization of emotional expression and nonverbal communication styles and skills. *Journal of Personality and Social Psychology,* 51(4):827–836.

Hammer, M. R., & Gudykunst, W. B. (1987). The effect of ethnicity, gender, and dyadic composition on uncertainty reduction in initial interaction. *Journal of Black Studies,* 18:191–214.

Hecht, M. L., Collier, M. J., & Ribeau, S. A. (1993). *African American Communication.* Newbury Park: Sage Publications.

Hecht, M. L., & Ribeau, S. (1987). Afro-American identity labels and communicative effectiveness. *Journal of Black Studies,* 21:501–513.

Holt, G. (1975). Metaphor, Black discourse style and cultural reality. In R. L. Willams (ed.), *Ebonics, the True Language of Black Folks.* St. Louis: Institute of Black Studies.

Ickes, W. (1984). Composition in black and white: Determinants of interaction in interracial dyads. *Journal of Personality and Social Psychology,* 47:1206–1217.

Jeffers, L. (1971). Afro-American literature, The conscience of man. *The Black Scholar* (January 1971): 47–53.

Jenkins, A. H. (1982). *The Psychology of the Afro-American: A Humanistic Approach.* Elmsford, NY: Pergamon.

Johnson, F. L., & Buttny, R. (1982) White listeners' responses to "sounding Black" and "sounding White": The effects of message content on judgments about language. *Communication Monographs,* 49:33–49.

Kochman, T. (1981). *Black and White Styles in Conflict.* Chicago: University of Chicago Press.

LaFrance, M., & Mayo, C. (1976). Racial differences in gaze behavior during conversations: Two systematic observational studies. *Journal of Personality and Social Psychology,* 33:547–552.

Mbiti, J. S. (1970). *African Religions and Philosophies.* Garden City, NY: Anchor Books.

Middleton, D., & Edwards, D. (1990). *Collective Remembering.* London: Sage.

Nobles, W. (1972). African philosophy: Foundation for Black psychology. In R. L. Jones (ed.), *Black Psychology.* New York: Harper & Row.

Nobles, W. (1976). Black people in White insanity: An issue for community mental health. *Journal of Afro-American Issues,* 4(1) (Winter): 21–27.

Ransford, H. E., & Miller, J. (1983). Race, sex and feminist outlooks. *American Sociological Review,* 48:46–58.

Redmond, E. (1971). The Black American epic: Its roots, its writers. *The Black Scholar* (January): 15–22.

Robinson, C. R. (1983). Black women: A tradition of self-reliant strength. *Women & Therapy,* 2:135–144.

Rose, L. F. R. (1982/1983). Theoretical and methodological issues in the study of Black culture and personality. *Humbolt Journal of Social Relations,* 10:320–338.

Schneider, D. (1976). Notes toward a theory of culture. In K. Basso & H. Selby (eds.), *Texts of Identity.* Albuquerque: University of New Mexico Press.

Seymour, H. N. & Seymour, C. M. (1979). The symbolism of ebonics: I'd rather switch than fight. *Journal of Black Studies,* 9:397–410.

Smith, A. (1983). Nonverbal communication among Black female dyads: An assessment of intimacy, gender, and race. *Journal of Social Issues,* 39:55–67.

Smith, E. (1974). Evolution and continuing presence of the oral tradition of Black America. Doctoral dissertation submitted to the University of California, Irvine.

Smitherman, G. (1977). *Talkin' and Testifyin': The Language of Black America*. Boston: Houghton Mifflin.

Spillers, H. (1971). Martin Luther King and the style of the Black sermon. *The Black Scholar* (September): 14–27.

Stewart, W. A. (1970). Toward a history American Negro dialect. In F. Williams (ed.), *Language and poverty*. Chicago: Markham Publishing.

van Dijk, T. A. (1987). *Communicating Racism: Ethnic Prejudice in Thought and Talk*. Newbury Park, CA: Sage.

White, J. L. (1984). *The Psychology of Blacks: An Afro-American Perspective*. Englewood Cliffs, NJ: Prentice-Hall.

White, J. L., & Parham, T. A. (1990). *The Psychology of Blacks: An African-American Perspective*. Englewood Cliffs, NJ: Prentice Hall.

Willis, R., Reeves, D., & Buchanan, D. (1976). Interpersonal touch in high school relative to sex and race. *Perceptual and Motor Skills*, 43:843–847.

6

SPEECH AND LANGUAGE DISORDERS VERSUS DIFFERENCES

Chapter Overview

Upon reading this chapter you will gain understanding of:

- The definition and characteristics of common speech, language and hearing disorders
- Whether a child is speaking African American English
- Which African American children should be speaking African American English
- Variation in prevalence of specific communication disorders among African American children
- The process of language acquisition in African American children

This chapter will make a clear distinction between features of African American communication and factors considered pathological communication that warrant treatment. The following topics will be addressed: normal acquisition of speech and language in children, language acquisition among African American children, descriptions of speech and language disorders, some causes of communication disorders, the manner in which speech and language disorders are manifest among African American children, and how linguistic differences of African Americans are confused with disorders of communication.

NORMAL LANGUAGE ACQUISITION

Part of being human is to acquire a language. "The simple phrase or sentence uttered by a child represents an exquisite constellation of skills that are universal for humans" (Meyerson 1995). This means that most people learn to talk, understand spoken language, and communicate with other people in their linguistic community. The linguistic community is the environment composed of people among whom the individual spends the greatest amount of time during waking hours. African American children acquire both verbal and nonverbal systems of communication that reflect their culture and interactional styles. Variation exists between the linguistic styles of Black children and the educational system that results in miscommunication and conflict. The result is that often the advancement of Black children through the formal schooling process is limited.

Language is acquired sequentially, according to a biological timetable. The timetable is determined by the genetic constitution of the individual and evolves with consistent exposure to the adult linguistic form. There is tremendous variation in acquisition rates of language, even children in the same family do not acquire language skills at the same pace. Although the velocity of language acquisition varies, the sequential stages are similar across languages and cultures, overlap each other, and vary among individuals. Rarely do children fail to acquire the language of the community. However, when it does occur, the problem is usually conspicuous and easily identified by the speakers of the language. It is not unusual for members of the family and peers to report that a particular child "talks funny," or acts as if he or she does not understand what other people say.

Children grow up in a specific linguistic community and extract all needed information from the language around them to become competent in language. Linguistic competence is the ability to use and understand a language, that is, "to know the specific rules of a language" (Berko Gleason 1993, p. 20). All linguistically competent individuals must acquire the vocabulary, syntax, phonology, and pragmatics of at least one language. While the typical American English-speaking child acquires only one language, millions of children throughout the world acquire more than one language at the same time. In the case of many African American English-speaking children, AAE is the first and only language they acquire and many never master standard English.

Although people of the world live in different cultures and speak many different languages, human beings use language in similar ways and must acquire similar linguistic information in order to be linguistically competent. Linguistic competence is attained by the time most children reach adolescence. They proceed through predictable sequential stages.

Children acquire the language of their community despite the variation in linguistic environments, or amount of environmental stimulation, encouragement, or reinforcement. In some families, little oral communication takes place between adults and children, and other families are verbal. While differences may exist among children in linguistic verbosity, creativity, and flexibility, both groups of children achieve linguistic competence with very few exceptions. Those exceptions constitute the communicatively impaired group.

Language Acquisition among African American Children

The universality of language development is well known and should make a discussion of variation based on ethnicity unnecessary. However, the reliance on normative data by speech-language pathologists for the assessment and diagnosis of communication disorders obliges a discussion of the developmental stages of surface structures of each linguistic group. Some researchers attempt to explain how and when Black children acquire those linguistic features that separate African American English and standard English. Although the purpose of such research is to document the appearance of phonological and grammatical rules of African American language, such data emphasize an implied model of deficit communication development. Reference is made to "deletion" or "omission" of speech sounds, words, and syllables, and "substitution" of one sound or word for another. It is inaccurate to assert that Black children who say "bafroom" are substituting the /f/ for /θ/, since there is no /θ/ sound in that word in the child's linguistic system, nor has there ever been. Black children are not attempting to say /θ/ and failing. They are simply following the rules of their phonological system. The English word "bathroom" is a variant in which a labiodental sound /f/ occurs instead of the interdental /θ/ sound that occurs in the standard pronunciation.

Little is known about the acquisition of specific superficial features of the language in Black children. It is for this reason that Stockman (1986) examined eight research studies that described the acquisition of African American language. Six general conclusions were drawn from the results.

- Black children develop language within a time frame.
- Semantic categories increase with age. The semantic categories of action and existence are acquired early, while the categories of causality and coordination are acquired later. This conforms to results of cognitive development studies.
- Pragmatic categories exhibited before three years of age included (1) commenting on the environment (e.g., see doggie) and (2) persuading others to do something (e.g., gimme cookie).
- The mean length of response increases with advancing age, similar to that in other groups.

- Features of African American English are not prominent before age three years. Features increase as the children become older.
- Individual variation exists in language acquisition in Black children. The category of "normal" is widely varied and a group of normal children can present a myriad of linguistic levels and behaviors. Some Black children enter school without knowing their formal name, school language, or behavior. Others enter kindergarten reading. By the third or fourth grade, the children may be quite similar.

The practice of researching language acquisition of children from different cultures suggests that language acquisition may vary with ethnicity. Some studies often compare Black and White children on specific features of standard English. Such data are meaningless since they provide little information that is relevant to the development of the features of African American English.

To determine whether school experience affected the use of the features of African American English between kindergarten and second grade, Toliver (1971) observed that second graders did not use significantly fewer African American linguistic forms than children in kindergarten. Samples of spontaneous connected speech were collected from 150 kindergarten, first-, and second-grade African American children who lived and attended school in a predominantly African American community in Northern California. It was concluded that school experience during the first three years had no major effect on the language used in conversation by Black children. In addition, the children failed to identify the same items on a vocabulary test regardless of age. Words such as transportation, ceremony, and web were missed consistently on the test by a significant number of the children.

Ramer and Rees (1973) completed a study similar to Toliver (1971) in which the authors noted that African American children in a low-income community in New York used increasingly more standard English morphological forms as they advanced from preschool to eighth grade. The results further showed that the subjects knew and used increasingly more rules of morphological construction of both African American English and standard English as they advanced in age. In addition, as the children increased in age, they used more standard English forms, but did not give up the African American English forms. There was a positive shift from African American English toward standard English between preschool and eighth grade.

The phonological system develops in a sequential fashion programmed neurologically and auditorily and follows the ability to discriminate speech sounds and the physiological ability to produce them. The coordinated movement of the mechanism for articulation evolves as a process of neuromuscular maturation, which is similar in all human beings. In each language in which the /m/ sound occurs, for example, the children acquire it early, as the first meaningful word in many languages begins with /m/. Menyuk (1971) divided speech sounds into "easy" and "difficult" categories based on facility of production. She reported that easy sounds are produced with the tongue in a resting position and acquired early (e.g., /m/, /b/, and /w/), followed by sounds produced in which the tongue tip is raised and touching another oral structure (e.g., /d/ and /n/). The most difficult sounds are produced when the tongue is thrust forward or when the tongue tip is raised without touching another oral structure (and therefore, acquired later). On the basis of Menyuk's observations, it is obvious that children who speak different languages may employ similar speech sounds in their conversational speech at similar ages, and may have difficulty producing sounds that have comparable coordinated oral movements across languages. In other words, the /r/ sound is acquired late by children who speak Arabic, Spanish, and other languages that contain that sound.

In response to the quandary regarding the acquisition and use of the /θ/ sounds by African American children, Seymour and Ralabate (1985) examined the development of the /θ/ sound in low-income African American children. The authors demonstrated that Black children between first and fourth grades were able to discriminate between the /f/ and /θ/ sounds, but did not use the /θ/ in conversational speech. They further observed that the use of the /θ/ sound increased with age, so that fourth graders employed the sound in isolated words and in conversation with greater frequency than did first graders. The significance of this study is to illustrate that variation and inconsistency in production and use of sounds believed to be absent in African American English show inconsistency in use by children at various ages. This may occur because of teacher correction and the overlap of phonological features of standard and African American English.

Stockman (1996) summarized research on phonological development in African American children and made the following tentative conclusions:

- The phonological system of African American children changes as children grow older and varies with socioeconomic class and geographical region.
- With few exceptions, African American children produce the same phoneme inventory as standard English-speaking children.
- The variation of final consonant deletion is rule-governed and cannot be described as "open syllables."
- African American children use alternative ways to mark tense when the final consonant is absent, such as lengthening or nasalizing the preceding vowels.
- Standardized articulation tests vary in items sensitive enough to reveal the presence of final consonant variations among African American

speakers. Such tests are likely to show persistence in the use of deletions beyond the age when such forms are developmentally appropriate in standard English speakers.

Linguistic differences in academic English (English used in textbooks) are a major problem for many African American children. While they can participate easily in conversation with a speaker of standard English and have no difficulty understanding speakers on radio and television, many Black children frequently have difficulty understanding and using standard English as the medium of learning. Black children at this stage are similar to second language users who have acquired the Basic Interpersonal Communication Skills (BICS), but have not acquired the Cognitive Academic Language Proficiency (CALP). Does this mean that African American children are considered Limited English Proficient? In a sense, Black children who speak African American English are often limited in their knowledge of academic language and have difficulty following directions, responding to questions, and deciphering the content of textbooks. When the textbook vocabulary is so different from the lexicon of the student and the syntax varies remarkably from the sentences heard commonly in the community, children have problems gaining the knowledge intended by the class curriculum. Children need to be taught academic language as a part of the classroom instruction. It is possible for them to fail classes in history, geography, and even mathematics when they are unfamiliar with the language being used to teach the subject. African American children may have difficulty following instructions because of the vocabulary and grammar. Vocabulary such as "compare and contrast," "discuss," and "explain" may present problems, as will sentences such as "Under what circumstances would General Grant order his troops to advance forward?" Learning becomes easier, however, when the language being used is taught before requiring the children to use it, particularly in test-taking.

According to Cummins (1985), a new language user requires about two years to achieve adequate proficiency in BICS. On the other hand, acquiring CALP takes approximately five years. Thus, African American children entering school who are introduced to standard English for the first time cannot be expected to be using it for academic purposes within the first five years of school without being taught the language. Black children and their parents tend to believe that their children comprehend standard English and can use it at will. The Ann Arbor court case (discussed elsewhere in this text) illustrates that the language of the Black children in Detroit was different enough from the classroom English to warrant special instruction.

Black children who speak African American English enter school speaking a language that may be as different from standard English as Latino children who speak Spanish-influenced English or Vietnamese children who speak Vietnamese-influenced English. These children have the ability to engage in conversation with a standard English speaker with little difficulty because of contextual cues. On the other hand, teachers become confused when the same children experience difficulty following both oral and written directions in the classroom, responding to questions asked, and in general, experiencing academic problems related to language. The children are then referred for speech-language testing. When the same children fail the language assessment, it is mistakenly confirmed that they are language disabled and in need of therapy.

Among the reasons why the children fail the language tests is the fact that standard English is being tested, a language the children do not speak. They do not have a language disability, but have a need to learn standard English for the purpose of learning academic material. When groups of the children from any one ethnic group fail the speech and language tests, it becomes clear that English as a second language needs to be taught to all of them. African American children need to be taught English in formal classes as do the other limited English speaking children to establish the ability to understand and use standard English in order to make the learning of academic subjects easier and more meaningful.

COMMUNICATION DISORDERS

Communication is defined as the process of information exchange. It takes place when a message is sent to another person, received, and interpreted. There are many media of communication. However, in this section, oral language is the focus.

Communication disorders are those disabilities affecting the individual's capacity to transmit or receive information due to problems in speech, language, cognition, or hearing. Earlier in this book, a distinction was made between speech and language. Language is defined as a systematic code that is used for communication and includes words, speech sounds (letters for written language), syntax, and rules. Speech is a physiological process of vocalization, resonance, and articulation. The development of speech and language are dependent upon the ability to hear and process auditory signals.

Speech Disorders

Included among speech impairments are difficulties in the production of vocal and speech sounds, or disturbance in the rate or rhythm of speech flow. According to Van Riper, speech is considered to be disordered "when it deviates so far from the speech of other people that it calls attention to itself, interferes with communication, or causes the speaker or his listeners to be distressed" (Van Riper & Emerick 1990, p. 34). The part that is missing from this definition is the issue of diversity. To be disordered, the speech of the individual should deviate from that of other people in the linguistic community. Taylor offered a more comprehensive definition of a communication disorder that included the culture and community of the speaker. According to Taylor (1986), the communication of the individual:

> *can only be considered defective if it deviates sufficiently from the norms, expectations, and definitions of (the) indigenous culture (or language group); that is, if it is*
>
> *(a) considered to be defective by the indigenous culture or language group,*
> *(b) operates outside the minimal norms of acceptability of that culture or language group,*
> *(c) interferes with communication within the indigenous culture or language group,*
> *(d) calls attention to itself within the indigenous culture or language group, or*
> *(e) causes the user to be "maladjusted" as defined by the indigenous culture (p. 13).*

The prevalence of speech disorders is unknown among African American English speakers. However, statistics show that African Americans represent a larger percentage enrolled in speech therapy in schools than their representation in the general population. The 1990 census data show that African Americans constitute 12.1 per cent of the United States population (Statistical Abstracts 1990). In a report compiled and distributed by the Office of Multicultural Affairs of the American Speech-Language-Hearing Association (1996), 16 per cent of the children enrolled in speech therapy in the public schools nationally in 1990 were African Americans.

Speech can be disordered in any aspect of vocal production, resonance, rhythm, articulation, or a combination of two or more of these elements. Among the most common speech disorders in children are speech sound disorders. Speech sound disorders are errors in the articulation of sounds and phonological rules of the language. *Articulation* is the physiological production of the speech sounds of the language (i.e., consonants and vowels). Most children have acquired all of the speech sounds and rules and can make themselves understood by people outside the family by the time they enter school. The teacher should have no difficulty understanding what a kindergarten child says, although occasional errors may be noted, particularly with unfamiliar words. Normally developing children experience difficulty producing speech sounds as they acquire the phonological system of the language. They may omit speech sounds (e.g., "ee" instead of "see"), substitute one sound for another (e.g., "tootie" for "cookie"), add extra sound (e.g., "scat" instead of "cat"), or distort the target sound. Many children who have impaired articulation experience difficulties similar to those of younger children. However, in cases where children have hearing loss or anatomical/physiological/neurological defects, the speech sound errors may be very different from the articulation of younger children.

African American children have similar articulation errors to those observed in other children. Their phonological system contains most of the same speech sounds that occur in standard English, although they sometimes occur in different combinations in particular words. Although the /θ/ occurs in words like *thick*, in some dialects of African American English, it tends not to occur in other words where it would be expected in standard English, for example *bathroom*, pronounced *bafroom*; *mouth*, pronounced *mouf*; and *teeth*, pronounced *teef*. Variation occurs in these characteristics according to geography, community, and socioeconomic level. In communities where these patterns occur and the majority of the children employ them, there is no need to enroll the children in therapy to modify these features.

In some African American communities in Southern states, including parts of Louisiana, North Carolina, South Carolina, Texas, and Georgia, the consonant blends /skr/ and /kw/ occur in certain words where /str/ and /tw/ occur in other dialects. The words *street* and *string* are pronounced *skreet* and *skring*, and *twenty* and *twelve* are pronounced *kwenty* and *kwelve* respectively. These standards should be employed in determining the presence of an articulation disorder in the appropriate communities. However, they cannot be expected to occur outside their respective communities except in cases where migration from one community to another has occurred. In addition, the standards of low-income Black communities should not be used as a basis of comparison for children in other neighborhoods where the standards are different.

The prevalence of articulation disorders among African American children is unknown. When studies that count phonological differences of Black children as errors are eliminated, there is no evidence to suggest that African American children experience more articulation errors than other children. Although many Black children receive speech-language therapy to help them use the standard /θ/, /v/, final consonant clusters, and /er/, this practice is not recommended except on a voluntary basis. To help the speech-language pathologists determine their role in the diagnosis and treatment of communication disorders in linguistic minority groups, the American Speech-Language-Hearing Association (ASHA) adopted an official position for the profession.

It is the position of the American Speech-Language-Hearing Association (ASHA) that no dialectal variety of English is a disorder or a pathological form of speech or language. Each social dialect is adequate as a functional and effective variety of English. Each serves a communication function as well as a social solidarity function. It maintains the communication network and the social construct of the community of speakers who use it. Furthermore, each is a symbolic representation of the historical, social, and cultural background of the speakers (Position Paper 1983, p. 23-24).

The position paper specifies the role of the speech-language pathologist in the diagnosis and treatment of communicative disorders in "nonstandard dialect" speakers.

The speech-language pathologist must have certain competencies to distinguish between dialectal differences and communicative disorders. These competencies include knowledge of the particular dialect as a rule-governed linguistic system, knowledge of the phonological and grammatical features of the dialect, and knowledge of nondiscriminatory testing procedures. Once the difference/disorder distinctions have been made, it is the role of the speech-language pathologist to treat only those features or characteristics that are true errors and not attributable to the dialect.

Aside from the traditionally recognized role, the speech-language pathologist may also be available to provide elective clinical services to nonstandard English speakers who do not present a disorder (Position Paper 1983, p. 24).

Teachers sometimes confuse articulation disorders with phonological disorders. While both are speech sounds disorders, phonological disorders involve linguistic rules in either reception, expression, or both. In the receptive area, the child may have difficulty perceiving the patterns of the phonological system. This means that the child may have difficulty discriminating speech sounds, remembering the patterns, or gaining meaning from the sounds heard. A hearing loss is a common cause of such difficulties, although many individuals who have perceptual problems do not have hearing loss. In addition to receptive problems, phonological disorders may be expressive. In some cases, the child omits syllables or sounds or substitutes sounds for other consonants that do not resemble the target sound. Some children, for example, substitute the /t/ (a stop sound—the airstream is totally blocked and exploded) for many other sounds. They may say "I tee tomebody looting in my hout" for "I see somebody looking in my house." Another child may continue to delete unstressed syllables beyond the age level when such speech behaviors are expected. Such children might say "They have many puters in tucky" for "They have many computers in Kentucky." Other children delete all final consonant sounds described as *open syllables*. When children have difficulty with the phonological system, articulation may be impaired related to the violation of rules of the phonological system of the language. An example of a rule violation is the omission of the initial /s/ in the word *smoke*, a manifestation of consonant cluster reduction. In other words, a phonological disorder is more involved than the individual simply substituting, deleting, or distorting individual sounds. In order to determine the extent of the phonological disorder, samples must be taken of the child's comprehension and production of speech sounds at a variety of levels, including individual words, syllables, and sounds in context.

Intelligibility

Intelligibility refers to the ease of the listener in understanding the speech of the talker. The number, type, and frequency of occurrence of misarticulated sounds affect the clarity of the child's speech. Children who have a large number of errors on frequently occurring sounds will be less intelligible than children who have a small number of errors, or errors on infrequently occurring speech sounds. In addition, large numbers of omitted sounds and syllables affect intelligibility significantly. Listeners unfamiliar with the language, dialect, or accent of the speaker will judge the speech unintelligible because they do not understand it. This does not mean that other people experience the same difficulty. Teachers sometimes refer children for speech assessment because they find the children's speech unintelligible. A question teachers can ask is "Do the other children from the culture or the family members notice any problems in intelligibility?" Family members and friends, particularly the child's mother, are able to discern whether the child's speech is different enough from that of the other children in the neighborhood to warrant referral to the speech-language pathologist. If the teacher finds that the intelligibility problems are unique to the teacher, the speech-language clinician can help. More will be said on this topic later.

Articulation disorders have many causes, including temporary or permanent hearing loss, structural defects of the articulators (the oral or nasal structures used to produce speech sounds), neurological impairment that limits the range of motion and speed of the articulators, and learning from speech models who have articulation disorders. Articulation errors caused by learning from inadequate speech models are the easiest to correct, particularly when the child is appropriately motivated to modify speech habits and there are no anatomical or physiological disabilities. Typically, showing the child how to produce the correct speech sound and allowing time for practice produce favorable results within a short amount of time.

Structural defects of the oral and nasal cavities include clefts of the lip and palate, ankyloglossia (tongue tie), macroglossia (abnormally large tongue), microglossia (abnormally small tongue), dental and occlusal problems, and obstructions of the nose such as enlarged adenoids. *Cleft lip* (the structures of the upper lip fail to unite in utero leaving a lip that is perforated) can affect the closure of the lip required for the production of labial sounds such as /b/,

/m/, and /w/. Cleft lip is usually repaired surgically when the child is very young, commonly during the first few months of life. Articulation disorders that result from cleft lip are sometimes caused by the presence of scar tissue resulting from surgical repair. In some cases, growth defects occur as the children grow larger, producing an upper lip that may be too short for closure. *Cleft palate* (failure of the hard or soft palate to unite at the midline in utero leaving a hole in the roof of the mouth) is diagnosed at birth and corrected surgically when the child is young. In some cases, several surgeries are required to create a structure and function to produce normal speech. Many children born with clefts of the palate have no speech problems after the surgical repair. On the other hand, many children have significant speech problems despite competent surgical repair at an early age. The quality of the child's speech is affected by the structure and function following the palatal repair. Speech affected by a cleft of the palate tends to be hypernasal with nasal emission of speech sounds and compensatory errors. The hypernasality is caused by the child's inability to occlude the nasal cavity to produce oral sounds. Other errors may be produced when the child attempts to compensate for the lack of nasal occlusion.

Cleft lip and palate are reported to occur less frequently among people of African descent than among other groups (Chavez, Cordero, & Bacerro 1988; Cole 1980; Millard & McNeill 1965; Siegel 1979). In a study of South African patients, Kromberg and Jenkins (1982) reported a significantly lower incidence of cleft lip and palate children within the Black African population (0.30/1000 births) than in the White African population (1.61/1000 births). The South Africans labeled Colored showed a rate lower than the White group, but significantly higher than the Black group (1.4/1000 births). In interracial families where the mother was White, there was a higher incidence of clefts than when the mother was Black. Children who had two Black parents had a lower incidence of clefts than either of the interracial groups (Khoury, Erickson, & James 1983). These results suggest that the race of the mother had a stronger influence for producing clefts than the race of the father.

Other studies have identified significantly more clefts in the presence of major malformations among Africans and people of African descent. Siegel (1979) noted that in a group of cleft lip and palate Black and White children in Philadelphia, the Black group had more multiple anomalies than the White group, and Black girls showed a higher incidence of clefts than Black boys. This is the opposite in White groups, where cleft lip and palate occur more frequently in males.

When economically poor Black children are compared to middle-class Black children, differences have been noted. Altemus (1966) reported a higher incidence of clefts among lower socioeconomic Black children in Washington, D.C. compared with Black middle-class children in the same city. The incidence of clefts appeared to be related to a number of factors, including gender, type of cleft, birth weight and order, and age of the mother (Altemus 1966). The highest incidence of clefts occurred in males, first born, to mothers between the ages of 13 and 30 years. Fewer clefts were found in babies weighing 5 pounds, 8 ounces or less.

Tongue tie is a concept that is common to the general public. While the layperson uses the term to refer to all articulation disorders, tongue tie is really a problem in which the lingual frenulum (a fold of mucous membrane extending from the floor of the mouth to the midline of the under surface of the tongue) is short enough to restrict the movement of the tongue tip. Most children who have short lingual frenula do not exhibit speech problems. In extreme cases, the children are unable to raise the tip of the tongue high enough to produce sounds that require the tongue tip be raised to touch the gum ridge, such as the /t/ and /d/ or thrust forward, such as /θ/. Surgical treatment is rarely recommended for the correction of tongue tie. Several years ago, surgery was offered when children experienced major speech disorders, regardless of the sound errors exhibited. Brembry (1987) reports no differences in the articulation of children before and after the frenulum was surgically severed.

Neuromotor problems are observed in children who have major as well as minor neurological impairment. In such cases impairment in the central or peripheral nervous system creates problems in which the articulatory structures may be affected by paralysis or weakness, resulting in slow, labored speech and imprecise articulation. Drooling may also be observed. Children who have cerebral palsy generally have such problems.

English as a second language speakers may have difficulty producing the sounds of their new language when such sounds did not occur in their first language. When the first language has speech sounds that are different from the sounds of English, interference will occur. Many second language speakers have difficulty producing the /θ/ sounds or the English /r/. Such speakers tend to use a sound from their first language that is closest in phonological features to the English sound. Frequently the speakers use the /f/ or /s/ in English words that contain the /θ/. Clearly such differences are not considered errors for African American English speakers.

Voice disorders occur when the quality, pitch, and loudness differ from other individuals of similar age, sex, cultural background, and geographical (Stemple 1984). Voice disorders are impairments in vocal sound production (phonation) or sound modification (resonance). Vocal sound is produced by the vibration of the vocal folds set into motion by the neurological processes and supported by the exhalation of air pressure from the lungs. The process of producing vocal sound is known as phonation. The vocal folds can be lengthened, shortened, tensed, or relaxed to modify the pitch and loudness of the voice. The voices of men and women are different from each other because of the length and mass of the vocal folds and the shape and size of the cavities of the head and neck. Disorders of phonation are produced when there is structural damage to the vocal folds, when the neurological mechanism responsible for movement and tension is damaged, or when emotional difficulties cause impairment of vocal function. Structural damage to the vocal folds is often caused by abuse related to the misuse of the voice. The most common result of vocal abuse is the creation of small pimple-like growths on the vocal folds called *nodules*. Screaming, yelling, speaking, and singing at the wrong pitch can create nodules. Nodules are common in young males, particularly boys who sing at the wrong pitch, engage in loud "rapping" at the wrong pitch, or make noise that forces the vocal folds to perform in a fashion that place undue stress and friction on them. Vocal nodules create a hoarse, breathy voice quality, although they may not prevent the speaker from talking or singing at very loud levels.

Disorders of phonation may be caused by vocal fold paralysis or paresis (weakness) resulting from accident or disease. A single vocal fold may be paralyzed or weakened, or both folds may be involved. When one or both folds are paralyzed in an open position, the voice may be weak in loudness, low in pitch, or totally absent, called *aphonia*.

Hoarse voices among children are commonly caused by extra mass on the vocal folds created by mucous resulting from allergies or colds. The good news is that such problems are temporary and go away when the condition subsides.

Racial and ethnic differences are observed in the epidemiology of voice disorders. De Jarnette and Holland (1993) described research studies that showed a substantial difference between the incidence of voice disorders in Black and White children. Black children had fewer cases of vocal modules and the male to female ratios were different.

Resonance is the modification of vocal sounds by the cavities of the head and neck. The shape of the oral and nasal structures of the head, along with the structure and function of the vocal folds, are responsible for the distinctive quality of the human voice. Thus, each individual voice is distinctive and recognizable by friends and acquaintances. The structural make up of individuals is genetically determined with similarities among relatives. This phenomenon explains why mothers, daughters, and sisters sound similarly on the telephone.

Disorders of resonance occur when there is damage or obstruction in the structures of the oral and nasal cavities. Most speech sounds are resonated by the oral cavity, while a small group of sounds (m, n, and /wg/) is resonated by the nose. Obstructions of the nasal cavity (e.g., clogging created by mucous or enlarged adenoids) can result in a resonance disorder called *denasality*. At the opposite end of the spectrum is *nasality* or *hypernasality*, in which too many sounds are resonated by the nose. Cleft palate and other forms of velopharyngeal incompetence (e.g., palatal paralysis or short soft palate) cause nasality related to the inability of the speaker to close off the nasal cavity, which would prevent resonance by the nose. Cleft palate was also discussed in the articulation disorders section because substitution of nasal sounds for oral sounds and the other types of errors observed in cleft palate affect articulation as well.

Finally, *fluency* disorders are impairment in the flow of speech. Such speakers may speak too rapidly, too slowly, or may experience interruptions in the continuity of speech. The most common disorder of fluency is *stuttering*. Stuttering is defined as a disorder in which the rhythm of the speaker is characterized by repeated speech sounds, words, and phrases, unusual pauses, and prolonged sounds. Van Riper and Emerick (1990) argue that stuttering "occurs when the forward flow of speech is interrupted abnormally by repetitions or prolongations of a sound, syllable, articulatory posture, or by avoidance and struggle behaviors" (Van Riper & Emerick 1990, p. 294). The speaker struggles to reduce the occurrence of the disfluencies by employing unusual postures, vocalizations, facial expressions, and bodily movements. In addition, people who stutter are fearful of certain words and situations and use specific avoidance behaviors, such as circumlocutions and word substitutions. There may be a notable amount of groping and searching for words that do not contain the feared sounds.

Culatta and Goldberg (1995) suggest that the definition of stuttering requires more than a statement of the characteristics of the speech acts. They argue for a "four-factor" definition of stuttering. The four factors include (1) stuttering is a developmental disorder of childhood, (2) the cause is unknown, (3) people who stutter view communication differently than normal speakers, and (4) people who stutter have abnormal overt or covert communication behaviors. Culatta and Goldberg also suggest that there are six different types of disfluency, which have different causes and manifestations. The six types of disfluency include normal disfluency, stuttering, neurogenic disfluency, psychogenic disfluency, language-based disfluency, and mixed fluency failures. Mixed fluency is a combination of fluency types. The individual may have stuttering, for example, and neurogenic disfluency.

Stuttering exists throughout the world, but appears at different rates and varies based on gender and ethnicity. Racial differences have been observed in the prevalence of stuttering in the United States, but little documentation is available.

The cause of stuttering is unknown, but explained by numerous theories. Sheehan (1970) suggested that stuttering is caused by a conflict within the individual between the need to speak and the avoidance of stuttering. The person who stutters wants to speak, but cannot because he or she is likely to stutter. The conflict between speaking and stuttering renders the individual's speech disfluent. Another theory, the learning theory, suggests that stuttering begins with normal disfluency in which the child learns to be disfluent because of the response of adults to the disfluency (Johnson 1961). According to Johnson, stuttering begins, not in the child's mouth, but in the head of the child's parents. Johnson indicated that disfluency in young children is observed between the ages of two and six years of age. The children repeat sounds, words, and phrases and exhibit unusual pauses and periods of silence. Disfluency of this nature usually disappears with age and needs no intervention. Parents and peers should not try to intervene with helpful hints, such as, "slow down," "take a deep breath," or "stop and start over." Such comments are not helpful and may be damaging by causing the child to make attempts to prevent the disfluency, which creates further disfluency. The need to prevent disfluency by the children creates a vicious cycle of fear for the children, which leads to disfluency, which leads to fear, which leads to disfluency, and so on. The one factor that perpetuates stuttering is fear, which causes the speaker to avoid speaking and to use techniques to prevent disfluency. The techniques selected and used by the person who stutters often become bizarre mannerisms that exacerbate the speech disorder. It is therefore, necessary for teachers, family, and friends to avoid calling attention to the disfluencies of the young disfluent child because of the possibility that great damage can be done to create the more serious disorder of stuttering.

Van Riper and Emerick (1990) believed that stuttering has many causes, many sources, and that the causes are not as important as the forces that maintain the condition once it has started. An eclectic approach suggests that, since the maintaining cause is the most important factor, working toward reducing the effects of the maintaining causes is important for the effective treatment of stuttering.

Stuttering among African Americans has been sporadically studied. The phenomenon among both Africans and African Americans has been compared with stuttering among White Americans. One of the earliest studies that reported the prevalence of stuttering among African Americans was conducted by Carson and Kantner (1945) who found that stuttering was 60 percent more prevalent among Black children than among White children. Cooper and Cooper (1993) report a study by Pritchett, who also found more stuttering among Black children. Gillespie and Cooper (1973) found four times more stuttering in Black high school students than among White children, and Conrad (reported in Cooper & Cooper 1993) also found more stuttering among Black people. In addition, the male to female ratio of stuttering prevalence is different in African American populations than in White populations, approximately 4 males to 1 female in White groups compared to 2 males to 1 females in Black groups (Conrad 1988; Goldman 1967).

In the studies presented, the criteria for determining the presence of stuttering varied from one study to the next, the methods of data collection varied, and the race of the examiner varied. There is no evidence in these studies that cultural or linguistic variation might have accounted for deviations. In the

Gillespie and Cooper study (1973), for example, the criteria for determining the presence of stuttering were the same for all speech disorders. Specifically, speech was considered "defective if it was sufficiently deviant from the speech patterns of the region to attract attention to the speech act, or to affect adversely either the speaker or listener" (Gillespie & Cooper 1973, p. 743). In other words, the criteria for determining the presence of a speech disorder were the same for both Black and White speakers.

The study by Leith and Mims (1975) did consider the effects of culture in the presentation of stuttering by disfluent African American speakers. They noted that Black people who stutter tended not to manifest overt stuttering. They tended to attempt to mask stuttering or exhibit silence when stuttering could not be masked or prevented. The Black speakers who stutter tended to be more "tense and anxious and seemed less willing to tolerate the occurrence of overt repetitions and prolongations" (p. 461).

The authors hypothesized that Black individuals who stutter are behaviorally different from White people who stutter, resulting from cultural differences. Thus, the Black speakers react differently to their disfluency than White speakers who stutter. One cultural influence on the Black stutterer is the high emphasis Black Americans place on oral communication. Young males who stutter, especially, are required to participate in competitive verbal games, such as rapping, playing the dozens, and sounding. A second cultural influence that affects the behavior of Black people who stutter is the need to be "cool." That is, Black males are expected to speak without struggle or excitement. These cultural factors would cause the person to do everything possible to hide disfluency.

Whatever differences that exist in the prevalence of stuttering in Black and White populations are difficult to explain. Perhaps explanations may be based on physiological, cultural, or sociological differences between Black and White people. Since a fully supported etiology of stuttering has never been found, whatever explanation for racial differences is generally speculative. A multifactorial etiology is a possible explanation and includes genetic predisposition, which might explain prevalence. Perhaps questions about prevalence are less important than answers about appropriate diagnosis and treatment. If stuttering among African Americans takes a different form due to cultural issues, it is appropriate that treatment focus on utilizing this information to treat people who stutter in different cultural groups. Conrad (1988) observed that Black people who stutter used more part word repetitions and prolongations than did White people who stutter. Leith and Mims (1975) noted that while Black people who stutter exhibited fewer disfluencies than White individuals who stutter and more secondary features including eye blinks, head movements, and facial contortions.

The reaction of listeners to stuttering varies among cultural groups. Stuttering is somewhat common among males in the Grand Bahamas Islands

(Gibson 1988). However, it does not bear the same stigma as it does in the United States. In the Bahamas, efforts to enroll stuttering males into speech therapy are often countered with resistance by the child and the parents since stuttering is not considered a serious disorder. Stuttering, according to some Bahamians, is a physical trait, similar to short stature, or large feet. Thus, there is no need to fix it.

Language Disorders

Language disorders are impairments in the ability to use the vocabulary of the language, form sentences, or communicate ideas in a fashion that is acceptable for the child's age or community. The capability to hear is needed for communication to take place and requires the capacity to receive and interpret auditory signals.

Language is considered disordered when the receptive and/or expressive presentation is inappropriate for the developmental level of the individual or the community. In other words, language is considered defective when the skills of the child are below the level of the peers. Problems may exist in semantics, syntax, or pragmatics. Many problems of language have no known cause, however, chronic otitis media (OM) and resultant temporary hearing loss are suspected in many cases.

Some African American children are enrolled in speech-language services because they do not speak standard English. They do not speak standard English because they have had little opportunity to use the language in their communities. Watching television and understanding the language used by the characters does not provide the stimulus to inspire the use of standard English in the children's neighborhood. Language used by television characters, in the minds of the children, is confined to the television and is not relevant to their lives. They may extract a phrase or word and use it to express some ideas. Such elements, however, do not become a permanent part of the children's language. Children develop the vocabulary, phonological system, pragmatics, and syntax needed to communicate effectively within their own communities.

Vocabulary

Children acquire all of the vocabulary they need to communicate effectively in their environment, but do not learn words they do not need. Vocabulary continues to grow as the needs change and exposure is enhanced. Some African American children arrive at school without knowing their full name, numbers, positions in space, or answers to obvious questions. However, they will learn everything required of them when they are taught. Teaching school vocabulary is the responsibility of the classroom teacher, not the speech-language pathologist. A disorder would be identified when the child's vocabulary is inadequate to communicate effectively within the home community or fails to expand with increasing exposure.

Grammar
Grammatical differences, similarly, cannot be considered language disorders. The grammar of Black children is determined by the linguistic community and the children cannot be expected to know the rules of standard English when they have had no opportunity to learn them. The role of the school is to teach children everything they need to learn in order for them to be considered educated, which includes the teaching of grammar. The caseloads of public school speech-language clinicians sometimes include African American, Latino, Asian, and other minority group children to whom standard English grammar is being taught. Osom (1997) observed that Black children enrolled in speech-language therapy in a school district in northern California received intervention for features of African American English, such as subject-verb agreement and variations of the verb *to be* in addition to intervention for errors that were considered defective. Some children in Osom's study were enrolled in speech-language therapy to modify only the features of their African American English.

Pragmatics
Pragmatics refers to the manner in which language is used within a particular linguistic group. Rules of pragmatics determine how people interact during communication. Included in pragmatics are rules for using idioms, turn taking, topic maintenance, topic termination, and nonverbal issues. Children learn how to use the language within their community, but make mistakes when they enter unfamiliar situations outside their neighborhoods. Many idioms customarily used in White communities are often unknown to the Black children.

Problems in pragmatics are observed when children and adults cross cultural lines and fail to recognize the rules of pragmatics in the new culture. Such rules, in time, are generally learned by observation. However, in the classroom, school pragmatics should be taught by the teacher to make the child's transition between the home culture and the school move faster. Schoolroom culture is separate from mainstream American culture but similar in some ways. Unlike mainstream culture, children have to raise their hand when they want to talk, get up, or ask a question. On the other hand, turn taking in conversation and standing in lines to enter and leave a room are similar to the cultural expectations in mainstream culture. Adults in American culture stand in so many lines that they often line up to get on planes even when seats have been assigned in advance.

Developmental Language Delay
The most commonly diagnosed language disorder in children is *developmental language delay* in which the language emerges more slowly than in children of similar age and community. Such children tend to use language in a fashion that appears immature to the people who know the child. Among the characteristics of language delay are underdeveloped grammar, reduced vocabulary, and phonological errors. Language delayed children acquire language in the same sequence as do normally developing children; however, development begins later and/or proceeds more slowly (Johnson 1996). The good news is that these children eventually acquire the language of their community without residual effects. A common cause of delayed language development is hearing loss caused by chronic otitis media (middle ear infections). Delays are also caused by neurological impairment, emotional problems, developmental disabilities, and a myriad of multifactorial etiologies.

Aphasia
Aphasia is a language disorder caused by neurological impairment. Although aphasia is observed most frequently in adults suffering head trauma or disease, it does occur in children. The characteristics of the linguistic impairment are related to the location and extent of the damage to the brain. Among African American children, aphasia is commonly associated with sickle cell disease. Sickle cell disease is a genetically transmitted condition that affects the shape of red blood cells in the body. It affects approximately 50,000 North Americans of African ancestry (Wasserman, Wilimas, Fairclough, Mulhern, & Wang 1991). In sickle cell disease, the red blood cells lose oxygen and assume an elongated shape that resembles a sickle. The condition is characterized by "hemolytic anemia, increased susceptibility to life-threatening infections, and painful vaso-occlusive crises" (Crawford, Gould, Smith, Beckford, Gibson, & Bobo 1992, p. 349). There is also damage to the organs of the body, particularly the spleen, brain, and ear. Children suffering from sickle cell disease are absent from school frequently because of illness, and therefore academic problems have been noted, particularly for subjects such as mathematics where consistent attendance is required (Wasserman et al. 1991).

Neurological manifestations of sickle cell disease and damage to other organs of the body occur frequently in sickle cell patients. Young children with sickle cell disease are at risk for cerebrovascular infarction (Prohovnik, Pavlakis, Piomelli, Bello, Hilal, & De Vivo 1989; Swift, Cohen, Hynd, Wisenbaker, McKie, Makari, & McKie 1990) with the incidence peaking during childhood. Strokes occur in 6 out of 10 of patients with sickle cell disease (Wasserman et al. 1991). Approximately 80 percent of the patients suffer strokes before 15 years of age with an average onset of six years. As a result of strokes, children suffer from hemiplegia, seizures, speech-language impairment, and visual problems (Wasserman et al. 1991).

The first stroke of sickle cell patients results in death or permanent neurologic disorders in fewer than half the patients. Most of the children survive the first stroke and recover most gross neurologic function and presenting symptoms within a few days. Ohene-Frempong (1991) examined 59 sickle cell patients who had suffered their first stroke. One 14 year-old patient died, however, 37 patients suffered no residual neurologic effects. Twenty-one of the subjects whose residual neurologic effects of the stroke did not resolve completely, continued to suffer from paresis and paralysis of limbs, seizure disorders, and permanent cerebellar signs (problems with balance). Left hemiparesis (weakness of the left arm and leg) was the most common residual symptom. The patients who recovered completely were older (average age of 10.0 years) than the patients who did not recover completely (average age of 7.3 years). It was concluded that younger patients had more residual effects than older patients following CVA.

Strokes are likely to recur in sickle cell children, usually within 12 to 24 months of the original stroke (Ohene-Frempong 1991). However, recurrence can be prevented with transfusion therapy. "The only therapy currently known to be effective in preventing recurrent stroke in SCD is transfusion therapy" (Francis 1991, p. 90).

Differences versus Disorders

Children who have moderate to severe language disorders are very different from their peers. They exhibit many of the disabilities described earlier and the need for intervention is obvious. Children with language disorders may speak in shorter utterances than their peers, use fewer words, and may have difficulty understanding the language that neighborhood children have mastered. They may be unable to name or point to objects common to the people in the community and respond slowly or not at all to questions or directions. Some tend to be very quiet, or if they are talkative, speech may be difficult to understand. The process of communication may be arduous, with the children appearing uncertain as to when or how to respond to their communication partners. They appear confused when given complex directions or long questions. In the classroom, linguistically impaired children may watch and copy the behaviors of other children when the teacher gives complicated directions. Mattes and Omark (1991) identified characteristics that separate linguistically impaired children from their normal peers. They report that language-impaired children (1) rarely initiate verbal interaction with peers, (2) do not respond verbally to oral communication of peers, (3) may use gestures to communicate, or (4) cannot use language to direct the behaviors of peers. Bloom and Lahey (1978) identified five types of language disorders, found in children who (1) have difficulty learning the linguistic rules of phonology, morphology, and syntax, (2) have difficulty conceptualizing and formulating ideas about events, objects, and relations, primarily in the area of semantics, (3) have difficulty adapting language to correspond to the situation or audience, (4) have difficulty integrating form, content, and use; and (5) exhibit delayed language development.

Hearing Impairment

Disorders of hearing have many causes and can affect people at all ages. Some children are born with hearing loss (congenital), and others acquire problems as a result of accident or disease.

Hearing loss varies from mild to profound. In many cases mild hearing loss requires no assistive devices and can be managed with instruction on appropriate positioning for listening and aural rehabilitation. Parents and teachers must be provided information regarding the nature and characteristics of the hearing problems with suggestions for assisting the child within family activities and the classroom.

There are three main types of hearing loss related to sensitivity of hearing and auditory perceptual disorders observed among children. The three types of sensitivity hearing loss include conductive, sensorineural, and central. Conductive hearing loss is a condition in which the loss is relatively flat, affecting all frequencies equally. Conductive hearing loss is caused by damage or obstruction in the outer or middle ear. Sensorineural hearing loss affects mainly high frequencies and is caused by damage to the inner ear or auditory nerve. Central hearing loss is caused by damage to the temporal lobe of the brain.

The most prevalent type of hearing loss observed in children is conductive hearing loss caused by chronic otitis media (OM). Otitis media is inflammation of the middle ear and is common in young children. It is so common that almost all children experience at least one ear infection in early childhood. "Approximately 70 percent of children in the general population have one or more episodes of OM by 5 years of age" (Buchanan, Moore, & Counter 1993). Prevalence varies depending on age, sex, and ethnicity. Black children reportedly have a significantly lower incidence of otitis media than White children, regardless of socioeconomic level (Robinson & Allen 1984; Robinson, Allen, & Root 1988).

Robinson and Allen (1984) conducted a study to examine the rate of occurrence of middle ear dysfunction as measured by tympanometry in Black and White middle-class children. Subjects included males and females between the ages of 30 and 48 months of age. Using a pass/fail scoring technique, the children were grouped on the basis of age, sex, and ethnicity. Results showed no significant differences between Black and White children who had definite middle-ear infections (11.1% of the White children and 10% of the Black children). There was a difference, however, between Black and White children whose impedance scores fell into the "suspected" category

(13% of Black children and 25% of the White children). Black children were represented at a significantly higher level in the normal category (77%) than White children (63.9%). The results of this study showed an overall significant difference between Black children (23.3%) and White children (38%) between the ages of 30 and 48 months.

In a followup study, Robinson, Allen, and Root (1988) used tympanometry to determine racial difference of children between the ages of six and thirteen months. Results showed a significant difference between Black and White infants in tympanometric failure rates. Thirty-three percent of the Black infants failed the test, implying middle ear pathology, while 57 percent of the White children failed. These results are consistent with those of earlier studies conducted with older children.

Hearing loss is observed throughout the life span and has varied causes. In children, the biological factors that affect the hearing may occur before or after birth. Before birth, etiological factors may be genetic or teratogenic (external factors that affect the fetus in utero). In these cases, the hearing loss is typically congenital (present at birth). After birth, hearing loss can be caused by accident or disease, although genetics may be the etiological factor that causes hearing loss in adults (e.g., otosclerosis). Common diseases that cause hearing loss in childhood include otitis media and high fevers caused by conditions such as meningitis.

Ethnic differences are observed in the prevalence of hearing loss. Prevalence varies as a function of etiology. Otosclerosis (a condition that causes an abnormality of the bones of the middle ear, resulting in conductive hearing loss) and presbycusis (hearing loss related to aging) are more prevalent in White people. Hearing loss related to conditions that are observed mainly in African Americans, such as sickle cell disease, is more common in Black people (Buchanan, Moore, & Counter 1993).

When compared with individuals who have normal hemoglobin, the sickle cell patients show a higher incidence of hearing loss. In a study of 83 sickle cell and normal individuals in Jamaica matched for age, Todd, Sergeant, and Larson (1973) found 22 percent of the sickle cell patients suffered varying degrees of sensorineural hearing loss compared to only 4 percent for the normal subjects. Older sickle cell patients had an even higher percentage of loss. According to Todd, Sergeant, and Larson there appears to be a relationship between the number of sickle cell crises and the prevalence of hearing loss. In a similar study in 1980, Friedman, Luban, Herer, and Williams noted a higher degree of hearing loss among children with sickle cell disease (12% for sickle cell children and 0% for the control group). The author of this study concluded that hearing loss of sickle cell children may be related to central nervous system involvement, as sickle cell patients are at greater risk for cerebrovascular accidents. The author also suggested that sickle cell disease may be causing damage to the inner ear that may be difficult to detect using the most sophisticated procedures for testing hearing. Crawford and colleagues (1991) noted that the prevalence of hearing loss in adults with sickle cell disease was 41 percent, greater than the prevalence in the general population.

Sensorineural hearing loss is the most common type of loss in sickle cell disease. Morganstein and Manace (1969) reported that the cause of sensorineural hearing loss was damage to the inner and outer hair cells in the inner ear due to the occlusion of the blood vessels that serve those structures. They observed that those blood vessels, as well as the venous and capillary channels of the temporal bone, were filled with sickled cells. The cochlea is highly susceptible to disruption in blood flow as it reduces the oxygen supply (Crawford et al., 1991). In the Crawford study, the prevalence was determined for adults rather than children. Both reversible and permanent hearing losses have been associated with sickle cell disease.

Sudden hearing loss has been described in several studies (O'Keefe & Maw 1991; Orchik & Dunn 1977; Urban 1973). Urban (1973) was the first to report on a case of a 20-year-old sickle cell patient who exhibited a severe sensorineural hearing loss for several weeks following a sickle cell crisis. On the 46th day, hearing returned to normal for pure tones, although problems remained in the understanding of spoken language. In 1977, Orchik and Dunn reported similar observations in an 18-year-old patient. In this patient, a severe sensorineural loss remained after the crisis in one ear, although hearing returned to normal several days following the crisis in the other ear. O'Keefe and Maw (1991) indicated that sudden deafness in a 25-year-old patient was not reversible and their subject remained deaf one year after the initial onset. These three case studies demonstrated the consequences of a temporary occlusion of blood vessels leading to the inner ear that may result in oxygen deprivation to the hair cells causing hearing loss. Such losses are sometimes, but not always, reversible.

SUMMARY

In this chapter normal and deviant speech and language development were discussed. The common disorders were described and known prevalence data were presented. Although limited research data are available that distinguish between Black and White speakers, some reports were described. It is reasonably clear that some speech, language, and hearing disorders occur differently in Black and White children. The prevalence rate of articulation and language disorders is unknown, and confusion remains regarding the prevalence of stuttering.

Speech, language, and hearing disorders are complex conditions. The causes are varied, which make it difficult to show clear-cut evidence of conditions that affect speech, language, and hearing of children of different ethnic groups. Regardless of the prevalence or etiology, it is evident that language acquisition follows a predictable sequence that appears to be biologically determined. In addition, the diagnosis of speech and language disorders in African American children requires special consideration to insure that an appropriate plan is developed for intervention. In other words, the speech-language pathologist must be able to distinguish between a language disorder and African American communication.

The conditions that cause speech and language disorders occur throughout the world, although the effects of these problems on communication vary in expression. There are many biological conditions that affect the processes involved in the production and use of oral language, as noted earlier. In many cases, the effects of chronic otitis media may linger for many years, resulting in speech, language, and academic disorders. The legacy of the otitis media remains far longer than the ear infections themselves.

African American children suffer from many of the problems that result in speech and language disorders. In addition, Black children are exposed to a number of menacing conditions that plague their communities. Pediatric AIDS, sickle cell disease, prenatal drug exposure, low birthweight, and exposure to lead toxicity affect African American children at higher rates than other children.

It is often assumed that a greater proportion of Black children experience communication disorders than other children. There is no evidence to support this assumption. Teachers and speech-language pathologists need to be objective when making referrals or testing for speech-language disorders. Objectivity is required to resist the judgment that the language of the African American community is impaired and needs to be altered.

PRACTICAL APPLICATION

Speech, language, and hearing disorders may be obvious or subtle. The child may be difficult to understand, respond inconsistently to auditory signals, repeat, hesitate, or prolong speech sounds, words or phrases, or experiences difficulty using or understanding language. When the teacher suspects a speech, language, or hearing disorder, he or she should refer the child to a speech-language pathologist. The following are suggestions for teachers who suspect that a child has a speech, language or hearing disorder.

Signs of a Speech Disorder

1. The child has difficulty pronouncing words that children in the same age group and culture can pronounce.

2. The child's speech is difficult to understand by people within the community and family who know the child well.
3. The child struggles to talk. The speech flow is interrupted by repeated sounds, words or phrases, hesitation, and prolongation of sounds.
4. The child's voice is hoarse, high or low enough in pitch as to be noticeable, excessively nasal, or denasal (sounds like the child has a constant stuffy nose).
5. The child's speech is too loud or too soft.
6. The child's speaking rate is too fast or too slow.
7. The child appears to be too shy to talk.

Signs of a Receptive Language Disorder and Hearing Loss

1. The child's responses to verbal stimuli are slow. When instructions are given, for example, the child does not respond immediately. Instructions have to be repeated several times in different ways, and the child may watch other children to determine which instructions are given.
2. The child's response to questions is inappropriate in a variety of contexts, such as at home, in the classroom, or on the playground.
3. The child has difficulty understanding conversational speech.
4. The child becomes distracted and active during group listening activities such as story telling.
5. The child appears distracted and is often accused of daydreaming.
6. The child's speech or language may be impaired.

Signs of an Expressive Language Disorder

1. The child's sentences are noticeably shorter than other children in the community.
2. The child has difficulty expressing ideas. Sentences may be sequenced in such an unusual way as to render the language difficult to understand.
3. The child does not have enough words to express ideas or uses wrong words.
4. There may be many false starts, corrections, and interjections of vocal sounds, such as "um," "huh," and "uh."

Signs of Problems in Pragmatics

1. The child has difficulty using language to communicate different messages. For example, the child may not be able to ask questions, ask for information, relate information, describe events, or ask for help.
2. The child has difficulty maintaining the topic of conversation.
3. The child's responses may be delayed or inappropriate.

4. The child may not demonstrate the ability to initiate conversation with family members, peers, teachers, and people who speak the language and familiar to the child.
5. The child may not understand or use idioms that are appropriate for the child's language and culture.

This list of characteristics of speech, language, and hearing disorders is not exhaustive. However, the school speech-language pathologist is available to answer questions and accept referrals from teachers. Below are recommendations for the school speech-language pathologist.

1. Offer in-service training for teachers and staff on a regular basis and describe linguistic diversity of African American children.
2. Make referrals easy for the teachers by providing an easy, comprehensive, referral process.
3. Communicate regularly with teachers to increase their familiarity with you and the referral process.
4. Talk with children on the playground and in the cafeteria to identify children who have not been referred by teachers or parents.
5. Become familiar with African American English and culture so that it becomes easy to isolate those problems that are diagnosable disorders rather than linguistic differences. Each time the speech-language pathologist talks with African American children, he or she becomes more familiar with the language and the culture.

REFERENCES

Altemus, L. (1966). The incidence of cleft lip and palate among North American Negroes. *Cleft Palate Journal*, 3: 357–361.

Baran, J., & Seymour, H. (1976). The influences of three phonological rules of black English on the discrimination of minimal word pairs. *Journal of Speech and Hearing Research*, 1: 467–474.

Berko Gleason, J. (1993). *The Development of Language*. New York: Macmillan.

Bloom, L. & Lahey, M. (1978). *Language Development and Language Disorders*. New York: Macmillan.

Brembry, A. (1986). Relationship between frenotomy and speech: A case study. Unpublished Master's Thesis, San Jose State University.

Buchanan, L., Moore, E., & Counter, A. (1993). Hearing disorders and auditory assessment. In D. Battle (ed.), *Communication Disorders in Multicultural Populations* (pp. 256–286). Boston: Andover Medical Publishers.

Carson, C., & Kanter, C. (1945). Incidence of stuttering among white and colored school children. *Southern Speech Journal*, 10: 57–59.

Chavez, G., Cordero, J., & Bacerro, J. (1988). Leading major congenital malformations among minority groups in the United States, 1981–1986. Reports on selected ethnic groups. Atlanta: U.S. Department of Health and Human Services.

Cole, L. (1980). Blacks and orofacial clefts: The state of the dilemma. *Asha*, 22:557–560.

Conrad, C. (1988). Fluency in multicultural populations. Unpublished paper presented at workshops on Communication Disorders in Multicultural Populations, American Speech-Language-Hearing Disorders.

Cooper, E., & Cooper, C. (1993). Fluency disorders. In D. Battle (ed.), *Communication Disorders in Multicultural Populations* (pp. 189–221). Boston: Andover Medical Publications.

Crawford, M., Gould, H., Smith, W., Beckford, N., Gibson, W., & Bobo, L. (1991). Prevalence of hearing loss in adults with sickle cell disease. *Ear and Hearing*, 12 (5): 349–351.

Culatta, R., & Goldberg, S. (1995). *Stuttering Therapy: an Integrated Approach to Theory and Practice*. Boston: Allyn & Bacon.

Cummins, J. (1985). *Bilingualism and Special Education: Issues in Assessment and Pedagogy*. San Diego: College-Hill Press.

De Jarnette, G., & Holland, R. (1993). In D. Battle (ed.), *Communication Disorders in Multicultural Populations* (pp. 212–238). Boston: Andover Medical Publications.

Francis, R. (1991). Large-vessel occlusion in sickle cell disease: Pathogenesis, clinical consequences, and therapeutic implications. *Medical Hypotheses*, 35: 88–95.

Friedman, E., Luban, N., Herer, G., & Williams, I. (1980). Sickle cell anemia and hearing. *Annals of Otology, Rhinology, and Laryngology*, 89: 342–347.

Gibson, A. (1988). Prevalence of stuttering in the Bahamas. Paper presented at the annual meeting of the National Black Association for Speech, Language, & Hearing, Nassau, Bahamas.

Gillespie, S., & Cooper, E. (1973). Prevalence of speech problems in junior and senior high schools. *Journal of Speech and Hearing Research*, 16: 739–743.

Goldman, R. (1967). Cultural influences on the sex ratio in the incidence of stuttering. *American Anthropologist*, 69: 78–81.

Gould, H., Crawford, M., Smith, W., Beckford, N., Gibson, W., Pettit, L., & Bobo, L. (1991). Hearing disorders in sickle cell disease: Cochlear and retrocochlear findings. *Ear and Hearing*, 12 (5): 352–354.

Heath, S. (1983). *Ways with Words: Language, Life and Work in Communities and Classrooms*. Cambridge: Cambridge University Press.

Johnson, B. (1996). *Language Disorders in Children*. Albany, NY: Delmar Publications.

Johnson, W. (1961). *Stuttering and What You Can Do About It*. Minneapolis: University of Minnesota Press.

Khoury, M., Erickson, D., & James, L. (1983). Maternal factors in cleft palate with or without palate evidence from interracial crosses in the United States. *Teratology*, 27: 351–357.

Kromberg, J., & Jenkins, T. (1982). Common birth defects in South African blacks. *South African Medical Journal*, 62: 599–602.

Leith, W., & Mims, H. (1975). Cultural influences in the development and treatment of stuttering: A preliminary report on the black stutterer. *Journal of Speech and Hearing Disorders*, 40: 459–466.

Mattes, L., & Omark, D. (1991). *Speech and Language Assessment for the Bilingual Handicapped* (2nd ed.). Oceanside, CA: Academic Communication Associates.

Menyuk, P. (1971). *The Acquisition and Development of Language*. Englewood Cliffs: Prentice-Hall.

Meyerson, M. (1995) Communication development and disorders of children with prenatal alcohol and drug exposure. In K. D. Lewis (ed.), *Infants and Children with Prenatal Alcohol and Drug Exposure: A Guide to Identification and Intervention* (pp. 229–250). North Branch, MN: Sunrise River Press.

Millard, D., & McNeill, K. (1965). The incidence of cleft lip and palate in Jamaica. *Cleft Palate Journal*, 2: 284–288.

Morganstein, K., & Manace, E. (1969). Temporal bone histopathology in sickle cell disease. *Laryngoscope*, 79: 2171–2180.

Ohene-Frempong, K. (1991). Stroke in sickle cell disease: Demographic, clinical, and therapeutic considerations. *Seminars in Hematology*, 28 (3): 213–219.

O'Keefe, L. & Maw, A. (1991). Sudden total deafness in sickle cell disease. *Journal of Laryngology and Oncology*, 105: 653–655.

Orchick, D., & Dunn, J. (1977). Sickle cell anemia and sudden deafness. *Archives of Otolaryngology*, 103: 369–370.

Osom, U. (1997). Current speech and language services in Northern California public schools for African American children who speak African American English. Unpublished Master's Thesis, San Jose State University.

Office of Multicultural Affairs. (1990). Unpublished paper. Rockville, MD: American Speech-Language-Hearing Association.

Office of Multicultural Affairs. (1996). Unpublished paper. Rockville, MD: American Speech-Language-Hearing Association.

Position Paper: Social dialects and implications of the position on social dialects. (1983), *Asha*, 25: 23–27.

Prohovnik, I., Pavlakis, M., Piomelli, M., Bello, J., Hilal, S., & De Vivo, D. (1989). Cerebral hyperemia, stroke, and transfusion in sickle cell disease. *Neurology*, 39: 344–348.

Ramer, A., & Rees, N. (1973). Selected aspects of the development of English morphology in Black American children of low socioeconomic backgrounds. *Journal of Speech and Hearing Research*, 16: 569–577.

Robinson, D., & Allen, D. (1984). Racial differences in tympanometric results. *Journal of Speech and Hearing Disorders*, 49: 140–144.

Robinson, D., Allen, D., & Root, L. (1988). Infant tympanometry: Differential results by race. *Journal of Speech and Hearing Disorders*, 35: 341–346.

Seymour, H., & Ralabate, P. (1985). The acquisition of a phonologic feature of Black English. *Journal of Communication Disorders*, 10:139–148.

Sheehan, J. (1970). *Stuttering Research and Therapy*. New York: Harper & Row.

Siegel, B. (1979). A racial comparison of cleft patients in a clinical population: Associated anomalies and recurrence risks. *Cleft Palate Journal*, 16:193–197.

Statistical Abstracts of the United States. (1990). Washington, DC: U.S. Department of Commerce.

Stemple, J. (1984). *Clinical Voice Pathology*. New York: Merrill.

Stockman, I. (1986). Language acquisition in culturally diverse populations in O. Taylor (ed.), *Nature of Communication Disorders in Culturally and Linguistically Diverse Populations.* San Diego: College-Hill Press.

Stockman, I. (1996). Phonological development and disorders in African American children. In A. Kambi, K. Pollock, and J. Harris (eds.), *Communication Development and Disorders in African American Children* (pp. 117–154). Baltimore: Brookes.

Swift, A., Cohen, M., Hynd, G., Wisenbaker, D., McKie, K., Makari, G. & McKie, V. (1989). Neuropsychologic impairment in children with sickle cell anemia. *Pediatrics*, 84(6): 1077–1085.

Taylor, O. (1986). Historical perspective and conceptual framework, In O. Taylor (ed.), *Nature of Communication Disorders in Culturally and Linguistically Diverse Populations.* San Diego: College-Hill Press.

Todd, G., Sergeant, G., & Larson, M. (1973). Sensorineural hearing loss in Jamaicans with sickle cell disease. *Acta Otolaryngologica*, 76: 268–272.

Toliver, G. (1971). Measurement of speech and language of Black children. Unpublished doctoral dissertation. Ohio State University. Columbus, Ohio.

Urban, G. (1973). Reversible sensorineural hearing loss associated with sickle cell crisis, *Laryngoscope*, 83: 633–638.

Van Riper, C., & Emerick, L. (1990). *Speech Correction: An Introduction to Speech Pathology & Audiology.* Englewood Cliffs, NJ: Prentice-Hall.

Wasserman, A., Wilimas, J., Fairclough, D., Mulhern, R., & Wang, W. (1991). Subtle neuropsychological deficits in children with sickle cell disease. *American Journal of Pediatric Hematology and Oncology*, 13 (1): 14–20.

7

DIAGNOSIS OF COMMUNICATION DISORDERS OF AFRICAN AMERICAN CHILDREN

Chapter Overview

Upon reading this chapter you will gain understanding of:

- The commonly used assessment procedures for the diagnosis of communication disorders
- Biases in assessment procedures used with African American children
- Recommended procedures for referral of African American children by teachers
- Recommended procedures for use with African American children
- Evaluation of important aspects of speech and language

The evaluation of speech and language disorders of African American children continues to be difficult for many speech-language pathologists. The difficulties stem from the perplexity within the profession that promotes the practice of maintaining the community language patterns while insisting on teaching a "standard" variety, based on the premise that the standard is necessary for success in school. Further discussion of linguistic diversity with some speech-language clinicians is countered with "yes, but the children need to learn standard English for educational purposes and the speech-language pathologist is the most qualified professional in the school system to make this possible." While it is true that African American children need to learn to read, write, and speak standard English, it is not the responsibility of the speech-language pathologists, regardless of qualifications, to teach it to a selected number of African American children. Responsibility rests in the hands of the classroom teachers who have access to all of the children in their classes. This issue is discussed further in later chapters.

The perplexity is further illustrated in the literature where it is proposed, on the one hand, that linguistic differences are acceptable, while encouraging speech and language intervention to modify the "problem" on the other. Adler (1990) recommends that special assessment procedures be used to insure that misdiagnoses do not occur with African American children. However, he indicates that speech and language intervention is recommended to help African American and limited English speakers "to be effective cultural code-switchers" (p. 137) and that speech-language clinicians should "be more aggressive regarding their consultancy role in the development of effective language arts programs for multicultural students" (p. 138).

The evaluation of communication disorders in African American children should not be more difficult than the identification of problems in other children. Definitions and characteristics of speech and language disorders remain the same, but the standard or target should vary with the linguistic community. For Black children, the target speech sounds, grammar, vocabulary, and pragmatics are not standard English, but the geographic and social variety of African American language used within the community by its educated members. The syntax and vocabulary of formal (educated) African American English is the same as standard English. This means that phonology, prosody, rhythm, inflections, and vocal quality continue to be different from standard English. In addition, the Black speaker identified as African American based on speech patterns will continue to be perceived as a Black speaker.

The most important part of speech-language intervention is the diagnosis of the disorder. Identification involves the naming of the problem, determining the severity, planning a treatment program, and making a prognosis. At each of the phases of the assessment plan, a comparison is made with a standard or "normal" sample of the behavior. Standards of normalcy should always be the speech and language patterns of other children in the neighborhood who do not have impairments or disabilities. Thus, speech or language disorders exist when a comparison is made between the client and other children in the community who are developmentally similar, speak the same language, and observed to be different. It is inappropriate to compare the Black client with people, languages, or ages that are outside the developmental range or community.

THE ASSESSMENT PROCESS

The speech-language examination is a choreographed assembly of procedures and methods designed to measure a broad range of skills and abilities in communication. The characteristics of each part of the appraisal are determined by the purpose of the assessment and the individual to be studied. The assessment procedure is composed of individual fragments constructed to explore each aspect of language, including comprehension and use and the collection of a case history. The case history is an ensemble of facts about the child, the development of the problem, the parents' and teachers' perception of the problem, what the family is willing to do to improve the situation, and the expected outcome. The individual aspects of language to be examined include speech sounds, grammar, vocabulary, and pragmatics. Skills in pragmatics do not need to be tested directly, but can be observed while other testing is taking place (James 1989). Features of pragmatics, such as turn taking, topic maintenance, modification of style, relevance, and language function can be observed during the collection of the language sample. The standard of appraisal continues to be the child's community and language. The examination of phonology, syntax, and semantics can be accomplished informally or using standardized procedures as long as the child's language is judged according to the rules of the African American culture.

Recognizing Speakers of African American English

Not all African American children speak African American English and those who do not must not be judged by the standard of the Black community. A 12-year-old, middle-class, African American child living outside the African American community who produces the /f/ in the middle of the word "bathroom," when no one in the community uses that form, must be judged by the standard of the community in which the child lives and needs to receive treatment for that problem. On the other hand, an African American child whose peers also use this pattern should not be identified speech disordered. Similarly, a 12-year-old Black child attending school in a low-income, predominantly Black community should not be placed in therapy because of the use of multiple negative forms or /s/ morpheme in third person singular verbs that conform to the rules of African American English.

Mislabeled Black Children

The mislabeling of communication disorders begins in the classroom with the referral by the teacher who designates children for speech and language testing for many reasons. According to Mehan, Hertweck, and Meihls (1986), the most frequent referrals are related to the child's behavior or perceived psychological state. Since the root of the problem is typically believed to be within the child, the school system establishes a procedure to determine what is wrong with the child and creates a plan to remediate it. The referral sources and the speech-language clinician tend to focus on the child rather than the environment that may be creating and maintaining the problem, such as the teacher's perception of the child and the child's language.

Black children inaccurately identified to be communicatively impaired are mainly children in low-income communities whose parents do not challenge the label. Children are labeled with disabilities that are observed only at school with some parents surprised that such disabilities have been noted. "Once such children leave school, many will never be identified in these ways again" (Mehan, Hertweck, & Meihls 1986, p. 161). In the case of speech-language therapy, many children diagnosed with subtle disorders remain unnoticed by people in the community. It is not unusual for Black parents to report that they failed to recognize the presence of a language disorder and maintain that the client is no different from the other children. Mehan, Hertweck, and Meihls write that "the main difference between normals and deviants is that the deviants have been apprehended by formal institutions, while the so-called normals have not been caught, even though normals and deviants have committed similar acts." Thus, "deviance is to be found not in the acts or characteristics of people, but rather in societal reactions to people's behaviors" (Mehan, Hertweck, & Meihls 1986, p. 160). Some African American children enrolled in speech and language therapy are similar to other Black children who are not enrolled in therapy except that those who are enrolled typically have behavioral and/or academic differences as well. Parents are often willing, however to allow clinicians to provide therapy because the parents believe that the clinician knows more about the topic than the parents. In other words, parents trust the clinician and want whatever is good for the child.

To further illustrate that children placed in special education as children grow up to blend into the community, Records and colleagues (Records, Tomblin, & Freese 1992) found that adults treated for specific language impairment as children experience a similar quality of life and satisfaction as comparable adults who were not so diagnosed. Tests showed that the language-impaired subjects continued to exhibit lower language test results. However, no significant difference was noted in personal happiness, satisfaction with life, and satisfaction with the life domains of job, social position, and family. Similar results were affirmed in studies of educable mentally retarded children, leading to their characterization as the "six-hour retarded" (Edgerton 1979, p. 72). The term was coined by Edgerton because the children placed in classes for the mentally retarded adapted well to life outside the school. "If children are disabled only at school, then it is possible to say that the school itself creates or generates the handicaps" (Mehan, Hertweck, &

Meihls 1986, p. 161). Edgerton argues that "once they leave school many will never be identified as retarded again" (p. 72).

Questions to Ask about the Child, Family, and Culture

When faced with a situation in which the clinician is unsure of the child's background, a number of questions can be asked to determine how to use the standards.

1. Who is this child? Who is the family? What is the culture of the family? What languages do they speak? Some of these answers can be obtained indirectly in the case history, but others have to be asked directly. On the other hand, questions about culture and ethnicity should be included in the case history. Clinicians must be cautioned that the idea of African American culture is not uniformly embraced by Black people, and that many would be offended by the term "Black English." Clinicians should never tell parents that their children speak Black English. A more appropriate phrase to use is "The child's language is similar to that of the other children in the neighborhood and is not considered a disorder." The clinician can then offer examples and explain that such linguistic patterns can be modified with help from the clinician on an elective basis. This means that the parents must choose to have the intervention take place, the child is not considered disabled and is not counted among the children with disabilities.

2. What are the occupations of the parents? What are their educational levels? Children whose parents are college educated tend to have different language experiences than people from the same culture who are not. Many educated African Americans live in culturally diverse neighborhoods and may be considered bicultural, share values with members of other cultures as well as their African American relatives and friends, and their children have experiences different from African Americans who have less formal education. In addition, educated parents tend to offer their children more opportunities to socialize with people from other cultures. Exceptions are observed, however, in all situations where people and behavior are concerned.

3. Where does the child live? With whom? Where does he or she spend most of the time when awake? More important than where the child lives is where he or she goes to school. The peers are usually other children who attend the school and after school care, rather than the children who live next door. Often when children attend school away from their home community, they develop friendships with the children in their classes,

regardless of ethnic affiliation. Thus, when the children play with friends, they often have to leave the neighborhood.

4. Where does the child attend school? Some children may list their permanent address in a deprived area, although they spend most of their time in a different community. Their address may have little influence on their language. In a predominantly White school in the hills of Los Angeles, the three African American children enrolled probably do not speak African American English. It is inappropriate to make assumptions about the children until more information is gathered.

5. Is the child's linguistic development different from that of the peers? It is not necessarily important for the child's linguistic performance to resemble that of his or her parents. It is, however, important that the child's language matches that of the other children in the environment.

Role of the Teacher

Teachers play an important role in the diagnosis of speech and language disorders in African American children. Many children selected for speech-language intervention are referred by teachers who are usually the first to notice a potential problem. Teachers are in a unique position to observe the speech and language of a child through daily interaction in a diversity of situations. Such situations include academic subjects, particularly reading, where the child speaks aloud in front of the other children. The teachers also observe the interaction of children with their peers throughout the day and can compare their performance with that of other children.

Teachers need instruction in communication development, linguistic diversity, and communication disorders. Such instruction, provided by the speech-language pathologist, improves the accuracy of referrals. In addition, the process must be efficient and require a minimum amount of paperwork. A simple checklist is the most effective. Teachers, despite the number of pressures on them, are willing to assist with the identification and, ultimately, treatment of the communication disorders of the children in their classes.

The checklist should include the teacher's perception of the type of disorder, examples of the manner in which the problem is exhibited, and how the teacher wants to see the problem resolved. Figure 7.1 shows a sample checklist.

Teachers often ask the speech-language pathologist to "listen to" a child. The request to listen to someone offers no clues regarding the type of problem the child may have. The clinician needs more specific information in order to select the appropriate assessment procedures to identify the child's problem. Occasionally, teachers are so frustrated and confused with the child's behavior that they simply want the child removed from the classroom, if only for a few minutes during the day. The referral form is a good

Child's Name _____ Teacher _____

Grade _____ Room _____ Date_____

Please provide the appropriate information requested. Please provide as much information as possible so the clinicians may select the most appropriate assessment procedures and to aid in efficiency.

1. What type of evaluation is requested?

   A. _____ Speech

   _____ 1. Articulation (speech sound production)
   _____ 2. Hoarseness   _____ 5. Denasal
   _____ 3. Nasal   _____ 6. Stuttering
   _____ 4. Drooling   _____ 7. Other (describe)

   B. Language

   _____ 1. Comprehension
           _____ a. vocabulary
           _____ b. directions
           _____ c. questions
           _____ d. choices
           _____ e. other (specify)

   _____ 2. Expression
           _____ a. vocabulary
           _____ b. grammar
           _____ c. coherence
           _____ d. explaining details
           _____ e. giving directions

2. In which subject(s) is the child having difficulty?

   _____ A. Reading   _____ D. Mathematics
   _____ B. Writing   _____ E. Spelling
   _____ C. Social Studies   _____ F. Other (specify)

3. Please give an example of a typical problem the child is experiencing.

4. How would you like to see this problem resolved?

   _____ A. Child receive assistance while remaining in classroom
   _____ B. Teacher assisting the child with consultation with specialist
   _____ C. Child removed from class
   _____ D. Other (please specify)

Date Received _____ Action _____

FIGURE 7-1   Sample Checklist

way to have the teacher identify the specific problem of concern. Sometimes, a child is referred to the speech-language pathologist for problems observed when reading, such as disfluency only when reading. Through conversation about the assessment process, the teacher is able to identify the problems of concern and determine how help can be provided in the classroom.

Classroom teachers who are unfamiliar with African American English sometimes refer children for speech-language evaluation. Sometimes the teachers realize that the communication differences are dialectal, but seek intervention anyway because of their own difficulty understanding the child. They may also project that others will have similar problems. Such projected uncertainty may or may not be accurate, as the teachers' observations and judgments may be unique.

Knowledge of linguistic diversity will help teachers to work effectively with the multicultural nature of the American classroom. When they have an appreciation for cultural and linguistic diversity and a program for teaching school language to the children, they are more willing to work closely with the speech-language clinician. The speech-language pathologist is familiar with the phonological, grammatical, semantic, and pragmatic variation among cultural groups and is capable of assisting the teachers to insure that all children acquire the linguistic skills required for academic success.

Effective Assessment

Effective assessment is a process of using the most valid and appropriate assessment tools and skills to gather the most useful information to obtain an accurate diagnosis. Richard and Schiefelbusch (1990) indicate that effective assessment is comprehensive; involves other members of the child's family; and is inclusive, multidisciplinary, ecologically valid, nondiscriminatory, and dynamic.

Comprehensive assessment must incorporate the important dimensions of language in a variety of settings because language competence is dynamic and exhibited differently in distinct situations. Assessment procedures must acknowledge the fact that the sample of language exhibited in the assessment process may not represent the total picture, but a snapshot only. Children's language varies with the audience and the setting. Ideally, a sample of language should be collected in a variety of settings, but is not practical. The speech-language pathologists who work in the schools may be overwhelmed by the expectations of the families they serve, the administration, teachers, and the paperwork that must be completed for all of the children at several schools. It may be inappropriate to expect assessments to be an ideal process. However, assessments are enhanced by the inclusion of information provided by informed observers including teachers, parents, and other people who know the child.

Informed observers are employed to provide useful information for the evaluation and, ultimately, the intervention program. "The assessment process should send a clear message to the caregivers that they are valued members of the team and their perspective and priorities are of central importance" (Richard & Schielelbusch 1990, p. 111). Family members are very familiar with the child and have observed him or her in many situations. Therefore, when parents disagree with a diagnosis, it is possible that they are accurate.

A variety of assessment procedures should be used and include samples of communication behaviors and naturalistic observations. Diagnoses should not be made based on the results of standardized testing only, but must include a variety of procedures and should always include a language sample. Assessments are done by a team of professionals and family members of the client, each offering and receiving information used to draw conclusions and develop an intervention program.

Ecologically valid assessment considers the home, environment, and the culture of the child and family. Language testing uses information from the child's background as part of the process. When language testing is performed outside the realm of culture and language, errors in assessment are made.

Effective assessment does not discriminate against people because of race, religion, ethnic affiliation, gender, or sexual orientation. Standardized tests that examine linguistic information that is irrelevant to the child's background are discriminatory. Similarly, tests that are translated into other languages are also discriminatory because the examiner takes linguistic information from one language and applies it to a totally different language.

Finally, effective assessment is capable of being updated over time. This means that assessment is a dynamic process and results can be modified and updated to show progress over time.

ASSESSMENT PROCEDURES

Language assessment procedures can be divided into two distinct types: testing and observation. Testing is a process of eliciting the desired types of behaviors through direct questioning, showing pictures, toys, or written words, and presenting a myriad of stimuli including identification, associations, analogies, opposites, completion tasks, instructions, and so forth. Testing may include standardized procedures; criterion-referenced, informal, developmental scales; language sampling and interviews. Observations may be naturalistic or structured. In naturalistic observations, the examiner is unobtrusive and stays away from the subject to obtain samples of behaviors that are typical in the setting. In structured observations, the examiner does not interfere, but modifies the environment to encourage a specific type of behavior. The examiner may place the child in a room filled with objects and people with which the examiner wants the child to interact. A comprehensive assessment includes both testing and observation.

Testing

Testing can be divided into standardized, dynamic, informal, and criterion-referenced. All of the methods can be used to some degree, but no one method should be relied upon as a sole means of assessment. Each procedure has value and can be used at different times, with different clients, and by different clinicians to obtain information that cannot be obtained in other ways. In this section several types of testing will be discussed. Suggestions will be made regarding methods that are more useful for identifying language disorders of African American children.

Standardized Testing

One of the most debated topics in the profession of communication disorders is whether to use standardized tests to examine the communication of African American children (Cole & Taylor 1990; Seymour & Miller-Jones 1981; Taylor & Payne 1983; and Weddington 1987). Treatment decisions, however, continue to be made on the basis of information obtained through standardized testing. Arguments for continuing to use such tests emphasize the need for scores and percentiles for special class placement and the need for a "standard" to which comparisons can be made. Such arguments are based on the notion and belief by clinicians and school districts that there is only one standard and that all children must learn standard English for success (Seymour & Miller-Jones 1981).

Arguments against the use of standardized tests indicate that the children are tested on information that they have had no opportunity to learn and that the results obtained have no value. In addition, Seymour and Miller-Jones (1981) challenged the format of standardized testing for language assessment as "unrepresentative of natural language" and "purports to assess aspects of communication in the absence of communication" (p. 234). Danowitz (1981) added that "formal tests of language have serious limitations for assessing the form and content of expressive language and are entirely unsatisfactory for assessing the use and comprehension of spoken language" (p. 103).

Taylor and Payne (1983) identified four types of bias in standardized tests when applied to African American children: situational bias, format bias, value bias, and linguistic bias. *Situational bias* is present when there is a "mismatch. . . between the clinician and the client with respect to the social rules of interaction" (p. 12). The behaviors of Black children that are acceptable within their own community may be misinterpreted in a testing situation, particularly when the examiner comes from another culture. Silence, according to the authors, can be an important communicative device, but is often interpreted by unfamiliar examiners as a sign of impaired language function. Seymour, Ashton, and Wheeler (1986) observed that test scores of African American children improved when the race of the examiner was the same. Fuch and Fuch (1989) also noted that "examiner familiarity improved the test scores of African American children." It is a common practice for speech-language clinicians, who have never met the children, to be assigned the task of examining communication, a skill that is best exhibited in familiar situations where the children know the rules of interaction. They should also be familiar with the individual who expects them to share private and personal information.

Format bias is present when clients are requested to interact in a fashion that is foreign to them. African American children have little experience with adults requesting obvious information from them. Directions such as "repeat after me" "show me x," or "wait until I have finished, then say what I say," are confusing, particularly for children who are unfamiliar with the culture of testing.

Value bias is present when a "correct response requires knowledge or acceptance of a value that may be unfamiliar or unacceptable to the respondent" (p. 13). When asked to make a value judgment such as, "What would you do if you found a stamped, addressed letter on the ground?" The expected response is, "Mail it." An inappropriate response is, "Nothing." To do nothing might be a requirement of the child's culture, therefore scoring it incorrect penalizes the child for responding according to the rules of the child's own culture.

Linguistic bias occurs when the test examines knowledge of linguistic rules that are unfamiliar to the child. Black children who speak African American English achieve lower scores on standardized testing because their language is different from the one being tested. This type of bias results in inaccurate conclusions about the language performance of the African American child, when in fact, the child's native language has not been examined at all. Another language, generally standard English, was tested instead.

To reduce bias in testing, Taylor and Payne (1986) indicated that it is incumbent upon the clinician to gather as much information as possible about the language and culture of children to be examined. The following information will prepare the clinician to work effectively with children from different cultures. The clinician should gather information about the following:

Cultural values; preferred mode of communication; nonverbal communication rules; rules of communication interaction; Who communicates with whom? When? Under what conditions? For what purpose; child rearing practices; rituals and traditions; perceptions of punishment and rewards, what is play? fun? humorous?; social stratification and homogeneity of the culture; rules of interaction with nonmembers of the culture; preferred forms of address; preferred teaching and learning styles; definitions of handicapped *in general and* communicatively handicapped *in particular; and taboo topics and activities, insults, and offensive behavior (p. 15).*

Placing children into speech or language therapy based on results obtained from standardized testing results to "remediate" linguistic structures that are not present in the home language should only be done on an elective basis. The speech-language pathologist is responsible for informing the child and family that the linguistic differences of African American children are not disorders. However, the clinician has the skills to teach new linguistic information to assist the children in their future careers, that is, to teach standard English as a second language. In this case, the family and the child (if old enough to make that decision) are in a position to make a choice to accept or reject the help. If the help is accepted, the clinician should not count the children in second language training as disordered, and therefore, should not be funded by resources designated for the disabled. Children enrolled for second language training should not be isolated in a special class called "special education." The label "special education" unfortunately, has a lasting effect on the child that is difficult to outlive. Mehan and colleagues (1986) noted that schools serve the purpose of placing the students into social groups. "Students are sorted and stratified in such a way that differential educational opportunities are made available to them" (Mehan et al., 1986, p. 171). For many African American children, special education is perceived to be a one-way street, in which students are placed without the opportunity to return to a non-special education status. Once placed into special education, some students are isolated for their entire educational lives so that there is no chance to obtain the skills needed for successful employment in adulthood.

Standardized procedures include materials developed to examine specific skills of a particular group of individuals with established correct responses. The test is then administered to a group of individuals from whom norms are established. It is these norms to which all people who take the test are compared. The common practice of including a representation of African American children in the normative sample does not negate the fact that the information sought by the test is exceedingly different from the linguistic information Black children have acquired.

Dual scoring is a technique designed to provide a contrast between the standard English performance requirement of standardized tests and the language of the child. Cole and Taylor (1990) examined the articulation of African American children using three standardized tests of articulation (*Arizona Articulation Proficiency Scale— Revised, Templin-Darley Tests of Articulation,* and the *Photo Articulation Test*). The results indicated that test scores of African American children increased significantly when scoring for their language was used instead of the scoring by the test. When the phonological features of their language were considered errors, varying numbers of children were diagnosed impaired depending on the individual tests. The authors noted that 21 per cent of the items of the Templin-Darley were biased; 14 percent of the items of the Photo Articulation Test; and 19 percent of the Arizona items. The results of this study "clearly show that a failure to take the issue of dialect variation into account substantially increases the likelihood of misdiagnosing normally speaking African-American children as having articulation errors" (p. 174).

Washington and Craig (1992) used a dual scoring procedure for examining the articulation of African American children in the northern part of the United States. Contrasting the results of this study with those of Cole and Taylor (1990), who tested Black children in Mississippi, Washington and Craig observed no significant differences in the scores obtained using the test scoring procedure and the scoring using adjustments for African American English. The authors concluded that the Arizona Test does not require alternative scoring methods for northern African American children.

Modification of standardized tests is a practice used to meet the needs of the individual client, linguistic community, or disabling conditions. "Modification is necessary because children are different from one another in test-taking skills, willingness to answer obvious questions, and interest in interacting with the speech-language clinician" (Weddington, 1987). Some children are impulsive and respond without evaluating options carefully. It is common for speech-language pathologists to make adjustments in the administration, scoring, and interpretation of tests to accommodate the problems of the clients being examined, often without reporting it. This is one of the reasons why different clinicians testing the same client with the same tests obtain different, and often contradicting, results. Salvia and Ysseldyke (1981) identified two types of test modification customarily utilized in assessment: (1) modification of stimulus demands and (2) modification of response requirements. While such modifications raise the scores of individuals tested, the established norms can no longer be used as a standard of comparison. The norms cannot be used validly or reliably with African American children anyway, therefore, alteration does not make the tests less valid, but may provide valuable information about the child's communication abilities.

Modification of Stimulus Demands

- Changing instructions by repeating them in different words, repeating them more than recommended, or using sign language.
- Changing the pronunciation of test items to reflect the language of the child's culture. Some words are missed on vocabulary tests because the client is unfamiliar with the pronunciation of the clinician. The standard

pronunciation of "wasp," "horse," and "ambulance" may not be recognized by the African American child even though these words appear in the lexicon of their language.

- Using different pictures. When the examiner finds that the pictures of a test do not elicit the expected responses, it may be necessary to use different pictures. Some outdated pictures and pictures inappropriate for the culture, such as freckles and skis, fail to elicit desired responses from Black children.
- Including additional items, modifying item wording, and probing during testing offer a better chance that the child will demonstrate skill in language.
- Explaining the reasons for testing. Testing for disabling conditions is a very serious matter with consequences. Children need to know why they are being tested and that they must perform as well as possible. The children also need to know that the clinician is there to help, but only when help is actually needed.
- Allowing the parents or other trusted adults to administer test items.
- Administering only a portion of the test.
- Completing the test in several sessions.
- Telling the child when an item is missed and explaining the correct responses.
- Using bribes, threats, or rewards to encourage the child to respond.
- Omitting items the examiner believes to be difficult for the client because of language, culture, or handicapping conditions.
- Modifying items, such as translating into another language, or offering more explanation than recommended.
- Repeating the stimuli.
- Failing to establish a basal and continuing the administration beyond the ceiling.
- Offering additional clues or examples.

Modification of Response Requirements

- Allowing more time than recommended by the test.
- Accepting responses that are different from allowable responses, but appropriate for the language or culture.
- Allowing the client to change responses.
- Allowing the client to clarify responses or ask questions.
- Allowing the client to respond using sign or foreign language or gesture.

When clinicians alter standardized tests, they must indicate such modifications in the report, decline to present scores and percentiles, and utilize the findings in the diagnosis. If the clinician chooses to use standardized tests, the modification can help the clinician learn whether the child has the skill that may be concealed due to failure to understand the instructions, impulsivity, or haste. Sometimes children are able to demonstrate the target skill when allowed more time, given additional instructions, provided reinforcement, or allowed an opportunity to ask questions. The goal of assessment is not to trick a child into making a quick and often incorrect response, but to learn as much about the child's linguistic system as possible. The questions to answer include: "Does the child have the skill tested, regardless of whether the skill is part of the child's home language?" If the child does not have the skill, the clinician is responsible for determining the reason. When the reason is cultural or experiential, the next question is, "Can the child acquire the skill?" One way to determine whether the child is capable of acquiring the skill is to attempt to teach it. Teaching new information to a child will offer the clinician a chance to determine the amount of time and effort needed for the child to acquire the skill. When the clinician feels compelled to use standardized tests, the suggestions below may offer an alternative that may assist the clinician in making an appropriate diagnosis.

- Administer each standardized test item according to the rules of administration.
- After each item administered that is incorrect, ask the child why the response was chosen.
- Teach the child the correct response by clarifying which answer is correct and explaining the reasons.
- Generalize by presenting a similar question. This technique is called probing.
- If the second presentation is answered correctly by the child, this means that the child may not know the correct response because of life experiences and exposure. However, if the child demonstrates the capacity to learn the skill, it shows that the skill will be acquired easily and perhaps quickly with little instruction.
- If teaching is not effective during the second administration of the test item, this may represent a disorder.

Dynamic Assessment

Dynamic assessment is a term coined by Reuven Feuerstein (1979) that considers assessment a dynamic process to examine mutable behaviors. Unlike static assessment that determines what the child knows, dynamic assessment examines the child's *capacity* to learn. Rather than "measuring a single performance before and after intervention, dynamic assessment measures the change that is constantly created by the assessment process itself" (Peña 1996). According to Feuerstein (1979), using the Learning Potential Assessment Device (LPAD) model, dynamic assessment is done for the following purposes:

- To determine how easily the behavior can be changed.
- To determine how much time needs to be invested to create a change in behavior.
- To determine if the teaching strategies developed to teach a particular skill can be transferred to other teaching situations.
- To determine areas of strengths and weaknesses.
- To determine whether errors observed represent a disorder or a difference.

Although dynamic assessment was not designed for assessing language, the process and notion of testing are applicable. The accepted process used in assessment in communication disorders is a static one that examines a behavior at a particular point in time and may not necessarily be generalized to other situations. Static language assessment suffers the same flaws as stagnant psychological testing, particularly with African American children, by taking a snapshot of linguistic behavior to make assumptions about knowledge and make predictions about future development. Language use is a dynamic process and is not amenable to a one-shot approach to evaluation. Viewing language as a static process is similar to looking at the world through binoculars. You can see small parts of many things, but have no opportunity to see the big picture.

Research studies of language testing using dynamic procedures are few; however, Peña (1993) used a test-mediate-retest approach to differentiate gains in language learning of two groups of preschool African American and Puerto Rican children. Subjects who received mediation following initial testing performed significantly better than subjects who received no mediation. Children who were language disordered failed to benefit from the mediation. It was therefore concluded that change in performance following mediation was diagnostic and separated those children who had disorders from those who did not. Normally developing children are capable of acquiring new linguistic skills. While disordered children can acquire new skills, their learning is slower and they may need a variance of stimuli and input modes.

Peña (1996) argues that dynamic assessment provides an opportunity for the examiner to observe the learning process. "This observation yields authentic, valid information about the child in the process of learning" (p. 297). The goal of dynamic assessment is to identify problems that require intervention and "describe how to support the intervention" (p. 297).

Informal Testing

Informal testing is conducted using materials that may either be developed by the examiner or taken from other sources, such as standardized procedures, without employing the standard requirements for administration, scoring, and interpretation. When informal measures are used, the examiner is in a position to select items from a variety of sources to obtain the amount and type of information desired. The stimuli can yield specific linguistic forms of African American English and ignore patterns from languages outside the African American linguistic community. Informal testing may be time-consuming because the examiner does not have a script to follow, no normative comparisons can be made, and results are descriptive.

Criterion-Referenced Testing

As part of the language assessment, criterion-referenced testing seeks information about the child's ability to understand or use specific linguistic information. The testing does not compare the performance of children to other children or a norm, but "utilizes knowledge about the sequential order of language and cognitive development as its reference" (Seymour & Miller-Jones 1981). Criterion-referenced assessment establishes a "criterion level that represents mastery of a given linguistic structure and examining the child's use of the structure to determine whether it meets the established criterion" (Washington 1996, p. 47). Examining the child's language and comparing it to developmental expectations for the linguistic community would make diagnosis more accurate than comparing the child's development to norms utilized in conventional standardized tests. Therefore, the results would not indicate whether a particular linguistic form was identified on a single presentation, but the number of times or consistency the skill was observed with multiple presentations would be provided. Linguistic skills that are observed inconsistently are said to be emerging and may not need remediation. Such skills can possibly be stimulated and encouraged by the child's family or classroom teacher when directed by the speech-language pathologist. Using criterion-referenced testing, the clinician has no need to compare the African American child with standard English-speaking counterparts. The only information the clinician needs for comparison are developmental information based on the growth of Black children, and the salient features of the language of the children's community. Little is known about the language development of African American children, however:

> *Black children are likely to produce a higher incidence than white children of features that correspond with the adult black English form. A good many of these black English features are not unlike the developmental patterns found in standard English. Consequently, black English features that are more prevalent among black children are also found among young white children. There is greater influence within the black speech community to maintain these features beyond the developmental years. Therefore, many features that begin as developmental for both black and white children are retained*

by black children beyond the level of acquisitional mastery by standard English children. (Seymour & Miller-Jones 1981, p. 241)

Observation

Observation is a useful technique for obtaining information about language and behavior. Using naturalistic observation, the examiner is as unobtrusive as possible to describe the language use, comprehension, and communication within the context of a variety of settings. Ideally, observations should be conducted in more than one setting with varied companions, including, parents, peers, and teachers. Two types of observational assessments are discussed in this section, specifically, language sampling and portfolio assessment.

Language Sampling

Language sampling is used to obtain information about the client's ability to use language in context. "Language sampling is essentially an observation of spontaneous language use in a low-structured setting" (Richard & Schiefelbusch 1990, p. 130). The sample must be collected in many settings and must be long enough to illustrate the varied linguistic structures the child has acquired. It is customary for 50 to 100 utterances to be collected to obtain a complete picture of language skills. James (1989) suggested that a sample of spontaneous connected speech can be analyzed for phonology, semantics, grammar, and pragmatics. Although James made no reference to the assessment of African American children, it is necessary to use the reference of African American language as the standard.

- Phonology: The child's use of speech sounds can be examined to determine which speech sounds are produced correctly and in what context. The phonological analysis can be completed using the sample to determine the types of phonological processes used and the phonological rules employed by the child.

  The errors the child makes in the use of speech sounds conform to a set of rules that are unique to him or her. Thus, the child who says "wook" for "look" is employing the rule to use the /w/ for /l/ words that the child is unable to say.
- Semantics: The child's vocabulary can be evaluated by using a variety of techniques including conversation, naming and pointing to pictures, and defining words. As the conversation proceeds, the child can be asked about selected words used by the clinician and the child. The clinician may ask "what does ____ mean?" or "Tell me another way to say that."
- Syntax: Mean Length of Utterance (MLU) is an accepted technique used as part of the syntax analysis procedure for young children up to approx-

imately age five years. MLU is the average length of utterances, measured in morphemes. It is a crude measurement of syntax development up to an MLU of six morphemes, but it cannot provide a clear picture of syntax development. While it may be clear that a five-year-old child who uses four-word utterances to communicate is delayed in language development, it does not describe how the child is using the words or which parts of speech are being employed. A five-year-old child who says "Me wanna go bye-bye" is using a four-morpheme utterance, as is the child who says, "I respect my mother." The two four-morpheme utterances are distinctly different. The latter child is far more advanced than the former. James further suggests that syntax analysis should include analysis of grammatical morphemes (e.g., plural and possessive nouns, verb tense, adjectives and adverbs), clause structure, negation, and wh-questions.

- Pragmatics: James (1989) recommended that two aspects of pragmatics can be determined from the language sample: communication intentions and conversational ability. Intention refers to the ability to use the language to perform various communicative acts, such as describing, arguing, and responding. Conversational ability refers to the process of communicating with a partner and includes turn taking, topic maintenance, and relevance.

Language sampling for African American English-speakers can be difficult for speech-language pathologists who have little experience with African American English. Since there are no norms, the clinician must use his or her own experiences to determine the appropriateness of linguistic forms observed.

Portfolio Assessment

"Portfolio assessment is a collection of student work samples that reflect the student's achievements, growth, and efforts in one or more selected areas, such as, . . . reading, writing, listening, and speaking" (CSHA Task Force: Assessment of the African American Child, 1993). This approach is quite different from static and dynamic assessment procedures and provides evidence of linguistic skill or progress over time. The clinician, teachers, and children participate in the development of the portfolio. Such a portfolio may include samples of language, new words learned, new definitions of old words, specific language skills taught, and the speech sound learned. Rather than prepare a single report that includes scores and percentiles or percentages, examples of the child's actual performance are illustrated. Portfolio assessment is not typically used to identify a speech or language disorder, but can be used to show progress or provide historical information about the progression of the child's disability. As part of the assessment, the speech-language pathologist may use the child's school work and examples of other linguistic activity to assist in a decision regarding the presence or absence of a communicative disorder.

COMMUNICATING ASSESSMENT INFORMATION TO PARENTS

The speech-language pathologist is required to work with family members at all levels of the assessment and intervention process. "When working collaboratively with families, professionals must be prepared to encounter a variety of family structures, cultural traditions, gender role and status expectations, communication styles and norms, child-rearing practices, values, beliefs, attitudes, goals, and aspirations" (Campbell 1996, p. 86). In some families, both parents are involved in the assessment process while other families may rely on a grandparent to raise the children. Clinicians should not insist on talking only with the biological parents, but must communicate with the individuals who are involved the most with the child. "By knowing with whom the child interacts, the style of interaction, and the topics, professionals will likely develop appropriate goals and procedures that will fit into the family routine" (p. 86).

When the speech-language pathologist receives the referral from the teacher, a plan should be developed for the assessment. The most valid and reliable assessment procedures should be chosen to provide a clear picture of the child's language development. For Black children, it is incumbent upon the clinician to collect information from diverse sources, including history from informed observers, parents, teachers, and peers. Next, several types of procedures would offer the clinician a chance to collect a sample of spontaneous connected speech using contrastive analysis, criterion-referenced testing, and dynamic assessment. Each procedure can offer the clinician the opportunity to observe the linguistic forms used by the child, and a chance to teach new linguistic information to determine how quickly the child learns the skills taught. A portfolio procedure is helpful to show how the child acquires the skill over time, which is useful diagnostic information.

When the assessment plan is delineated, the family should be notified when and how the assessment will be completed, and exactly what information is being sought. A brief description of the procedures to be used, written in clear language, must be provided. Family members should be encouraged to telephone the clinician if they have questions. Prior to the assessment, requests are made for information from the parents and they are asked for their concerns for the child's difficulties. If the parents agree that a problem exists, it is easy for the clinician and parents to agree on an assessment plan to answer the questions of both the parents and clinician. When parents disagree that a problem exists, the clinician must determine the nature of the discrepancies. Parents might be concerned about issues different from the clinician which need to be considered when planning the assessment. In some cases the clinician might be concerned about the child's speech, while the parents are concerned about the child's reading. When the clinician considers the parents' interests and tries to accommodate their concerns, the assessment is more inclusive and the parents' questions may be answered. In addition, parents tend to be more cooperative when they believe that the child's needs are being met.

The primary complaint that parents have about speech-language clinicians is that they do not explain assessment information in terms that are meaningful to them. Parents should be told in clear, understandable language the problems that are evident in communication, what skills the children need, and how intervention will be accomplished. Also it should be indicated that both the SLP and classroom teachers will work together to help the child acquire the language needed for learning. For the skills that constitute a disorder, the same care should be taken to help the family understand the nature of the disability. They need to know what is planned for the child's remediation, and that their assistance is valuable. The clinician should tell the family that the clinician will keep them informed of progress through frequent communication.

Black families are concerned about their children and willing to help them in any way possible. Clinicians and teachers need to make the families feel as comfortable as possible and respect their opinions. Once they are convinced that the clinician is genuinely interested in doing whatever is necessary to help the children, they will offer support. The clinician should let the parents know that speech-language therapy has definite goals that can be accomplished within a manageable period of time.

COMMUNICATING WITH TEACHERS

Teachers are happy to make referrals when they believe that the clinician will act upon them. Often teachers are unsure of the significance of the problems observed and are seeking validation that their observations are appropriate. The clinician has a responsibility to help teachers understand what speech-language disorders are and how to recognize them. When the teacher refers children for linguistic differences, clinicians need to inform the teacher that such differences do not constitute a disorder. Such information must be provided honestly, clearly, and respectfully. The clinician must offer supportive, written evidence of the existence of linguistic diversity and provide assistance for teaching standard English to all of the children in the classroom. The speech-language pathologist must volunteer to collaborate with the teacher, for example, by teaching phonics and speech sound production as well as other language skills to the children.

THE WRITTEN REPORT

The written report should be informative and descriptive, providing examples of the types of differences and disorders noted. Scores should not be a part of the report but presented on a separate sheet and offered to the administrator as supporting evidence for special education placement. The scores should not be distributed with the report, since scores tend to be the first item reviewed by the recipient of the report while the most important information (descriptions of the responses) might be ignored. Scores are useless in making decisions regarding the specific skills that need to be remediated, how the skills would be taught, or the ease of teaching the skill and can only detract from the descriptive information presented.

The report should describe all responses that are different from those considered "correct" on the test, that is, responses that are consistent with the features of African American English. When teachers and others read the report and observe the children, they are likely to notice the differences and question the competency of the examiner and the validity of the assessment. Listing differences tells the reader that the examiner has noticed them, but does not consider them disordered communication.

The report should also explain how the child's responses on the test are appropriate or inappropriate for both African American English and standard English. Both types of information are important since they show the level of the child's language skills in both languages. When the reason for the child's responses (although incorrect according to the test), is clear to the examiner , he or she should explain the logic of the response.

When standardized test are administered, rather than discuss scores and percentiles, the speech-language pathologist should summarize each section of the test and give examples of the child's responses. If the response is similar to that of other African American children, the clinician should provide illustrations and indicate whether such responses are appropriate for the child's development. When modifications have been made to the administration or scoring to accommodate the child's linguistic differences, the clinician should report them and describe what was done.

The report should also include an identification of the problem and recommendations for treatment. The identification should never be "Black dialect." Labeling a language pattern *Black dialect* is not an identification or diagnosis of a disorder and should not be used in that way. However, the clinician may summarize the information by stating that the language "is appropriate for the child's chronological age and linguistic community."

SUMMARY

The issues of assessing the language of African American children for the diagnosis of speech and language disorders is complicated. A variety of methods has been recommended but none can be used in isolation of other procedures. The most important requirement for competent assessment is the knowledge of the culture and language of African Americans and respect for their abilities. The approaches used currently in the public schools have labeled far too many Black children and placed them into speech-language therapy for the purpose of remediating their linguistic differences. The suggestions identified in this section might reduce the number of children falsely identified with speech and language disabilities. Based on the information presented in this section, it is much more beneficial for the child to receive no speech or language therapy than it is to place a child into therapy who has no disabilities. Children without actual disabilities should not be placed in special education, because the evidence is not available that shows that such placement is more beneficial for the child than regular class placement. Perhaps special education placement is important for the teacher and classmates in a situation in which the child is disruptive. However, special education placement is inappropriate for language-different students, especially African American students who experience special education as a dead-end educational system. Special education tracks children, programs them for failure in the educational system, and creates lowered self-esteem.

PRACTICAL APPLICATION

In this section, practical procedures to be used for the gathering of information and assessment of speech and language by speech-language clinicians and classroom teachers are discussed. Campbell (1996) recommends an ethnographic interview and observations to uncover the culture of the home, classroom, and other places the child visits. Collecting information on a continuous basis will provide updated information beginning at the preassessment stage and proceeding throughout the intervention process. Campbell lists seven factors that must be considered during an ethnographic interview.

- The purpose of the interview should be presented clearly to the informant. At all times the informant should know why questions are asked and what use will be made of the information.
- The informant should understand why the interview is being conducted and to understand that the questioning is necessary for a clear understanding of the child's problem so that a treatment program can be developed and implemented.
- The interviewer should ask the most appropriate questions to the most appropriate informant so that the information gathered can be used in the most suitable manner.
- The interviewer must be attentive and respectful of the informant and the information being collected. The interviewer should never act surprised or astounded with any information divulged.
- Both the interviewer and informant should have a chance to ask and answer questions.
- Professionals must minimize the effects of perception and situational variables that might affect the success of the interview.
- The clinician must word questions on sensitive subjects carefully. The informant might feel comfortable when it is clear that such information is important and will be kept confidential. African American families might be unwilling to divulge sensitive information.

Case History

The case history information varies according to the age of the children and presenting problem. Information must be gathered from a number of people in the children's life, including the family members and teachers. Questions should be confined to the child's problems and not issues of privacy, unless it is absolutely necessary for the identification and treatment of the child's disability. Black people are reluctant to talk about personal information to strangers and may not divulge the details of their home lives. Since very little can be done about the home life, symptomatic therapy can be effective regardless of any unusual lifestyles the family may live. Save the prying questions for later when trust has been established.

Questions for Parents of Young Children

- Do you believe your child has a speech or language problem?
- Describe the problem as you see it.
- How long have you noticed that a problem exists?
- What does your child say when you ask a question?
- What happens when you give directions such as "Come here"?

- How does the child respond when you instruct him/her to "go to your room, look in the closet, and bring the red shoes"?
- Do you understand what the child says? Are there ever times when you do not understand the child? What do you do? How does the child respond? When you show the child how to say a sound, is he or she able to say it?
- Under what conditions is the problem the most noticeable?
- Why do you believe your child has this problem?
- What have you done to help?
- What type of specialists have you consulted on your child's behalf? (e.g., physician, speech-language pathologist, faith healer, etc.)
- How is this child's communication different from that of his family and friends?

Sample Questions to Ask the Teacher

- When is the child's problem the most obvious?
- Describe a situation when you have experienced the most significant communication problem.
- What happens when you give complex directions to the child?
- In which subjects does the child experience the most linguistic difficulty? The least?
- Are there times when the child is embarrassed to speak? (e.g., in front of the class, with certain groups)
- How is this child's communication different from other African American children you have known?
- In which class activities does the he or she participate the most?
- How serious does the child's problem appear to you?
- How do you help the child in class?
- Have the parents asked for your help?

REFERENCES

Adler, S. (1990). Multicultural clients: Implications for the SLP. *Asha*, 21: 135–139.

Bernstein, D. (1989). Language development: The preschool years. In D. Bernstein, & E. Tiegerman (eds.), *Language and Communication Disorders in Children* (pp. 95–132). Columbus: Merrill.

Campbell, L. (1996). Issues in service delivery to African American children. In A. Kamhi, K. Pollock, & J. Harris (eds.), *Communication Development and Disorders in African American Children* (pp. 73–94). Baltimore: Paul Brookes.

Cole, L., & Taylor, O. (1990). Performance of working class African American children on three tests of articulation. *Language, Speech and Hearing Services in the Schools*, 21: 171–176.

CSHA Task Force (1993) *Assessment of the African American Child*. Sacramento: California Speech, Language, and Hearing Association.

Danowitz, M. (1981). Formal and informal assessment: fragmentation versus holism. *Topics in Language Disorders*, 1 (3): 95–106.

Edgerton, R. (1979). *Mental Retardation*. Cambridge, MA: Harvard University Press.

Fuch, D., & Fuch, L. (1989). Effects of examiner familiarity on Black, Caucasian, and Hispanic children: A meta-analysis. *Exceptional Children*, 55, (4): 303–308.

Feuerstein, R. (1979). *Dynamic Assessment of the Retarded Performers: The Learning Potential Assessment Device, Theory, Instruments, and Techniques*. Baltimore: University Park Press.

James, S. (1989). Assessing children with language disorders. In D. Bernstein & E. Tiegerman (eds.), *Language and Communication Disorders in Children* (pp. 157–207). Columbus: Merrill.

Mehan, H., Hertweck, A., & Meihls, J. (1986) *Handicapping the Handicapped: Decision Making in Students' Educational Careers*. Stanford, CA: Stanford University Press.

Peña, E. (1993). Dynamic assessment: A non-biased approach for assessing the language of young children. Unpublished doctoral dissertation, Temple University.

Peña, E. (1996). Dynamic assessment: The model and its application. In K. Cole, P. Dale, & D. Thal (eds.), *Assessment of Language and Communication* (pp. 281–308). Baltimore: Paul H. Brookes.

Records, N., Tomblin, J., & Freese, R. (1992). The quality of life of young adults with histories of specific language impairment. *American Journal of Speech-Language Pathology*, 1 (2): 44–53.

Richard, N., & Schiefelbusch, R. (1990) Assessment. In L. McCormick. & R. Schiefelbusch (eds.), *Early Language Intervention: An Introduction* (pp. 110–141). Columbus: Merrill.

Salvia, J., & Ysseldyke, J. (1981). *Assessment in Special and Remedial Education*. Boston: Houghton Mifflin.

Seymour, H., Ashton, N., & Wheeler, L. (1986). The effects of race on language elicitation. *Language, Speech and Hearing in the Schools*, 17: 146–151.

Seymour, H., & Miller-Jones, D. (1981). Language and cognitive assessment of Black children. In N. Lass (ed.), *Speech and Language Advances in Basic Research and Practice* (pp. 203–263). New York: Academic Press.

Taylor, O., & Payne, K. (1983). Culturally valid testing: A proactive approach. *Topics in Language Disorders*, 3: 8–20.

Washington, J. (1996). Assessing language abilities of African American children. In A. Kamhi, K. Pollock, & J. Harris (eds.), *Communication Development and Disorders of African American Children*. (pp. 35–54). Baltimore: Paul H. Brookes.

Washington, J., & Craig, H. (1992). Articulation test performances of low income, African-American preschoolers with communication impairments. *Asha*, 23: 203–207.

Weddington, G. (1987). Language assessment of African American children. Unpublished paper presented to the Speech-Language Clinicians, Chicago, IL.

8

EDUCATIONAL ASSESSMENT PRACTICES AND AFRICAN AMERICAN STUDENTS

Chapter Overview

Upon reading this chapter, you will gain understanding of

- Cultural influences on assessment
- Problems associated with cultural insensitivity and assessment practices
- Linguistic assessment bias
- Legislated nondiscriminatory evaluation
- Significant court decisions regarding linguistic rights of Black children
- Informal measures of students' progress
- Linking assessment and instruction

Standardized assessment instruments, practices, and procedures used in American schools continue to be applied to African American students without regard to their cultural, experiential, and linguistic differences. Such practices are unfair and distort facts about the mental capacities, language abilities, and functioning of African American students. The basic contention here is that standardized tests that have been developed from Eurocentric perspectives and standardized on European American children should not be administered to African American children. The results of these tests do not represent factual performance results; instead, the results reflect, if anything, the differences between White and Black children based on cultural and experience differences. During the past twenty years, it is a well-documented fact that incongruences between the communication style or language of assessors and the children's assessed result in test bias (Taylor & Lee 1987). Furthermore, intelligence tests and other assessment procedures have been found linguistically and culturally discriminatory and upheld in several important court decisions (i.e., *Larry P. v. Riles*, 1972, *Diana v. State Board of Education*, 1970; & *Mattie T. v. Holladay*, 1977).

Contemporary investigators have challenged the deficit interpretation of Black–White differences in IQ and scholastic achievement and advanced what is termed the *difference orientations*. The difference orientation theorists believe that there are differences among children from different ethnic and cultural groups with respect to learning experiences, learning styles, language, learning attitudes, and achievement orientations as a result of the socialization provided by their families and communities.

Since standardized assessment tools are known to be an unfair means of measuring African American students abilities, why are schools placing so much emphasis on assessing students instead of teaching them?

It is important to remember that assessment, which often involves testing, is a highly subjective process that was in part developed and propagated by people committed to a particular social world view and cultural orientation (Hilliard 1987). Assessment practices are influenced by attitudes and expectations of the examiner, as well as the sociopolitical, cultural, and linguistic context. When these contextual variables are ignored, assessment of Black children cannot be considered an objective procedure. Limited awareness regarding the actual implications of cultural and linguistic diversity influencing assessment by psychologists, teachers, and other professionals results in invalid and potentially harmful evaluative conclusions and recommendations.

Because cultural and linguistic variables are important to the assessment process, it is crucial that all educators, administrators, counselors, and psychologists involved with assessment of Black children recognize the extent to which these variables affect assessment results and their interpretation.

This chapter focuses on current assessment practices with Black children from an educational perspective with particular emphasis placed on cultural and linguistic variables on the effects of assessment, interpretation of results, instructional impact, and student placement decisions.

CULTURAL INFLUENCES ON THE ASSESSMENT OF BLACK CHILDREN

Black children learn language and communication in their homes and communities where it is embedded in the cultural contexts that surround them.

These context structure interactions, assumptions, and expectations used in the development of their language form their knowledge of the world and the skills needed to survive and achieve comprehensibility. Therefore, it should not be difficult to understand that changes in the cultural context that are experienced by Black children when they enter school significantly affect them. As mentioned earlier, there is cultural incongruence between the home and school cultures. This mismatch has a profound impact on communication, motivation, and overall school performance of Black students. To compound the problem further, assessment practices in the schools broaden the mismatch even more by failing to consider issues of cultural diversity that complicate and influence test results and interpretation. By design, tests used in the assessment process are heavily biased against Black students who speak African American English and come from a cultural and socioeconomic background that is different from the expectations of school personnel. Black children from low socioeconomic inner cities suffer even greater consequences than many other children because they have to contend with prejudice and stereotypes associated with poverty, as well as those associated with racial, cultural, and linguistic differences. Assessments are done by trained examiners who are usually licensed and/or certified individuals. They administer tests, interpret the results, and make recommendations based on their interpretations. When mental measurements are desired, intelligence quotient (IQ) tests are administered. Intelligence test results are usually reported in the form of a standardized IQ score. The IQ standard score is usually expressed with a mean score of 100. The use of the mean IQ test score has resulted in inappropriate and disproportionate placement of African American students in special education classes for the mentally retarded, learning disabled, and seriously emotionally disturbed. How could this happen? Simply by ignoring the importance of culture, language, and background during intellectual assessment, African American and other students from diverse backgrounds are subjected to lower scores on these tests. Although these students are deemed intellectually and socially competent by their cultural and community standards, the single test score is often used incorrectly for diagnoses and placement into special education.

The most widely accepted definition of mental retardation is the one developed by the American Association on Mental Retardation (AAMR). Its earlier definition was incorporated into Public Law 94-142, the Education for All Handicapped Children Act (1973, and revised in 1983). The most recent definition is as follows:

Mental retardation refers to significantly subaverage general intellectual functioning resulting in or associated with concurrent impairments in adaptive behavior and manifested during the developmental period (Haring, McCormick, & Haring 1994, (p. 217).

Significantly below average is defined as an IQ below 70, however, the AAMR definition of 1983 gives some flexibility for IQ between 70 and 75. Although intellectual functioning involves more than a single test score (i.e., capacities to learn, solve problems, accumulate knowledge, think, and adapt to new situations), other aspects of intellectual functioning are often ignored when testing African American and other culturally different children.

Adaptive behavior is also to be determined as a part of the assessment process. Adaptive behavior refers to how well people cope with the demands of their immediate environment. According to Haring, McCormick, and Haring (1994), there can be a close relationship between intellectual functioning and adaptive behavior. There are two components of adaptive behavior: (1) level of skill development and (2) relationship of acquired skills to development and chronological age.

Assessing adaptive behavior is difficult because behaviors vary according to developmental age, situation context, and culture. People function in different roles at different ages and stages of their development across cultures. Behaviors are also strongly influenced by cultural factors and situational context.

A good example of cultural influence can be found in the area of child-rearing practices. African American families stress the importance of giving the child an opportunity to be a child and enjoy the care and protection of adults until such time that the child is ready for adulthood (Willis 1992). In contrast, among the strongest childrearing biases of European American family values are beliefs in education and independence. Their beliefs lead them to foster self-help and self-reliance skills at an early age.

When the cultural differences are examined in the example given, it is quite easy to see how an African American child's adaptive behaviors in the home and school may be judged inaccurately as immature for chronological age. This child may simply be enjoying and fulfilling an expected cultural value of being a child. On the other hand, through the eyes of European American cultural values and expectations, the Black child may be considered developmentally delayed, socially incompetent, or immature. Similar types of assessment problems occur with Latino, Puerto Rican, and Native American children because of their cultural differences. As a result, their difference orientations often result in misdiagnosis and misplacement in our schools as well. Cultural values, language, behavioral norms, and traditions are critical to the testing situation. These variables define who the children are, how they think, interact, behave, and view the world. These variables also shape their beliefs and ideas that structure their actions in and reactions toward the world. Therefore, *cultural differences* cannot be ignored during the assessment process. Culture consists of three primary categories: cultural behavior, cultural artifacts, and cultural knowledge (Spradley 1980).

When assessments are conducted with African American students, the examiner must be able to look beyond observable behaviors and artifacts and explore the child's internal knowledge. It is the internal knowledge that influences how children behave, how they learn, and how they use what they have learned. For example, cultural knowledge will determine how a child will respond when hit by another student. Will the student hit the other child back, walk away, tell the teacher, or threaten to fight the other child after school? The responses will be determined, in part, by the student's cultural knowledge and cultural values. When examiners fail to consider cultural knowledge during the assessment process, the resulting diagnosis will likely be inaccurate. For example, differences in communicative style interfere with the validity of performance observations because standardized test protocols are typically based on eliciting a communicative style that requires verbosity and stating of obvious information. When there are variations from the expected communicative style, judgment of low performance or ability often results (Taylor & Lee 1987). Another example relates to differences in storytelling among children. Heath (1982), Michaels (1981), and Michaels and Collins (1984) report that the communicative styles used to tell stories vary across sociocultural groups. Michaels (1981) has delineated features associated with two communicative styles used to tell stories—topic-centered and topic-associating.

The topic-centered style is the style most often expected in standardized tests. This style is characterized by: (1) structured discourse on a single topic, (2) elaboration upon the topic, and (3) lack of presupposing shared knowledge (Michaels, 1981). The topic-associating style is not the expected communicative style for storytelling for most standardized tests. This style is characterized by: (1) structured discourse on several linked topics, (2) presupposition of shared knowledge, and (3) lack of consideration for detail. The topic-associating style is preferred among most working class African Americans; however, it is not regarded as storytelling ability by standardized tests.

When African American children use the topic-associating communicative style in test situations, they are often viewed as disorganized. As a result, their stories are devalued and considered pointless because of differences that conflict with the expected style of standardized tests. Such conflicts often result in misdiagnoses of language disorders or learning disabilities. These examples illustrate that within and across cultural groups, consideration for variance is a critical factor that must be considered in the development of standardized tests. Otherwise, the tests will remain an invalid source of information for many students.

Interpreting Assessment Results

Since culture plays a major role in the assessment process, it is very important that Black students' responses be interpreted through a cultural filter. This means that factors that can influence performance must be considered when administering and interpreting test results. For example, the examiner, test items, and testing situation are factors that can influence behavior and responses; however, these factors are seldom considered when evaluating student performance.

Four major problems have been identified by Hamayan and Damico (1991) as causes of cultural insensitivity by examiners in the assessment process. The first problem is misinterpretation between the Black student and the assessor. This means that the student and the examiner have different understandings regarding their roles and expectations during the assessment process. When both parties lack a clear understanding of their roles in the testing situation, this can lead to perceived or actual poorer performance by the student. For example, a Black student's inexperience with tests may result in failure to perceive the testing activity as related to school, learning, or promotion, thus not behaving in the expected manner in testing situations. The examiner, on the other hand, expects and looks for certain types of behaviors from the student. When such behaviors are not exhibited, the student may be perceived as inattentive or disinterested. Misperceptions of students' behaviors can result in inaccurate test interpretations, thus resulting in inappropriate recommendations for intervention. Many recommendations are for placement in special education or compensatory programs. This is an example of perceptual incongruence resulting from different culturally based experiences and knowledge between the student and examiner.

A second problem that may occur due to cultural insensitivity during assessments is the process of cross-cultural stereotyping (Tannen 1984). Cross-cultural stereotyping is the lack of awareness of cultural differences; thus, groups may be stereotyped as possessing intrinsic traits, when, in fact, they are merely exhibiting behaviors that are appropriate in their own culture. For example, Black students may give a verbal response to a question asked by the teacher without first holding up a hand to be called upon. This type of call-and-response behavior represents a cross-cultural difference that is a part of the Black experience in the church and the home. Because this type of behavior is incongruent with the teacher's classroom behavioral expectations, calling out answers without holding up a hand first, then waiting to be called upon to speak by the teacher, could result in harsh consequences. Blurting out answers, whether correct or incorrect, is usually perceived as rude, aggressive, and disrespectful by individuals who are unaware of the call-and-response practices in African American culture, homes and churches. These are acceptable cultural practices that result in positive interactions between family members and friends. When these instances occur early in an African American child's school experience, teachers should instruct the child to use the classroom rule of holding up the hand first, being acknowledged by the teacher, then speaking. The children will learn this expected behavior, which will become a part of their expected behavioral repertoire for school. As their mainstream American behavioral repertoire expands, African American children learn how to switch behaviors between home and school and use them appropriately. African American students learn expected behavioral norms of two cultures—theirs and mainstream America.

The third problem that arises from cultural insensitivity is miscommunication. When the examiner and student do not share the same background and lack understanding of the interaction patterns exhibited in each other's cultures, there is a likelihood that misinterpretations will occur while attempting to communicate. This will likely result in confusion and misinformation, especially if the miscommunications are not recognized. Black children do not typically share the same communication patterns and culture of their teachers. Therefore, when teachers give examples in class to clarify information based on their own cultural experiences and knowledge, Black children may become confused due to cultural, linguistic, or perceptual differences and interpretations about what is being communicated. In this regard, information that is supposed to aid the student's learning may, in fact, serve as a barrier.

Many examples of examiner misinterpretation and miscommunication occur with African American children and their parents. One common example relates to how the examiner discusses test results with parents, often assuming they fully understand tests and measurement jargon because the parents appear polite, quiet, and very observant of what is going on around them. Their behavioral patterns and body language may be signaling high levels of discomfort and intimidation because of differences associated with the environment and the examiner's language pattern and technical vocabulary.

In these types of situations, the parents' body language and behavioral patterns may be interpreted by the examiner as total parent cooperation and attentiveness, when in fact, the parents may be feeling anxious, overwhelmed, and inattentive because they do not understand what is being communicated to them. In situations like these, cultural clashes are often abundant. African American parents often feel left out of the conversation and barriers to effective communication are apparent. When this occurs, the parents are usually anxious to leave.

The fourth effect of cultural insensitivity is assessment bias. This problem occurs when educational personnel and other professionals involved in the assessment process do not take into consideration cultural differences when assessing Black and other diverse students. Tests used for assessment have biasing factors that should be taken into account. These factors are both extrinsic and intrinsic to the tests (Miller 1984). Extrinsic biasing factors are child rearing and schooling differences, sociocultural position and role of the test population within society as a whole, attitudes in test-taking and response styles, the value of competition in the student's culture, and adjustment to the artificiality of the testing situation. Biasing factors that are intrinsic to the tests include the use of culture-bound stimuli, background knowledge not accessible to the student, language and conceptual differences, and selection practices for determining normative samples (Miller, 1984).

In America, most tests are normed on the mainstream population, or the White middle-class. Even when tests include culturally diverse populations in the standardization process, these populations are included in such small ratios that the results are insignificant. This practice may also merely serve to further bias the test validity. Examiners should be aware of this problem when testing and interpreting results obtained for Black children. Examiners need to learn more about the impact of cultural differences on test results in order to begin interpreting students responses appropriately and fairly. Unless they have this type of cultural understanding, they will not be able to make appropriate interpretations or recommendations for Black children.

There is clearly a need for a variety of culturally and linguistically sensitive assessment instruments that can be used with different cultural and linguistic groups. The availability of such instruments would certainly help diminish current practices of assessment bias and child and instrument abuse.

It has only been recently that increasing efforts are made to use tests normed on samples of ethnic minority students. There is also evidence of the growing use of dynamic testing methods resulting from the pioneering efforts of Professor Reginald Jones, who was teaching at the University of California at Berkeley when he published a casebook of nondiscriminatory assessment of minority group children (Samuda & Kong 1989).

Prior to Dr. Jones' development of the casebook of nondiscriminatory assessment of minority group children, another group of researchers worked on Afrocentric assessment instrumentation. The earliest work in this area was conducted by Dr. Robert L. Williams during the early 1970s. Through his research, the first Afrocentrically sensitive psychological measures were developed (Hilliard 1987). A total of five Afrocentric measures consisted of the following: (1) The Black Personality Questionnaire, (2) The Black Preference Inventory, (3) The Black Opinion Scale, (4) The Themes of Black Awareness Test, and (5) The Themes Concerning Blacks Test. Of these five instruments, the Black Personality Questionnaire has been used on a limited basis. Additional research, data collection, and analysis are still underway on all of the measures. At this stage of development, the actual usefulness of these various measures of Black personality assessment remains to be determined in the future (Hilliard 1987).

There are many facets of culture that affect assessment outcomes of African American students. The one cultural variable that continues to dominate the literature and create much debate is African American language or linguistic influence on assessment. Because there are differences within cultures as mentioned elsewhere and because all Black people are not African

American, assessment practices and results cannot be generalized to all Black children.

Linguistic Assessment Bias

One of the most serious problems related to the assessment process is the assumption by examiners that all Black students' language preference is mainstream American English without checking first to verify the students' language and cultural status. It is a common assessment practice to examine students without consideration of the following linguistic influences that definitely impact assessment results: (1) student's primary language, (2) language difference, (3) language loss, (4) code-switching, and (5) dialectal variation. The direct impact of these language variables are discussed in this section as they relate specifically to African American students and the assessment process.

Students' Primary Language

There are many first languages spoken in America's schools by students. In California, for example, over 50 different languages are spoken among its student population. In any one school district it is not uncommon to find over twenty different languages spoken, with English as the second language. In view of the changing demographics of the nation, standard English is not the first language for a large percentage of the population. Therefore, language difference and language choice of students are essential considerations when planning assessment activities.

With respect to Black children, examiners should not make any assumptions about their primary language. A child's primary language cannot be determined by skin color. It is not uncommon for examiners to test Black children using mainstream American English to discover after the fact that the child is from another country, continent, and culture—thus, a different primary language. When situations like this occur, it creates major problems for the students, especially when the test results are used in making instructional and placement decisions. Depending on the integrity of the examiner, the results in such cases may be used as valid or invalid when making recommendations to the school about instructional needs. Since examiners' interpretations and recommendations about children are seldom questioned or challenged, their assessment reports are often used as the basis for academic decisions.

Language Difference

As mentioned throughout this text, the majority of African American children learn and speak African American English prior to coming to school. The majority of them have acquired the skills in pragmatics to use situational cues to switch between home and school languages by the time they are in the third grade (Wofford 1979). In other words, most African American children learn by grade three how to code-switch from their home language to the school language based upon situation and context. Fishman (1968) suggested that numerous factors interact to determine the actual language or register that a speaker selects when interacting with others (e.g., setting, purpose, audience, political views, or emotional state).

As mentioned previously, the majority of Black children learn fairly quickly upon entering school that the English language spoken at school sounds different from the language they speak at home. Thus begins a "language use pattern conflict" for Black children. The teacher may expect one type of language use patterns from the children when they begin school, when, in fact, young Black children may be able to produce only the language and language patterns learned at home. In these situations, the teacher is usually unaware of code-switching skills and the need for most Black children to learn and master these skills in order to fulfill the teacher's pragmatics and expectations.

The same occurrences take place when examiners conduct formal assessments with young African American children. If they assume that the children's language—particularly pragmatics—are the same as their own and proceed with the assessments, the children may fail the tests miserably. In situations like these, the children are placed at a disadvantage and usually encounter many testing difficulties. Their performance on linguistic tasks, such as story retelling, may result in conclusions that are incorrect about their language proficiency and pragmatics. Caution needs to be exercised when assessing Black children; particularly, comparing their language and testing results with those of monolingual English speakers. These types of comparisons too often result in misinterpretations about Black children's cognitive functioning and linguistic abilities. Inaccurate assessment conclusions made early in their education experiences can affect the rest of their schooling negatively.

Language Loss
Language loss refers to losing proficiency in a first language while still learning a second language. This variable is applicable to Black children. According to Baratz (1973), standard English for the speaker who uses African American language exclusively is for all practical purposes a foreign or second language. The following example demonstrates the variability of results that can be obtained when Black children are assessed over time. When most Black children begin kindergarten at age 5, they are generally proficient in African American language. By the time they are in the third grade or so, they have gained partial control of two languages—the home language and the school language. In the process of gaining mainstream American English, they tend to lose some of their African American language. As their main-

stream American English language skills increase, they gain the tool and ability to code-switch from one code (African American language) to the other code (mainstream American English) based on need.

Labov, Cohen, Robins, and Lewis (1968) indicate that Black children should not be expected to simply throw away their prior language experience. Their home language should be respected as a different language when teaching mainstream American English. Even though their different home linguistic experience may interfere initially with their efforts to read, write and speak mainstream American English, the lack of total correspondence between the two languages should not be considered an aberration of mainstream American English. Instead, teachers should concentrate their efforts on teaching and modeling the language (mainstream American English) that the children need to learn. The home language should be treated and respected the same as any other language that is different from mainstream American English. Today, efforts are made to assist bilingual children in maintaining their primary language while acquiring English as their second language; the same principles and understanding apply to African American children.

Language loss is a variable that creates a functional conflict for African American students because of how it is related to an identity function. Black children identify with their primary group and culture through a shared language. Learning a new language is often the first step toward cultural alienation. Labov and colleagues (1968) speculated that Black children may view standard English as "White" or alien to them and their culture; thus, to learn it and speak it exclusively may imply that they have to reject one of their most important cultural ties, their language. Children's language identifies them with their family, race, culture, peer group, and self. In this regard, Black children may be placed in the midst of a conflict that involves learning mainstream American English and possibly breaking a strong connection to their peers and their ethnic-family background.

This functional conflict seems to boil down to the question of not whether the Black child can learn to fully use mainstream American English, but whether the child wants to learn to use it (Wilson 1987).

There is general agreement with Labov's views that conflict between the different structures and functions of African American language is one of the major contributors to school failure for many Black children. This is especially true since public schools usually demand that mainstream American English be used exclusively in the classroom. Labov and colleagues (1968) also indicated that in order to fully understand the function of African American language, one has to know something about the value system and social structure that are the foundation of that language.

With respect to assessment, it is not difficult to see where numerous conflicts might arise. First, written or verbalized instructions may be partially lost when the Black child attempts to translate, understand, and perceive what it is that the examiner has said and expects. Secondly, some examiners may not be aware of the structural, situational, and functional differences between African American English and mainstream American English. Thirdly, the examiner may not be aware that Black children gradually learn to shift from their home language to mainstream American English based on situation and context. This means that African American students usually experience some "home" language loss while acquiring mainstream American English language.

During this period of language loss, many Black children experience emotional conflict in their efforts to sort out which language is expected at home and which one is expected at school. It is during this phase of mainstream American English learning and transitioning that Black children begin adapting their language usage to context and situation; thus, code-switching skills begin to develop. Black children soon learn that they need to know how to survive in both systems—their family system and the school system. This realization and acquisition of code-switching skills represent just another aspect of the Black child's duality of socialization in America.

Code-Switching
Code-switching refers to the ability to change from one language code to another language code based on situation and context. This means that a person can switch from one language to another based on environmental and linguistic expectations of that environment. Bicultural and bilingual children are forced to acquire code-switching skills in order to survive and achieve in two distinctly different cultural and linguistic environments.

In test-taking situations, code-switching may be viewed as a liability instead of an asset. This means that if the examiner does not understand the register into which the Black child has switched in response to a verbal or written question, the child may be scored wrong even though the response is correct. Until recently, few teachers and examiners were aware of code-switching; most thought that code-switching was an indication that the Black child had not developed standard English skills in accordance with chronological age and was therefore considered possibly "language delayed" or "learning disabled." They were unaware of the legitimacy of African American language and the fact that Black children during the "language transition phase" might respond to questions partially in mainstream American English and partially in African American language. In either case, the rules of both languages are usually maintained throughout code-switching.

Linguists have studied code-switching from a sociolinguistic perspective and have found that the way in which bilinguals code-switch is predictable and regular. Since assessment typically occurs in one language (mainstream

American English), there is no provision for Black students to regularly, predictably, and appropriately code-switch. This means that when African American students answer questions in African American language, the examiners are not usually sure how to score these responses. The responses may be penalized (as determined by the subjective judgment of the examiner), or the responses may be an underestimation of the student's ability. Recognizing these testing pitfalls for Black students, code-switching behavior may be viewed as a barrier by examiners instead of its known benefit to Black students.

Dialectal Variation

In the formal assessment process, dialectal variance is another linguistic consideration. Dialects vary in the way they are used depending on geographical location, social status, learning experience, and the contexts in which the language is used. In the testing situation, if the examiner's dialect is different from the student's dialect, or if the test was normed on a population that speaks a dialect different from the student being tested, the student's performance may be judged inadequately. This is particularly true when the student uses vocabulary and grammatical constructions that are different from the standards of middle-class, mainstream American English grammar. Students' performance on tests may also be hindered if they use the dialect with which they feel most comfortable and it differs from that of the examiner.

With regard to Black children, they can be viewed as being in a "double bind" when measured against the middle-class mainstream American English standards if they speak African American language and have a noticeable regional dialect. Dialectal difference is more apparent in the Black child who lives in a region where the regional dialect is noticeably different. For example, the Black child who is born and reared in the deep South is likely to have a noticeable dialect and language pattern difference than the Black child born and reared on the east or west coast.

In some testing situations, both the language difference and regional dialect can be used against the child in a testing situation (scoring and interpreting results) if the assessment environment, assessment tools, and examiner represent White, middle-class, mainstream American English standards.

Cultural and linguistic variables influence assessment outcomes. Teachers, examiners, school administrators, and other professional and paraprofessionals working with Black students should be made aware of the language differences that exist between mainstream American speakers and the majority of African Americans. Such knowledge is valuable in preventing inappropriate responses to the children's language and in making unwarranted referrals for speech and language assessments.

LEGISLATED NONDISCRIMINATORY EVALUATION

In 1975 Public Law 94-142, the Education of All Handicapped Children Act, passed and established some ground rules for state education agencies, local school districts, schools, parents, and children. Although this law was renamed in 1990 to the Individuals With Disabilities Education Act, the basic requirements and intent of the law remained the same.

The six basic requirements of the law are summarized below.

- Schools must educate all children with disabilities and may not exclude any school-aged children solely because of the disability.
- Nondiscriminatory evaluation is required. All schools must test and classify children fairly by administering non-biased tests in ways that do not put children to a disadvantage but allow them to show their educational strengths, abilities, and disabilities.
- An appropriate individualized education plan must be prepared that is tailored to meet the individual needs of the child.
- Least restrictive environment means that schools are required to educate children with disabilities with their peers to the maximum extent consistent with their educational and social needs.
- Procedural due process means that parents must be provided the opportunity to consent or object to their children's identification, classification, individualized education plan, or placement.
- Parent involvement means that parents of children with disabilities may participate in various ways in their children's education (Turnbull & Turnbull 1986, p.170)

Under this law, state education agencies and local school districts are required to establish procedures to ensure that testing, examination materials, and procedures used for evaluating and placing children with disabilities will be selected and administered so as not to be racially or culturally discriminatory. Each state education agency and school district must provide and administer such materials or procedures in the child's native language or mode of communication unless it is clearly not feasible to do so. The phrase *nondiscriminatory testing* applies to evaluation materials and procedures used with all children, as made clear in the regulations.

In response to the requirements for racially and culturally nondiscriminatory testing and evaluation, the law requires that

(a) Tests and other evaluation materials
(1) Are provided and administered in the child's native language or other mode of communication, unless it is clearly not feasible to do so;

(2) *Have been validated for the specific purpose for which they are used;*

(3) *Are administered by trained personnel in conformance with instructions from the producer.*

(b) *Tests and other evaluation materials include those tailored to access specific areas of educational need and not merely those which are designed to provide a single general intelligence quotient.*

(c) *Tests are selected and administered so as best to insure that when a test is administered to a child with impaired sensory, manual, or speaking skills, the test results accurately reflect the child's aptitude or achievement level or whatever other factor the test purports to measure, rather than reflecting the child's impaired sensory, manual, or speaking skills (except where those skills are the factors which the test purports to measure).*

(d) *No single procedure is used as the sole criterion for determining an appropriate educational program for a child and placement.*

(e) *The evaluation is made by a multidisciplinary team or group of persons, including at least one teacher or other specialist with knowledge in the area of suspected disability.*

(f) *The child is assessed in all areas related to the suspected disability, including, where appropriate, health, vision, hearing, social and emotional status, general intelligence, academic performance, communicative status, and motor abilities. (Turnbull 1990, p. 85)*

Public Law 94-142 also requires that before a child is initially placed in a special education program, a complete and individual evaluation of the children's educational needs must be conducted. This evaluation is supposed to draw upon information from a variety of sources, including aptitude and achievement tests, teacher recommendations, physical condition, social and cultural background, and adaptive behavior. Information obtained from all of these sources should be documented and carefully considered in the decision-making process.

Placement decisions are to be made by a group of persons, including persons knowledgeable about the child, the meaning of the evaluation data, and the placement options available. Finally, the placement decision is supposed to be made in conformity with the least restrictive environment rules of the law and with parents' informed consent (Turnbull, 1990).

The intent of this special education legislation is to insure that all children with disabilities receive a free, appropriate, public education in the least restrictive environment with their peers. Nondiscriminatory evaluation procedures are supposed to be followed to assure that testing, materials, and procedures are not racially or culturally discriminatory. Such precautionary practices are intended to prevent special education referrals and placements of students due to racial and cultural differences.

The first provision of nondiscriminatory evaluation requires that tests are administered in the child's native language. In order to comply with this provision, initial speech and language screening should be done by a speech-language pathologist who is familiar with the African American culture to determine the children's primary language and to determine if they have fully resolved any structural conflict that exists when acquiring the rules and language to speak, read and write mainstream American English. It should also be determined in advance of formal testing if the children have the skills to code-switch without difficulty. These informal types of preliminary screenings are important to their overall performance on tests administered during the assessment process.

The risk of misdiagnosing Black students is great from both a linguistic and cultural perspective. The examiner can help prevent misdiagnoses by exercising every precaution to prevent assessment violations that often result in misdiagnosis and misplacement of Black students.

Precautionary measures are necessary when assessing African American children because many African Americans speak standard American English as their first language, while many others, perhaps a majority, speak African American language. As mentioned earlier, African American language is, in linguistic terms, a fully developed language. Therefore, full recognition of this fact is critical to testing and academic outcomes for African American students.

Although schools are not asked to change the language of instruction or teach African American language, we must point out that most diagnostic mistakes are made due to limited awareness of this linguistic reality. Errors are made in the analysis and interpretation of test results in areas related to language, reading, and writing, that have caused many African American children to be falsely labeled mentally retarded, speech impaired, and low achievers. African American children should not be degraded, misdiagnosed, or classified as pathological in order to receive an appropriate education.

Several significant court decisions were made during the 1970s that were landmark cases relates specifically to the linguistic rights of children. In *Lau v. Nichols* (1974), the U.S. Supreme Court ruled unanimously in favor of the plaintiffs from San Francisco's Chinatown community that the absence of programs designed to meet their children's specific linguistic needs violated their civil rights. The plaintiffs argued further, and the Court agreed, that equality of education goes beyond the provision of the same buildings and books to all students to include intangible factors such as language. Because they could not understand the English language used in the classroom, the Chinese plaintiffs argued they were deprived of even a minimally adequate, and hardly equal, education (Taylor 1986).

Citing *Lau v. Nichols* and Section 1703(f) of Title 20 of the United States Code, a United States District Judge in Michigan ruled in 1979 on behalf of nine Black children in Ann Arbor, Michigan who claimed that the local school board had denied them their equal rights by failing to take their native Black English into account in the educational process. In this court case of *Martin Luther King Junior Elementary School Children, et al., v. Ann Arbor School District Board*, parents of eleven Black students ranging in age from 6 to 13 and living in Ann Arbor's Green Road Housing Project won a landmark decision.

The parents accused school officials at Martin Luther King Elementary School of insensitivity to the indigenous speech of Black students. These students had been classified as needing speech therapy or as learning disabled by the school. Parents demanded that school authorities recognize Black English as a formal and distinct dialect with historical and cultural basis and its own grammatical structure. The plaintiffs argued that, in the process of determining students eligibility for special education services, the Ann Arbor School District Board failed to ascertain whether learning difficulties stemmed from cultural, social, and economic deprivation—deprivations that, the plaintiffs alleged, prevented them from making normal progress in school (Bond & Chambers 1983).

> *In July 1979, after three weeks of argument, U.S. District Judge Charles W. Joiner ruled that the district must recognize Black English, the language most Black students speak at home. Joiner also ordered the district to develop a program to help teachers recognize this language and take it into account in teaching standard English. In so doing, he observed that there was a failure on the part of the school board to provide leadership and help for its teachers in learning about the existence of Black English as a home and community language of many Black students. (Bond & Chambers 1983, p. 98)*

In essence, Joiner recognized that some school children spoke "Black English" and ruled that their at-home language be the basis for at-school achievement.

In the case, *Martin Luther King Junior Elementary School Children, et al., v. Ann Arbor School District Board* (1978), Section 1703 (f) of Title 20 states:

> *No State shall deny equal educational opportunity to an individual on account of his or her race, color, sex, or national origin by . . . the failure of an educational agency to take appropriate action to overcome language barriers that impede equal participation by its students in its instructional programs. (Taylor 1986, p.6)*

This court ruling established the legitimacy of language differences and supported the use of African American children's native language in the educational process. Therefore, teachers and examiners should consider these court decisions in carrying out their work. Efforts should be made to become cross-culturally competent and respectful of cultural and language differences as a matter of ethical practice in classroom instruction and formal assessment. Equally as important is an understanding of why testing is done and for whose benefit. Testing is not done to improve student achievement; this idea has been disproved over the past twenty years. For example, in the 1970s, thirty-eight states had some kind of mandated testing program, and by the end of the 1980s, forty-seven states had such programs. But, student performance was just as inadequate (Hymes, Chafin, & Gonder 1991).

Furthermore, teachers should not rest the fate and future of their students on standardized test results. Teachers still have available everyday classroom practices that can be used as alternative assessment tools to measure their students' academic progress and to improve instruction. As a matter of fact, teachers will probably feel more comfortable and competent in using the following methods. These are sample activities that have been used quite effectively for years in classrooms.

OBSERVATION OF STUDENT BEHAVIORS

Many teachers observe the students at different intervals, chart their behaviors and make notations about the students performance and progress in each subject matter area, social skills, and communication. Ongoing observations and documentation over time provides enormous insight about students' needs and achievements.

Asking Questions

Asking students well-chosen questions to spur them into critical thinking is probably the oldest form of informal assessment of students' acquired knowledge and ability to process, analyze, and think critically. Asking questions enhances thinking skills by giving students a chance to think. It also gives the teacher information about how much information has been received, how it has been interpreted, and how it fits into the students' cognitive schemas.

Asking questions can be done in writing or orally. In either case, the nature of the questions can generate a lot of useful information for the teacher. Questions may be used for recall of facts (spelling or multiplication facts) or critical thinking.

Self-Evaluation

Simply asking the students how they are doing can provide insight into their progress. Ask about their understanding of the subject matter, their interpretation of it, and how useful or applicable the information is to them. Student feedback is useful for teachers in planning instructional activities and approaches. Students' self-evaluation will tell a lot about their academic progress.

Paper-and-Pencil Testing

Paper-and-pencil tests are an integral part of classroom assessment. However, the teacher should devote a lot of care in constructing these tests to differentiate between rote recall of facts and those designed to demonstrate higher-order thinking. Too frequently, teachers tend to construct paper-and-pencil tests that emphasize rote recall and memory skills. The intent of paper-and-pencil testing should be to capture and determine the mastery or success level of each student and not to compare students' scores. This type of testing is usually done after completing important units of instruction. These tests should vary in format depending on what the teacher is trying to assess.

With respect to thinking skills, the following classification system encourages teachers to use at least five categories of basic thinking skills. Table 8-1 illustrates the five categories: recall, analysis, comparison, inference, and evaluation. By using these five categories, the full range of thinking skills is covered in each assessment activity.

In keeping with education reform are new visions and trends for assessment, curriculum, and instruction. The most recent trends in assessment are: (1) changes from behavioral to cognitive views of learning, and assessment that focuses on the learning process, active construction of meaning, integrated and cross-disciplinary assessment, self-monitoring, and the application and use of knowledge; (2) shift to authentic assessment where emphasis is on complex skills, individual growth, contextualized problems, relevance and meaning to students; (3) use of portfolios for the assessment of students' work samples over time; (4) use of multidimensional assessments instead of single attribute assessments that allow for recognition of students' many abilities and talents and opportunities for students to develop and exhibit diverse abilities; and (5) use of group assessment whereby group process skills and collaborative products are assessed (Herman, Aschbacher, & Winters 1992).

Linking Assessment and Instruction

New visions of effective curriculum, instruction, and learning demand new attention to today's assessment practices. Learning is no longer considered a one-way transmission of knowledge from teacher to students. Instead, meaningful instruction engages students actively in the learning process. Good teachers draw on the knowledge of student culture, student learning, and child development principles. They use a variety of instructional strategies that actively involve students in hands-on projects, discussion groups, direct instruction, coaching, whole group and individualized activities. For each

TABLE 8-1   Categories of Five Basic Thinking Skills

If you want to measure:	Use these key words in the exercise:		Illustration
Recall	define identify label list name	repeat what when who	List the names of the main characters in the story.
Analysis	subdivide break down separate	categorize sort	Break the story into different parts.
Comparison	compare contrast	differentiate distinguish	Compare the themes of these two stories.
Inference	deduce predict infer speculate	anticipate what if apply conclude	How might we might make this character more believable?
Evaluation	evaluate judge assess appraise defend	argue recommend debate why critique	Evaluate this story. Is it well written? Why or why not?

Source: Hymes, D., Chafin, A. E., & Gonder, P. (1991) *The Changing Face of Testing and Assessment: Problems and Solutions*. Arlington, VA: American Association of School Administrators, p. 68.

student, specific learning goals are established as well as learning goals for the whole group.

Good teachers are able to utilize their knowledge and professional skills to integrate knowledge of intended goals, learning processes, curriculum content, and assessment. They know and use cognitive learning theories that support contemporary cognitive psychology, indicating that learning is not linear and is not acquired in bits and pieces. Instead, learning is an ongoing process during which students continually receive, interpret, and connect information with what they already know and have experienced—their prior knowledge (Herman, Aschbacher, & Winter 1992).

Contemporary learning theories support the importance of students receiving information that they are able to reorganize and revise in their internal conceptions of the world, which are called mental models, knowledge structures, or schema. These theories are congruent with the theory of discontinuity between home and school cultures. Most African American children's assessment and school experiences require learning new information and interpreting it, but they are not always able to connect it to what they already know and have experienced because of major cultural, linguistic, and experiential differences.

Recognizing these differences, teachers who are aware of the current intelligence theories will focus their teaching on the variety of talents and capabilities of African American students. Gardner (1993) argues that traditional schooling has emphasized only two abilities—verbal-linguistic and logical-mathematical—however, many other important intelligences exist.

Multiple intelligences theory pluralizes the traditional concept of intelligence and defines an intelligence as the ability to solve problems or fashion products that are of consequence in a particular cultural setting or community. The problem-solving skill allows one to approach a situation in which a goal is to be obtained and to locate the appropriate route to that goal. The creation of a cultural product is crucial to such functions as capturing and transmitting knowledge or expressing one's views or feelings (Gardner 1993, p.15). Gardner claims there are seven intelligences and all individuals have strengths in two or three of the areas. The seven intelligences are: visual-spatial, bodily-kinesthetic, musical, intrapersonal, logistical-mathematical, linguistic, and spatial intelligence. Gardner claims that instruction and assessment need to draw on more than the two traditional intelligences and subscribe to the assumption that all students can learn. Furthermore, curricula need to be reconfigured and adapted to the particular learning styles and strengths of students.

SUMMARY

Assessment practices in our schools work to the disadvantage of African American and other students from diverse cultural and linguistic backgrounds. Traditional practices do not take into consideration the inappropriateness of using standardized tests that have been normed on student populations different from those the tests are used to make educational decisions. Because of cultural and linguistic differences, African American students often perform poorly on standardized tests. Their performance on such tests are greatly influenced by major cultural and language incongruences inherent in the test, testing situation, and assessor. Because of test bias, African American children continue to be diagnosed and placed in low-ability groups, special education classes, and compensatory programs. Most teachers and assessors have not been trained on variables that contribute to assessment and interpretation biases. As a result, most perceive assessment outcomes as correct and view the student as having the problem.

Four major problems were identified and discussed as causes of cultural insensitivity by assessor. These four problems are: (1) misconceptions between the Black student and the assessor, (2) the process of cross-cultural stereotyping, (3) miscommunication, and (4) assessment bias.

Numerous conflicts arise when assessing African American students using standardized tests. Examples of these conflicts are cited throughout the chapter. In order to counteract the misuse of standardized test to misdiagnose African American and other students from diverse backgrounds, special education laws have passed stipulating that nondiscriminatory evaluation is required and that all schools must test and classify children fairly by administering non-biased tests in ways that do not put the students to a disadvantage but allow them to show their educational strengths, abilities, and disabilities. Several landmark court decisions that relate to inappropriate assessment and placement of children using standardized tests are presented. These cases are examples of how language and cultural differences were ignored in testing, diagnosing, and placing students in special education classes. In one landmark court decision, the *Martin Luther King Junior Elementary School Children, et al., v. Ann Arbor School District Board* in 1978, the judge ruled in favor of African American children's Black English by indicating that their at-home language be the basis for their at-school achievement. Equally as important, the judge ordered the district to develop a program to help teachers recognize the children's language and to take it into account in teaching standard English.

Several sample activities are discussed that teachers may use at different intervals to chart students' performance and progress in the classroom. In addition, a classification system with five categories of basic thinking skills that teachers can use in each assessment activity was presented. Some discussion is devoted to how teachers link assessment and instruction as well as how good teachers are able to utilize their knowledge and professional skills to integrate knowledge and intended goals.

PRACTICAL APPLICATION

It is very important that teachers and examiners become cross-culturally competent. Do not make assumptions about African American students' abilities or competence solely on the basis of a standardized test score. The following suggestions are recommended to increase awareness and sensitivity about cultural differences:

1. Use the references of this textbook to seek new knowledge and information about African American culture and language.
2. Observe African American children's interactional patterns and language style without passing judgment.
3. Become familiar with known variables that interfere with African American children's learning.
4. Utilize the classroom environment to teach and learn about the different cultural and language groups represented in the United States.
5. Enable all children to see their culture reflected in the classroom curriculum and activities every school day.
6. Do not prejudge students' abilities on the basis of their racial, cultural, and linguistic differences.

REFERENCES

Banks, J. (1988). *Multiethnic Education*. Boston, MA: Allyn & Bacon.

Baratz, J. (1973). Teaching reading in an urban Negro school system. In F. William (ed.), *Language and Poverty*. Chicago: Rand McNally College.

Bond, J., & Chambers, J. (1983). *Black English: Educational Equity and the Law*. Ann Arbor, MI: Karoma Publishers.

Community Crusade for Children (1993). Coordinated by the Children's Defense Fund. Washington, D.C.

Fatini, M. D. (1979). From school system to educational system: Policy considerations, In Doxey A. Wilderson (ed.), *Educating All of Our Children: An Imperative for Democracy*. Westport, CT: Mediax, pp. 134–153.

Fishman, J. A. (1968). *The Sociology of Language*. The Hague: Mouton.

Gardner, H. (1993). *Multiple Intelligences: The Theory in Practice*. New York: Basic Books.

Hamayan, E. V., & Damico, J. S. (1991). *Limiting Bias in the Assessment of Bilingual Students*. Austin, TX: PRO-ED.

Haring, N., & McCormick, L. (1991). *Exceptional Individual*. Columbus, OH: Macmillan.

Haring, N. G., McCormick, L., & Haring, T. G. (1994). *Exceptional Children and Youth: An Introduction to Special Education*. New York: Macmillan College.

Heath, S. B., (1982). What no bedtime story means: Narrative skills at home and school. *Language in Society*, 11:49–76 .

Herman, J. L., Aschbacher, P. R., & Winters, L. (1992). *A Practical Guide to Alternative Assessment*. Alexandria, VA: Association for Supervision and Curriculum Development.

Hilliard, A. G. (1987). Testing African American students. In *Special Issue of The Negro Educational Review*, 38 (2–3, April–July).

Hymes, D. L., Chafin, A. E., & Gonder, P. (1991). *Testing and assessment: Problems and solutions*. Arlington, VA: American Association of School Administrators.

Kong, S. L. (1991). *Assessment and Placement of Minority Students*. Toronto: Intercultural Social Sciences Publications.

Labov, W., Cohen, P., Robins, C., & Lewis, J. (1968) . A study of the non-standard English of Negro and Puerto Rican Speakers in New York City. Report on Cooperative Research Project 3288. New York: Columbia University.

Michaels, S. (1981) . Sharing time: Children's narrative styles and differential access to literacy. *Language and Society*, 10:423–442.

Michaels, S., & Collins, J. (1984). Oral Discourse Styles: Classroom interaction and the acquisition of literacy. In D. Tannen (Ed.), *Coherence on Spoken and Written Discourse*. Norwood, NJ: Ablex.

Miller, N. (1984). Some observations concerning formal tests in cross-cultural settings. In N. Miller (Ed.), *Bilingualism and Language Disability: Assessment and Remediation* (pp. 107–14). Austin, TX: PRO-ED.

Moore, E.G., (1987). Ethnic social milieu and Black children's intelligence test achievement, *Journal of Negro Education*, 86(1):44–52).

National Association for Black School Educators. (1989). A Report of the National Alliance of Black School Educators, Inc. Saving the African American Child. Washington DC: NABSE A Vision for American's Future.

Samuda, R., & Kong, S. (Eds.) *Assessment and Placement of Minority Students*. Toronto: Intercultural Social Sciences Publications.

Spradley, J. P. (1980). *Participant Observation*. New York: Holt, Rinehart and Winston.

Tannen, D. (1984). The pragmatics of cross-cultural communication. *Applied Linguistics*, 5:189–195 .

Taylor, O. L. (1986). *Nature of Communication Disorders in Culturally and Linguistically Diverse Populations*. San Diego, CA: College-Hill Press.

Taylor, O. L., & Lee, D. L. (1987). Standardized tests and African American children: Communication and language issues. *Negro Educational Review*, 38(2–3):67–80.

Turnbull, A., & Turnbull, H. R. (1986). *Families, Professionals and Exceptionality*. Columbus, OH: Merrill.

Turnbull, H. R. (1990). *Free Appropriate Public Education: The Law and Children with Disabilities*, 3rd edition. Denver, CO: Love.

Willis, W. (1992). Families with African American roots. In E. W. Lynch & M. J. Hanson (Eds.), *Developing Cross-Cultural Competence*. Baltimore: Paul H. Brookes.

Wilson, A. N. (1987). *The Developmental Psychology of the Black Child*. New York: Africana Research Publications.

Witkin, H. A., Moore, C. A., Goodenough, D. R., & Cox, P. W. (1977). Field-independent cognitive styles and their educational implications. *Review of Educational Research*, 47:1–64.

Wofford (van Keulen), J. E. (1979). Ebonics: A legitimate system of oral communication. *Journal of Black Studies*, 9(4):367–382.

9

TREATMENT OF SPEECH-LANGUAGE DISORDERS

Chapter Overview

Upon reading this chapter you will gain understanding of:

- The health care in African American communities
- Clinical and personal qualities required to serve African American speech-language impaired children
- Therapy goals for treating communicatively impaired African American children
- Recommended goals for the development of academic language of African American children
- Suggestions for working with teachers
- Roles of teachers and speech-language pathologists

The treatment of communication disorders in African American individuals requires knowledge of their language and culture and the flexibility of speech-language pathologists to provide treatment within a cultural context. This means that the clinicians should make every attempt to use materials and events that reflect the African American traditions and experiences in the Individualized Educational Plan (IEP). This does not mean that the clinicians need to speak African American English or generate novel sentences in that language. It does mean, however, that clinicians should be willing to suppress their own biases toward languages and cultures that are low in prestige and make every effort to ensure that the children develop the linguistic skills they need to be effective in school.

Suggestions were made in Chapters 7 and 8 for the valid assessment of speech and language of African American children to ensure that the children accepted into speech and language therapy have speech and language disorders. In this chapter, issues related to the treatment of communication disorders of African American children will be explored, followed by recommendations for working with the children, their teachers and families. Also included are inquiries into health care utilization in the Black community, application of assessment results for determining speech and language therapy goals, involvement of family members, responsibilities of the speech-language pathologist, and partnership with teachers. This chapter will elaborate on the treatment of the most common communication problems among school-age children, disorders of articulation and language.

SERVICE DELIVERY FOR AFRICAN AMERICANS

The low-income African American population is underserved in health care and resources in the United States (Freeman, Bernard, Matory, Smith, Whitico, Yancy, & Bond 1982). Health care is mostly unavailable, expensive and inaccessible. African Americans have a lower rate of physician contact than other groups and tend to seek medical care only when an emergency exists, or when the pain, bleeding, fever, or other symptoms become unbearable (Thomas 1981; Waldman 1992). Thus, when compared to other Americans, African Americans utilize the emergency room more (White-Means, Thornton, & Yeo 1989), because frequently there is no primary care physician. Thus, problems that are not life-threatening, uncomfortable, or unpleasant are left to resolve without services, or the individual learns to make adjustments. There is an acceptance of problems that are believed to be unchangeable or remain as "God created" the person.

Speech-language disorders are often associated with health conditions and financed by health insurance. Some speech-language services are funded on a limited basis by Medicaid in the public schools. Speech and language services are not considered vital; therefore, failure to receive them is not life-threatening. It would not be determined high enough in priority for families to take extraordinary measures to seek out such services, even if the parents were aware that such services were available.

Socioeconomic factors and health insurance are important considerations that influence the utilization of health care services by African Americans (Guendelman & Schwalbe 1986; Thomas 1981). Poor people tend to seek the assistance of religious healers, practitioners of folk medicine, home remedies, and over-the-counter medications before resorting to scientific medicine

(Snow 1981). Self-prescribed home medications are generally taken before seeking care from a physician and may continue after medication is prescribed without the knowledge of the physician. "African Americans tend to consult an alternative health practitioner primarily because of: (1) their attempt to cope with health problems within the context of (their) resources and sociocultural environment; (2) their belief that alternative health practitioners have some control over the forces that cause anomalies in a person's life, whereas westernized medical physicians cannot heal certain cases of illness and misfortune and (3) lower monetary expense associated with such treatments" (Bailey, 1991, p. 37). Alternative health practices are less costly and usually end in a reduction of symptoms.

Since speech-language therapy is a health-related service and often connected to medical centers, expensive, and frequently not funded by health insurance programs, poor people are not likely to believe that speech-language therapy is needed. Most families do not know anyone who failed to acquire speech and language, therefore, it may be difficult for them to believe that an individual child would need assistance learning to talk. Learning to talk, it is believed, is as natural as learning to walk or independent toileting, therefore everyone will develop the skill if parents wait long enough. Black adults can sometimes cite at least one example of an individual who failed to talk until five years of age or older, but began to speak in sentences one day. Such people, reportedly, grew up to be normal and needed no intervention for this very important human skill.

One reason why Black people are unfamiliar with speech-language pathology services is that speech-language pathologists are not visible members of the community. There are very few Black clinicians within the profession and rarely are children familiar enough to choose it as a career. Although every public school in the United States has access to speech-language pathology services, most parents and some teachers do not know the name of the speech-language pathologist that serves the school, or would not recognize her or him even on the school grounds. Often, the first time the Black family encounters a speech-language pathologist is when the message arrives requesting permission to test the child.

QUALITIES REQUIRED TO SERVE AFRICAN AMERICAN CLIENTS

Speech-language clinicians who serve low-income Black communities must develop competencies that render them effective. Meyerson and Weddington (1986) postulated that the SLP "should have an understanding of the culture and language of low income black people, their values, their needs for medical care of high quality, the effects of poverty on all aspects of their lives, and their strategies for coping with problems, handicaps and disabilities" (p. 417). They further offered suggestions for speech-language clinicians to deliver optimal services.

1. The clinician should learn as much as possible about the language of the African American community. Knowledge of the language provides the background data to which assessment results can be compared. Characteristics of the content, form, and use of the child's home language are delineated in the first five chapters of this book. In order to determine whether the child has a speech or language disorder, contrastive analyses must be conducted and completed. Speech and language characteristics that deviate from both African American and standard English are possible features of the disorder.

Most speech and language testing concentrates on linguistic form of the communication sample, rather than on content or use. This means that features of communication form, such as phonology and surface structure of grammar, are targeted for treatment. Some phonological disorders are exhibited as errors in articulation and affect the intelligibility of the message. However, speech therapy should be offered only for those articulation differences that do not represent phonological features of African American English. Deviations in syntax are treated the same as articulation errors in which the clinician determines whether the features are different enough from both standard and African American English to be considered a disorder. Word order errors and telegraphic speech are problems that would warrant intervention. Abnormally short utterances need to be examined further to determine whether the sample analyzed is an accurate prototype of the children's typical behavior in varied situations, and whether the length of the utterance is representative of personality or emotional differences, or possible disorders.

2. Judgments about content are based on the ability of language impaired children to communicate comprehensible messages, therefore, a number of questions need to be answered.
- Does the child have an acceptable number of words needed to communicate within the home environment?
- Does the child demonstrate the ability to learn new words and use them within a reasonable amount of time?
- Is the child able to retrieve the words in the vocabulary when needed?
- Assessment results should also offer information about comprehension of what is said in the home language.
- Does the child follow instructions quickly and accurately when presented in the home language?
- Does the child respond appropriately to conversational speech or questions?

- Under what conditions are the responses made?
- Is it necessary to repeat the stimuli a number of times?
- Is there a delay in the response? When a question is asked, the child is expected to answer within a specified period of time. When the child takes too long to answer, there could be a problem in auditory processing, auditory sensitivity, receptive or expressive language, or the language is unfamiliar to the child (i.e., a second language). It is not unusual for African American children to appear befuddled when questions or directions are presented in standard English. They may have difficulty with the phonological features of the language, vocabulary, grammar, or paralanguage.
- Are responses made only when the question is accompanied by gestures? Linguistically impaired children or children who do not speak the language may be dependent on the gestures to gain meaning. When the gestures are omitted, the children fail to respond appropriately.
- Are responses appropriate? Does the child answer questions asked? Follow directions given? Respond to conversation logically?
- Does the child say, "I don't know" to verbal stimuli in the home language? The response "I don't know" is typically used as a means of resistance, or the child is unsure how to respond. When forced to interact in an unfamiliar situation, the response of children is typically, "I don't know." Clinicians should not accept this response at face value and should either continue to probe, or request assistance from family members to explain the response. A litany of "I don't knows" is a sign that a problem in testing is indicated.

3. Discover resources in the community for referrals for additional services and treatment. Children respond better in familiar, relevant situations, therefore speech-language therapy is more effective when materials and contexts orginate in the child's community. In addition to involving the classroom teachers and teaching skills to support the educational process, the SLP should make every effort to find African American books and that can be used in speech-language therapy. Also, the clinician should determine the location of museums, bookstores, markets, and other African American establishments for field trips and rewards for good performance.

4. Develop a friendly relationship with other members of the educational team, which includes the teachers, resource teachers, psychologist, and family. The involvement of the SLPs with culture and language places an added burden on them to guarantee that such information is infused into the child's education and related services of disabled children. The SLP is able to offer consultative services to the members of the team and should solicit assistance from them as well. Family members can provide family treasures, books, and

other materials that can assist the clinician with the goal of making the speech-language services more meaningful.

5. Clinicians should be prepared to work with the extended family to enhance the effectiveness of the services. Varied members of the extended family are genuinely interested in the welfare of the disabled child. Older siblings are especially helpful as role models and peer teachers. The clinician can extend feelings of good will to all interested parties by inviting individual members to observe therapy and to work on specific skills with the child. The clinician should always offer suggestions when a family member asks, "What can I do to help?"

6. Clinicians should be flexible enough to allow for modification in scheduling, as low-income families may have difficulty meeting schedules due to transportation problems and other crises that develop in the lives of the client and family. Being poor and Black presents challenges to daily life that many middle-class professionals never have to face. Unreliable transportation, childcare problems, and other responsibilities routinely interfere with planned activities. Problems such as illness of the parent and family members and their responses to such illnesses result in missed meetings and appointments. The clinician needs to be as understanding and flexible as possible to avoid alienating the parents and thus diminishing their cooperation altogether.

7. The clinician should plan a treatment strategy that is important to the child. Speech-language clinicians spend hours of precious time creating and practicing drills to teach "is + verb + ing" to Black children. There are few things that are less meaningful for Black children than "is + verb + ing." Sometimes it is important to actually ask the disabled children and their parents about skills they or their family want to develop. Sometimes, the children may simply want to be able to say their own names correctly, or to be able to ask for something desired. Assisting the children with language-related school work not only helps the children succeed in school, but improves their use of standard English outside the classroom.

Using a similar approach to service delivery for African American children, Terrell and Terrell (1993) suggested a "nonbiased" approach to the management of communication disorders of African American clients. The management procedure would require the speech-language clinician to establish the native language as the basis for all assessments and treatment. The authors offered a series of recommendations to improve the services delivered to African American clients that would communicate respect for the culture, language, and community:

- Nonbiased assessment procedures should be administered.
- The clinicians must avoid negative judgments about the client and the family.

- Permissions for testing, questionnaires, and assessment results must be provided in person.
- Offer an escort to insure the safe and prompt arrival for assessment or intervention.
- Involve family members in intervention procedures.
- Adapt treatment materials to reflect the child's language and culture.

Terrell and Terrell (1993) suggest that once the speech-language clinician has conducted a self-study and has decided that working optimally with African American children is a viable choice, the clinician can begin to work with individual clients. Only clinicians who are willing to set aside their own biases, prejudices, and belief that the language of Black children is inferior to other languages and in need of remediation should treat the communication disorders of African American children. The decision to begin therapy should be made by the family of the children with assistance from the SLP and teachers.

DETERMINING THERAPY GOALS FROM ASSESSMENT RESULTS

When the speech or language disorder is diagnosed, the next step is to use the assessment results to determine the treatment goals. The goals will be determined by the age of the client, communication need, and the type of problem diagnosed. For speech-language therapy to be indicated, the disorder must be different enough from any noted features of African American English to render it conspicuous. At no time should a public school speech-language clinician enroll a Black child in therapy for linguistic differences, except on an elective basis (please see the ASHA Position Paper on Social Dialects summarized in Chapter 6).

Articulation: The goals selected for remediation of speech sounds can be determined by developmental sequence, sounds that occur frequently in the language, sounds that are stimulable, or sounds the child chooses to remediate. For African American children, it is important to insure that the goals selected are not speech sound differences between African American English and language. The clinician should look for those errors that are different from the phonological systems of both African American and standard English. Phonological disorders such as frontal and lateral lisps, w/r substitutions, p/f substitutions, and so on, are possible targets. A Black child tested recently for articulation disorders at a preschool program in Northern California exhibited unintelligible speech characterized by omitted syllables, substituted and distorted speech sounds, and rearranged sounds in words. The nature of the articulation disorder was easy to diagnose by the speech-language clinicians who had no knowledge of African American English because the errors were actually errors. Thus, when the child pronounced the word "potato," for example, "kapato," there was no doubt that such a production was strange. On the other hand, changing the /θ/ in the middle of words, final consonant clusters, and /ʒ/ (as in the word bigg<u>er</u>) goes beyond articulation therapy into English language teaching.

Language goals: The goals of language therapy should be designed to improve skills found to be impaired during language assessment. None of the features of African American English should be remediated. Usually the results of standardized language testing serve as the basis for developing IEP goals for children. Tests of vocabulary often yield errors in vocabulary and other tests point to needs for treatment in following directions, imitating sentences, generating sentences using selected words, analogies, irregular verb construction, absurdities, and a number of other skills. The speech-language clinician must be aware of the role vocabulary plays in all of these assessment tools and make sure that the children understand what is required of them to be successful in the assessment process. Often African American children fail in sentence construction because they are not familiar with the word or phrase to be used in the sentence. If the test is not a vocabulary test, the clinician must insure that the child knows the word. As discussed earlier in this text, assessment results for African American children often yield confusing results, particularly when a test has been given and it is not clear that the children understood what was required of them. It is for this reason that probing is necessary to determine whether the results obtained represent the child's linguistic knowledge rather than the inability to understand what is required.

Familiarity with African American English

Speech-language pathologists who work with Black children should be familiar enough with African American English to recognize deviation in phonology, syntax, semantics, and pragmatics. Since school-age African American children have been exposed to both African American English and standard English, their expressive language may be filled with inconsistencies. It is, therefore, the responsibility of the speech-language pathologist to make the distinction between language patterns and to recognize where interference occurs.

Many speech-language clinicians are unfamiliar with the characteristics of the language of the African American children with whom they work. A body of literature that spans more than thirty years is available in libraries, bookstores, and through various organizations, including the American Speech-Language-Hearing Association. In addition, workshops, lectures, and conferences are held throughout the country for clinicians who need to expand their knowledge of African American English. Also, school districts offer in-service training to teachers and speech-language clinicians in the school districts. There is no reason for speech-language clinicians to remain unknowledgeable of the language of the children they serve.

Regardless of the number of books, articles, and chapters the speech-language clinician reads or the number of workshops he or she attends, it is still necessary for the clinician to compare the language of the children he or she serves with the characteristics in the literature. Invariably, data collected for the research projects reported in the literature were collected from adolescents, adults, and sometimes children who live in different geographic regions. This means that the features of African American English observed in your region is likely to vary consistently from the ones reported. The clinician should look for consistency in the language of the children to determine what features are used by the children with whom the clinician works.

It is important for speech-language clinicians who work with African American children who speak African American English to learn as much as possible about the language in order to serve as a resource for teachers and families of children whether or not they have a speech or language disorder. No one expects the speech-language clinicians to use African American English, but they are expected to understand, translate (if necessary), and remediate speech-language disorders within a culturally rich environment.

How to Select Therapy Goals

The therapy goals selected by the speech-language pathologist are important for the intervention process. Goals must be appropriate, meaningful, and useful to the educational process.

Select goals that are meaningful for the child and family. All goals should reflect the needs of the child's home environment and the educational system. When a child has a limited vocabulary, for example, the words needed to be an effective communicator at home would be the first goals to consider. Names of important people in the home and community, events, objects, feelings, and concepts would be valuable additions to the language system. Vocabulary to be taught to the African American communicatively impaired child is not selected by the speech-language clinician according to vocabulary acquisition charts, but should be selected by the child, family, and teachers who will have specific needs for certain academic skills to be learned.

Select goals that emphasize classroom instruction. As the language skills develop, emphasis must be placed on preparing the children with language impairments to function in the classroom. Selecting vocabulary, instructions, problems, and language functions from the textbooks, workbooks, and classroom activities will serve a dual function. Not only will the children acquire the skill for communicative purposes, the skill is further reinforced through activities within the classroom, thus helping the children to be successful in school.

Select goals that emphasize content and use of language, de-emphasizing form . Seymour (1986) supported the notion that differences between African American English and standard English are in linguistic form, rather than content or use. Therefore, the teaching of linguistic form creates confusion between the two languages and promotes the teaching of standard English rather than remediating disorders. Content is the underlying meaning of the message, and use is the function the language performs. Although many children display errors or differences in linguistic form, they may still be effective communicators when the meaning and use are intact.

The methodology used to teach language skills to children with linguistic impairments should include meaningful information, presented in a manner that would be interesting to the children. The following suggestions will facilitate the language learning experience:

- Use meaningful stimuli from the culture. The clinician should select books, pictures, and games from the African American child's community. Books written for and about Black children offer them a chance to see pictures of themselves in books and read stories that may be familiar to them because of shared experiences with the characters in the books. When books are unavailable, the family photo albums can be a remarkable resource for teaching and practicing communication skills.
- Use multiple presentations. For each new skill being taught, the speech-language clinician should provide numerous opportunities for the child to experience it and numerous opportunities to practice it. For learning to take place, the two necessary ingredients are practice and opportunity. Daily practice in the classroom, during speech-language therapy, and at home will help the children to learn the skill faster. Each member of the team should encourage the children, provide opportunity to practice, and reward their attempts to employ the skill.
- Use stimuli in context. Context creates meaning for the language learner. "Repeated experiences using language in multiple natural settings will teach the child to make proper associations between utterances and the environmental events or stimuli they control" (McCormick & Schiefelbusch 1990, p. 193). The clinician should "use authentic, purposeful communication interaction to teach language skills" (Langdon & Chang, 1992, p. 272).
- Use interesting stimuli. Children should come to speech-language therapy with great excitement and interact with the clinician willingly. Talk with nondisabled African American children to determine what games they play, which heroes they appreciate, and what creates excitement. Using their suggestions, the clinician can re-create the activity within the

therapy program. Invite older children into therapy to demonstrate and participate in the activities.

- Use stimuli that involve activity. When speech-language pathologists observe Black children in the classroom, it is common to see them (particularly males) moving about. Teachers report that they experience difficulty having Black boys remain in their chairs. It is therefore necessary to encourage active involvement in the therapy session.

The discussion above relates to an "ideal" situation in which teachers are not overworked and available to perform all of the tasks suggested. It is incumbent upon the SLP to make every attempt to involve the teachers. On the other hand, when teachers are unavailable, the clinician should include teaching assistants, peers, volunteers, and whoever is available to assist with these situations. Clinicians must, however, keep teachers informed of what they are doing, whether in writing, in person, or by demonstration.

Role of the Family

The African American family is one of the most powerful institutions in the African American community. It serves as the source of strength for each of its members. The strong kinship bonds that encompass all of its members related by heritage, as well as individuals informally adopted into its folds, can involve any number of people. A single household may include numerous members of the extended family. The entire family is concerned with the welfare of each of its members, and each member is genuinely interested in the others. "The African American family's propensity to support one another during adjustment to disability may illuminate why so few African Americans who are disabled seek help from public or private rehabilitation agencies" (Turner & Alston 1992, p. 918).

It is uncommon for Black parents to seek speech-language services before the disabled children enter school, unless their language is different enough from peers to warrant it. In the schools, the parents first learn about the referral for problems when a request is made for permission to complete the assessment. The parents, believing that the speech-language pathologist has recognized a problem that might have an impact upon the child's education, offer their permission. Such permission is granted with the belief that the assessment will uncover problems that can be remediated, and thus make education more facile for their children.

Although the family members are willing to do what they can to help their children develop communication skills, they may not believe that they are capable of assisting children with their speech development. Occasionally parents themselves have been told by the schools that they had speech and language disorders as children, and have even been treated in special education. Under the circumstances, they are likely to believe that they are not capable of helping.

It is important for the clinician to explain to the parents what needs to be done, how it will be done, the expected outcome, and how the members of the family can help. In addition, the clinician should explain the potential consequences of failure to receive services. Families are more willing to participate when they understand what needs to be done and when they believe that they have something to contribute. It is the responsibility of the speech-language clinician to accept these important caregivers as significant members of the educational team.

Routinely, homework and progress reports should be sent home to keep parents informed. The clinician should not be disturbed when the homework is not returned, since keeping up with individual papers may be a major problem in some homes. When the parents see papers and notes from the speech-language pathologist, it shows them that the clinician is genuinely interested in the child and wants to help improve learning. Phone calls to the parents to report good performance are also appreciated. Invite the parents and other family members to observe therapy, but the clinician should not be discouraged when the parents fail to attend. Continue to invite them. They may surprise you with an unannounced visit.

Parents are likely to ask about the child's use of African American linguistic forms, referring to the language as "bad" English. Explain that children have a tendency to acquire the language of the people around them because it is heard the most frequently. Parents need to know that there is nothing wrong with African American English, that it is easier for the children to use because they are more familiar with it, and that it is an effective system of communication within the children's community. Explain that African American English is the children's native language and provides the basis for adding new languages. Assure the parents that standard English is being taught by the classroom teachers as part of the education curriculum.

Role of the Teacher

The teacher's role does not end when the child referred for language testing is enrolled in speech-language therapy. The work has just begun for the child, speech-language clinician, parents, and teachers. Included in the Individualized Educational Plan (IEP) should be recommendations for the teacher. Although the teachers have a complex role that can be very stressful, they are in the unique position to spend large blocks of time with the children.

Teachers should ensure that the speech-language clinician remains apprised of the skills being taught in the classroom. It is especially important for the speech-language clinician to be informed of language-related academic skills such as spelling words, reading themes and new words, mathematical concepts that need to be reinforced by the speech-language pathologist, and all workbook assignments. The clinician needs to examine the instructions in workbooks to ensure that the children are able to understand them, and therefore follow them. This also gives the speech-language pathologist a chance to incorporate classroom work into therapy, thus helping all of the children in the classroom, including those who receive speech-language therapy. This also gives the children one more chance to practice new skills and to use their new knowledge in the classroom.

The teacher should invite the speech-language clinician into the classroom to teach linguistic concepts to all of the children. In addition, the speech-language pathologist can teach phonics in the classroom and participate in reading groups to guarantee that children who are habituating newly learned speech sounds, for example, are reminded to use them while reading.

The teacher should meet routinely with the speech-language pathologist to discuss academic lesson plans, and also meet with individual students to develop proposals for activities that need to be performed in the classroom by the speech-language pathologist. In the schools, many of the contacts between the speech-language pathologist and teachers are initiated by the speech-language pathologist. The speech-language pathologist sometimes feels like an outsider and must make a special effort to communicate with teachers. Occasionally contacts are not well-received by the teachers, especially when there is resistance to having the children leave the classroom to go for speech therapy. When teachers reach out to the speech-language clinician, it shows that the teacher is willing to work with all members of the team for the benefit of the children. Additionally, when the teachers and speech-language clinicians work well together, the teachers are more willing to accept suggestions for developing programs to teach standard English and the SLP would be more willing to work with the teachers.

The teacher can be instrumental in helping the African American children who are in the minority in the classroom to accept their own communication styles and cultural patterns. Black children have been told in many ways by the dominant culture that they are "less" than other people and that their culture is inferior. When children enter school with negative beliefs about themselves, it is easy for teachers to add to feelings of inferiority unintentionally. How the teacher deals with the linguistic differences is critical for creating an atmosphere of acceptance of the children by the other students. Rejecting the children's language communicates a rejection of the children themselves, making it difficult for self-expression. The following suggestions will help the teacher communicate to the other children that cultural and linguistic diversity are positive realities.

- The teacher should emphasize diversity in the classroom, not dismiss it. Talk openly about similarities and differences. Read stories to the children and encourage all the children to read stories about various cultural groups.
- Discuss linguistic differences. Talk about different words in different languages and dialects with the children and give them a chance to hear differences. Explain that no language is better than any other language, but some languages have more social prestige than others. Encourage the children to learn other languages. Let the children know that all of them must master standard English for success in education and career.
- Teachers must accept the differences of the African American children. A policy of full recognition of African American English is the only way a teacher is able to transmit acceptance to the other children. Limited recognition communicates that the language is acceptable but has to be modified.
- Teachers should never "correct" the African American grammar or pronunciation in front of the other children in the classroom, even if all of the children in the classroom are African American and speak African American English. Such correction is ineffective and communicates disapproval by the teacher. Instead, the teacher should collect those examples of differences and use them for contrastive analysis during English classes.
- Set time aside for requiring the use of standard English skills that have been taught. Children learning new skills, whether they have a disorder or a difference, cannot be expected to incorporate them into conversational speech quickly or easily. Using new linguistic skills requires numerous opportunities and practice.

Oyer, Crowe, and Haas (1987) provide detailed suggestions for teachers of communicatively impaired children. These suggestions are applicable for linguistic diversity as well. They suggest that teachers should offer the following:

- The teacher should model appropriate speech and language within the classroom. This is a subtle way to transmit the message that good communication skills are desirable.
- The teacher should create an atmosphere in the classroom that encourages communication. Children should be able to express themselves in a nonthreatening environment.
- The teacher should accept (not tolerate) the children who have a communication disorder by allowing them to communicate without the threat that someone will interrupt or fail to listen to them.
- Encourage the other children in the classroom to accept the communicatively impaired child.

- The teacher should reinforce speech-language therapy goals in the classroom.
- The teacher should remind the child of therapy appointments.

Working with Children Who Do Not Qualify for SLP Services

Numerous African American school-age children are enrolled in speech-language therapy for the remediation of speech and language disorders in the absence of problems. Such treatment, in many cases, is directed toward the modification of recognized linguistic differences unrelated to disordered communication. In other words, the children are enrolled in speech-language therapy to learn English as a second language.

When African American children have no speech-language disorders, no speech or language therapy is required. In fact, no children should be labeled based on the unique linguistic features of the speech community. Only disorders should be treated as disorders, while standard English should be taught to all of the children in the classroom. Even standard English-speaking children need to learn the formal rules of the language that will allow them to write and speak it in formal settings. Language instruction for African American children can be done using second language acquisition procedures. When African American speaking parents insist that such linguistic differences used by the child constitute a disorder, it is clear that the parents do not accept the policy of full recognition and want their child to change enough to be perceived as using standard English. When this occurs, the clinician must make a decision to treat the child's difference on an elective basis (assuming that the clinician has room in the caseload), or to reject the student because no disorder is present. The speech-language clinicians who accept this role must realize that they have stepped outside their role as speech-language pathologists whose job is to remediate disordered communication, thus reducing the amount of time they are available to serve those children who are desperate for the services they provide.

Teaching Standard English as a Second Language

Teachers are responsible for teaching standard English to all of the children in the classroom. While it is clear that not all teachers speak standard English all of the time, we must assume that they know the rules and can apply them in the educational process. A teacher who is not familiar with standard English should not attempt to teach it. In this case, the administration of the school must decide how to insure that all of the children learn this prestigious language as part of the educational system.

A variety of second language teaching methods can be employed to help African American children acquire the rules of standard English. Some of these are discussed in the next chapter. Although the speech-language pathologists are not responsible for teaching standard English to nonhandicapped children, they can provide services indirectly by offering assistance to the teacher. Although the speech-language clinicians have no special expertise in second language acquisition, they do have experience teaching language and can serve as a resource for materials, information, and demonstrations.

African American English is similar to standard English in phonology, syntax, vocabulary, and pragmatics. On the other hand, significant differences exist (described earlier this book). When new language skills are taught to children, immediate habituation cannot be expected. This means that children cannot learn the rules of standard English one day and apply them consistently the next. Children need time to learn the rules and practice them in a non-threatening environment. It is therefore suggested that time should be set aside for the children to practice speaking standard English only at a certain level of consistency within a small frame of time. Children who are learning new linguistic information cannot be expected to apply it consistently throughout the day, particularly when the subject is history, for example. Teachers should not discourage classroom participation by interrupting the children to force them to use standard English rules.

Teachers often attempt to teach rules of standard grammar, for example, by "correcting" the patterns of the child's home language randomly and aggressively without explaining rules. The consequence of such teaching methods is confusion by the children. A second grade Black child I met never used the word "have" in conversation. Instead, she used the word "has" with both plural and singular nouns and pronouns. Accordingly, she created sentences, such as: "I has a ball," "you has a ball," "he has a ball," and "they has a ball." Such usage results from the child's conclusion that the word "have" should never be used. In response to the child's sentence, "John have the ball," the teacher corrected her by saying, "don't say have say has," so the child did. Correction, therefore, is among the least effective methods of teaching. This point is discussed further in Chapter 10.

Content of Instruction

Teachers and speech-language pathologists agree that African American children need to learn to read, write, and speak standard English. However, there is little agreement regarding the content or methods of instruction. There is also no agreement regarding the professional responsible for teaching standard English. The authors of this text believe that it is the responsibility of classroom teachers to teach English (preferably teachers of English as a second language) rather than the speech-language pathologist. Formal English is needed by all of the children in the classroom and should be taught in a positive manner.

It is clear that the children need to learn vocabulary, grammar, and pronunciation of standard English. In addition, they need to acquire the following:

1. **Effective communication:** To be effective, the speaker must be able to adjust communicative content and style to fit the situation and communicative partners (Hecht, Collier, & Ribeau 1993). In other words, the children must be able to use different levels of formality to meet the communicative need. They must speak at the most appropriate volume, use meaningful vocabulary, speak at the most suitable rate, and employ rules of syntax and pragmatics required in each situation. The children must also learn to communicate with the children in groups outside their own culture as well as with children within their own culture.

2. **Nonverbal behavior:** Children need to learn how to use their eyes with groups and individual listeners, when and how to touch communicative partners, the amount of distance between speakers and listeners, and how to listen both actively and passively according to the rules of the situation.

3. **Pragmatics:** Issues of topic initiation, maintenance, switching, and closing are important features of pragmatics to teach. In the early years of school, Black children need to be taught the rules of the classroom. Rules such as listening to the teacher, responding to the teacher, asking for help, requesting permission, taking turns in conversation, and so on. need to be taught.

4. **Figurative language:** Speakers of African American English often have an entirely different set of idioms from standard English. Common idioms such as "take a seat," "get in line," "raise your hand," or "line up" are typically not heard by Black children until they enter school. Teachers should pay attention to the idioms they use, since idioms are among the most confusing linguistic aspects needed for effective communication.

5. **Classroom rituals:** Hand raising to communicate the child's wish to answer questions asked by the teacher, to request permission, roll-call, entering and leaving the classroom are learned easily when the teacher teaches these rituals, if there is an expectation for the children to learn them.

INSTRUCTIONAL METHODS

The method of instruction is not as important as the atmosphere of acceptance in the classroom. It is crucial for the children to feel comfortable enough to make attempts to use standard English during the periods when it is required. Hamayan and Damico (1991) suggest that a "language usage plan" should be developed that allows the child increasing amounts of time to establish the new language (standard English). The usage plan includes the following:

- Educational support should be provided in the child's strongest language. It is not necessary for the instruction to be provided in African American English, but it is necessary for the children to understand what is going on in class.
- Children should never be separated from their most comfortable language.
- There is no need to choose a language. Black children should be able to use both languages both inside and outside the classroom. Children should be expected to use standard English only for those activities when standard English is being practiced and only at the level that is appropriate for the child's stage of learning. By high school, Black children should be able to speak in standard English in all of their classes if required. However, teachers should not expect them to continue to use this system in informal conversation with their peers.
- Create a language usage plan that will ensure that the children use standard English with expectations that are consistent with their stage of development. Do not expect more than the children are able to deliver.
- Provide an atmosphere in which children feel free to take risks in language use.
- Allow the children to make errors in standard English. Correcting children each time they make an error can be discouraging and may interfere with the willingness of the children to participate in oral activities.

Teachers can use a variety of techniques to teach standard English to African American children. Below are a few suggestions for using games and cultural practices observed in the African American community to make learning exciting because children are able to use cultural information to learn a new skill.

- **Rapping:** Rap is a stylish, rhythmic form of speaking in rhyme. The individual creating the rap selects a topic and develops poetry to a particular beat. In language training, the children can develop a rap as a group or each student can add a line. The bad news is that rap is seldom done in standard English, although this is possible. When using rap in language training, the children should be allowed to use African American phonology and intonation, but may be required to use a particular standard grammatical pattern.

- **Competitive language games:** African American children, particularly males, engage in competitive linguistic games that require comparative information. Games such as the dozens, sounding, and signifying (described earlier in this text) can be used in language teaching. The dozens requires the child to use comparatives and superlatives.

  Such comparisons can continue as long as the children can think of something to say, or are interested, or the teacher decides when the game is over. The dozens sometimes involves the use of profanity and is seldom played in standard English. However, the teacher determines the skills to be taught and can even determine the type of comparison to be made. The dozens can be a clean competitive game and does not have to include profane language. The teacher can collect material for the dozens from older children and the families.

- **Writing:** Journal writing is an effective method of teaching children to communicate using written language. Journals during the early grades are usually done in the children's language by teachers and read for the children. This allows the children to hear their own words read by someone else. The early journals are not translated into standard English, but written exactly as the children speak it. Later, the children can write their own journals, which can initiate discussion between the teachers and the children about their own vocabulary, spelling, and grammar. When the children read their own written language aloud, they often translate it into standard English for a White audience. At first, have the children read their journals aloud exactly as they have written them. After the teacher notes specific forms, the children can translate them into standard English. Teachers must be particularly carefully to communicate the message that both forms are acceptable, but different ways of communicating similar information (Hamayan & Damico 1991).

  Journals can be used by children to convey to someone else their feelings and thoughts. When read by the teacher, journal writing becomes an interactive process between the teacher and each child. Journals encourage children to communicate private information in a nonthreatening situation. African American children can be encouraged to use journals to learn and use standard English. They can be used to teach about a variety of topics. The journal begins with the child writing on a topic of interest. Teachers can respond to the child's messages, not the grammar. Each entry may be comments on previous entries, expansions, and various types of questions, including clarification questions. When the teachers fail to correct grammar, the children are encouraged to make longer entries.

It is believed that the children will eventually make fewer errors, write more, and eventually develop competence in writing in standard English.

- **Stories:** Storytelling is a well-established method of allowing the children to communicate in a language different from their own, as well as to communicate in a language similar to their own. Black children enjoy telling stories, particularly stories about events in the children's lives. In the Black community, children are encouraged to relate true stories, embellished for emphasis.

- **Thematic contexts:** Children may be taught language through the use of themes. Meaningful themes are developed by teachers over a period of time. During that time frame (perhaps a week or more), the children listen to, read, and tell stories on the topic, talk about it, write about it, view movies on the topic, and take field trips related to the theme. Themes should be meaningful to the children. If the theme is alligators, for example, the children can visit the zoo and learn about alligators through many sources. The concept of alligators can be combined with the teaching of syntactic forms, vocabulary, and other aspects.

SUMMARY

Black parents of communicatively disabled children do not tend to seek out speech and language services—the services usually come to them unsolicited. Health care is unavailable and inaccessible to Black families who live in low-income communities, therefore, speech-language services needed by the child are usually provided at school.

The speech-language pathologist is a member of a diagnostic and treatment team whose primary focus is the education of the child. Often the SLP is responsible for taking a leadership role to protect the child from other members of the team who choose to ignore the fact that the language and culture of African Americans are independent of the dominant American culture. The SLP may also have to assume a leadership role to work with parents and teachers to design a treatment plan that involves them in the selection and modification of therapy goals. The goals may include second language acquisition for African American children who do not have speech-language disabilities.

PRACTICAL APPLICATION

Speech-language pathologists and teachers must work together to ensure that African American children gain everything they need while in school. African American children are quite proficient in their home language when they enter school and should be encouraged to use it to express themselves in the classroom. It is clear that spontaneity and creativity are impaired when children are required to speak in an unfamiliar language in the classroom. When the children are taught standard English and provided numerous opportunities to use the language in non-threatening situations, they can eventually be required to employ standard English in all classes while at school. However, teachers should not expect them to use standard English outside the classroom. It is also clear that children cannot use standard English when it is not taught. Many African Americans have learned standard English on their own, but with a great deal of frustration and difficulty. Only the most motivated individuals accomplish this task, while many African Americans believe that they know it when, in fact, they do not. Such individuals apply the rules of grammar inconsistently and never master the phonological system. Teaching standard English can assist Black children to learn all of the contrasting features of standard English so they can apply the rules consistently and volitionally when needed.

Rather than enrolling African American children in speech-language therapy to learn standard English, it is more efficient for the skills to be taught by teachers in the classroom. This would provide teachers the opportunity to teach the language to all the children, including African American children.

Speech-language clinicians can serve as a resource for teachers by assisting them with lesson plans, themes, and even assistance in the classroom. In addition, when children have communicative disorders, the speech-language pathologist is the only professional prepared to teach the children their native language.

REFERENCES

Bailey, E. (1991). *Urban African American Health Care*. Lanham, MD: University Press of America.

Freeman, H., Bernard, R., Matory, W., Smith, F., Whitico, J., Yancy, A., & Bond, L. (1982). Physician manpower needs of the nation: Position paper of the surgical section of the *Journal of the National Medical Association*, 74: 617–619.

Guendelman, S., & Schwalbe, J. (1986). Medical care utilization by Hispanic children: How does it differ from black and white peers? *Medical Care*, 24: 925–940.

Hamayan, E., & Damico, J.S. (1991). *Limiting Bias in the Assessment of Bilingual Students*. Austin, TX: PRO-ED.

Hecht, M., Collier, M. & Ribeau, S. (1993). *African American Communication*. Newbury Park, CA: Sage Publications.

Langdon, H., & Chang, L. (1992). *Hispanic Children and Adults with Communication Disorders*. Gaithersburg, MD: Aspen Publishers.

McCormick, L., & Schiefelbusch, R. (1990). *Early Language Intervention*. Columbus, OH: Merrill.

Meyerson, M., & Weddington, G. (1986). Birth defects, communication disorders and Black children. *Journal of the National Medical Association*, 78 (5): 409–419.

Oyer, H., Crowe, B., & Haas, W. (1987). *Speech, Language and Hearing Disorders: A Guide for the Teacher*. Boston: College-Hill Publications.

Seymour, H. (1986). Clinical intervention for language disorders among nonstandard speakers of English. In O. Taylor (ed.), *Communication Disorders in Culturally Diverse Populations* (pp. 135–153). San Diego: College Hill Press.

Snow, L. (1981). Folk medical beliefs and their implications for the care of patients. In G. Henderson & M. Primeaux, *Transcultural Health Care* (pp. 78–101). Menlo Park, CA: Addison-Wesley.

Terrell, S., & Terrell, F. (1993). African American Cultures. In D. Battle (ed.), *Communication Disorders in Multicultural Populations* (pp 3–37). Boston: Andover Medical Publishers.

Thomas, D. (1981). Black American patient care. In G. Henderson & M. Primeaux (eds.), *Transcultural Health Care* (pp 209–223). Menlo Park, CA: Addison-Wesley.

Turner, W., & Alston, R. (1992). The role of the family in psychosocial adaptation to physical disabilities for African Americans. *Journal of the National Medical Association*, 86 (12): 915–918.

Waldman, H. (1992). Differences in the health status of black and white children. *Journal of Dentistry for Children*, 59 (5): 369–372.

White-Means, S., Thornton, M., & Yeo, J. (1989). Black and Hispanic use of the hospital emergency room. *Journal of the National Medical Association*, 81: 72–80.

10

FACILITATING STANDARD ENGLISH ACQUISITION FOR AFRICAN AMERICAN CHILDREN

Chapter Overview

Upon reading this chapter you will gain understanding of:

- The nature of standard English, taking into account the difference between formal and informal standards
- The difference between language learning and language acquisition
- The potential for harm in correcting, and other traditional methods of teaching standard English
- Effective ways of teaching standard English to speakers of other dialects based on language acquisition theory
- The merits of using methods associated with foreign language teaching for teaching standard English to speakers of African American English
- Harmless approaches to teaching reading and writing.

Upwardly mobile speakers of certain dialects sometimes seek to alter their native dialectal patterns to produce a more acceptable accent, or acquire a second, higher-prestige dialect for business purposes. Programs to develop bidialectalism in African American children often have the explicit purpose of giving the children a variety of English that will prove advantageous in adult life. Teachers facing the prospect of teaching AAE-speaking children are challenged to find effective ways of developing standard English skills in such children. In this chapter we shall explore that challenge in terms of its impli-

	comprehension	*production*
spoken	listening	speaking
written	reading	writing

FIGURE 10-1   Fourfold paradigm of language development.

cations for a policy of full recognition. The answers that we offer are derived from key implications of recent work in language acquisition theory, that is, that language is not taught, but acquired.

One of the most controversial aspects of a policy of full recognition of AAE is the belief that it neglects the development of proficiency in Standard English. Educators who advocate for full recognition accept and respect the native language of African American children and try to teach in a manner that fully exploits its educational potential. They are not opposed, however, to teaching African American children Standard English. What is distinctive about the policy of full recognition is its insistence on doing no harm to African American children in the process of teaching them.

The policy of full recognition may be fairly summarized as a policy of leaving AAE alone, especially in the sense of doing no harm. The policy of leaving it alone applies most strictly to spoken language. To a lesser degree it also applies to written language. As we proceed with the discussion of these points it will be convenient to think of language development taking place within a fourfold paradigm represented by Figure 10-1:

A working assumption will be that the spoken language that AAE-speaking children bring to the classroom is adequate for the initiation of instruction in all areas including reading and writing. Teachers do not have to engage in any classroom practices that overtly or by implication impose a negative evaluation upon AAE, or in some other way are potentially harmful. Such practices could include correcting AAE features of children's speech as well as classifying dialectal features as "bad," "substandard," or "incorrect." Some alternative "harmless" practices are suggested that promise to provide impetus to the development of AAE speakers' language skills in ways that will serve their present and future academic and career development.

STANDARD ENGLISH

It was pointed out in Chapter 2 that everyone speaks a dialect and that all dialects are equal. When we look closely at prevailing standards of English usage, however, it is clear that some dialects are more equal than others in that they favor members of certain ethnic groups and socioeconomic classes (Sedley 1990; Smitherman 1977). Dialects spoken by the dominant groups and classes of society are often labeled standard English. The dialects of poor and despised members of society, although technically equal to standard dialects, tend to be labeled *nonstandard dialects*, or *vernaculars* (Wolfram, 1991). The term standard English is also used in reference to a kind of English that is used mainly in writing.

To avoid confusion between the two uses of the term standard English, some linguists make a distinction between a *formal standard* and an *informal standard*. The formal standard is not spoken by anyone as a native language. It is not a dialect, but a style of English, reserved for use in written communication, and on special occasions where proper speech is expected. The formal standard conforms to prescriptive rules, including those that are frequently broken in informal standard speech, and contains lexical forms and syntactic patterns that do not often occur in spoken language.

The informal standard may be defined in terms of Chomsky's theory of linguistic competence as consisting of those rules and elements that specify what "sounds right" to educated middle-class speakers of the dialects in question. Although it is prestigious, the informal standard does not conform to all prescriptive rules. As noted in Chapter 2, certain rules, such as the preference of *whom* over *who* for objects and the prohibition against ending a sentence with a preposition, are frequently violated by the "best" speakers.

CORRECTING

One way of leaving AAE alone is to refrain from correcting children's speech when they are talking. The practice of correcting is traditionally associated with teaching standard English. There is a significant amount of linguistic evidence, however, that correcting is not very effective and probably is harmful (Krashen 1992). Children are frequently observed receiving corrective feedback from caregivers and repeatedly making the same error after every correction. Experienced classroom teachers frequently report cases in which they assign to second language learners the task of correcting all the errors marked on a written work, and then seeing the same kinds of errors occur, at the same frequency, in subsequent work. Correction given before learners are ready to benefit from it seems to be in vain. Based on such evidence, advocates of full recognition advise teachers to refrain from correcting students and acquire more effective methods of teaching standard English.

Calling upon teachers to desist from correcting students' language errors is not a call for acceptance of poor performance. More than anything, it is a call for teachers to be very careful not to miscommunicate to students a dislike or disdain for an integral part of their identity and self-concept. Many students learn, as a consequence of constantly being corrected by teachers and authority figures, that their speech and writing leaves something to be desired—not only persons of low socioeconomic status, but middle-and upper-class persons as well. Speakers of what are considered "better" varieties of English, however, may be able to endure the adverse effects of traditional instruction without suffering great damage. For them, the experience of being corrected by parents and teachers may serve as a positive incentive to learn and apply rules of correct usage. For children who already suffer from low self-esteem because of their position in society, however, the experience of being constantly corrected can be devastating.

While educators work in other ways to counteract the devaluing of African American children embedded in social reality, they may contribute to the continued devaluing of African American language by teaching a language arts curriculum based on the premise that the children's language is bad. Studies of Black self-concept suggest that African American children need experiences that boost their self-esteem, not lower it. Several ways of helping students improve their language output without damaging their self esteem are discussed below. The discussion presupposes a basic understanding of some general principles of language acquisition.

LANGUAGE ACQUISITION

Recent work in linguistics has focused on the problem of accounting for how individuals acquire their linguistic competence, that is, explaining how what we have been calling the grammar in your head gets there. It is important to keep in mind that the consciously taught prescriptive grammar discussed in Chapter 2 only accounts for a small part of what speakers know, and that most of what we know about our native language is unconscious and intuitive.

Scholars such as Krashen (1992) make an important distinction between language *acquisition* and language *learning*. Acquisition occurs automatically when speakers receive what Krashen calls *comprehensible input*. That is, when a new speaker is exposed to a token of the language in a context that makes it understandable, he or she acquires that much of the language. For instance, someone who does not know Spanish and hears the Spanish word *lobo* "wolf" uttered in connection with a picture of a wolf may comprehend its meaning, and thereby acquire that much of the Spanish language.

One important implication of language acquisition theory for teaching is that much of what we know of a language is not taught, but acquired. It was noted in Chapter 2 that the system of English grammar is so complex that no linguist has come close to a complete explicit description of it. Native speakers acquire a good part of the system before they begin their formal schooling, and parents lack the conscious knowledge of descriptive grammar necessary to consciously teach it to their children. Rather than teach children their native language, parents facilitate their acquisition of it by providing comprehensible input. The children see the parents *model* the language in contexts that makes it comprehensible, and they pick it up, so to speak, automatically. Perhaps teachers would be more successful if they were willing to facilitate their students' acquisition of standard English than to attempt to teach it to them.

In addition to the distinction between acquisition and learning, language acquisition theory makes several other claims that have important implications for teaching. One of them is the so-called *critical age hypothesis* (Lennenberg 1967), which attempts to explain why young children seem to be much more capable than adults and their adolescent peers of acquiring full proficiency in a language. Young bilingual children typically attain native-like control over both of their languages. That is, they speak either of two different languages fluently, unhesitatingly, and with no trace of a foreign accent. Individuals who attempt to master a second language after puberty may attain a high level of proficiency but rarely attain the capability to produce native-like, unaccented speech. The traditional place of foreign language instruction in the secondary school curriculum fails to take advantage of the special language acquisition capabilities of young children. In recent times, a program for teaching *Foreign Language in Elementary School* (FLES), designed to exploit those capabilities, has gained currency in some school districts.

The critical age hypothesis advances a biological explanation for the seemingly superior ability of young children to acquire language. The fundamental claim is that the area of the brain in which language is located atrophies around puberty with the result that the ability to acquire language is greatly diminished. Another explanation of the same phenomenon in social rather than biological terms is suggested by Krashen's claim that the effectiveness of language acquisition, given the availability of comprehensible input, depends crucially on the state of what he calls the *affective filter*. The basic idea is that, other things being equal, language acquisition is more effective when the learner feels good, or has a positive affective state. When the learner is in a state of nervousness, anxiety, tension, or some other affectively negative situation, the availability of comprehensible input is less likely to lead to acquisition.

The affective filter hypothesis may explain differences between children and adults in the success of their language acquisition by suggesting that young children are generally less inhibited by foreign language experiences than older persons. Rather than react with fear and apprehension to people producing what initially appears to be gibberish, children may respond with fascination and notice clues in the environment that make the language input at least somewhat comprehensible, gradually leading to their acquisition of the language. The idea that learning should be fun is basic and noncontroversial, although teachers are always challenged to maintain a curriculum that is affectively as well as intellectually rich. The affective filter hypothesis not only reinforces the challenge to infuse enjoyment into lessons, it also promises the reward of more effective language instruction.

Teachers seeking insights from language acquisition theory have developed a variety of methods that are consistent with what is known as the *natural approach* to language instruction. The basic idea is to structure classroom experiences that take cues from the way human beings naturally acquire their native language. As noted above, natural language acquisition occurs automatically, without any conscious effort of parents to teach or for children to learn. The idea of "picking up a language" aptly characterizes the way that language is acquired under natural conditions. Teaching methods following the natural approach discourage attempting to consciously instill correct patterns through memorization, drill, and corrective feedback, and encourage the use of visuals, games, and simulation of real-world communication situation.

One important insight derived from the study of natural language acquisition is the fact that comprehension develops ahead of production. Applied to the classroom, this fact suggests that students should be given opportunities to passively absorb the language, so to speak, before they are challenged to actively engage in dialogues. One method that facilitates such passive involvement is known as *total physical response* (TPR). Students are taught to understand the target language by learning to respond to commands such as "stand up," "raise your hand," "touch your nose," "go to the board," "write your name," and so on.

A method of teaching English as a second language using principles of the natural approach is known as *Sheltered English*. The basic idea of Sheltered English is that teachers are trained to teach academic subjects such as math and history to students with limited knowledge of English. Teachers skilled in this method are capable of delivering lesson content in comprehensible English without detracting from the academic quality of the instruction. Because the teacher's English is comprehensible, the students acquire English and develop their English proficiency at the same time that they are learning the academic content of the lesson.

We shall further discuss Sheltered English and other methods inspired by the natural approach to language teaching later in this chapter. Having raised the issue of correcting in the introductory section, and having provided some justification for discouraging it based on language acquisition theory in this section, we suggest in the next section a promising alternative to correcting based on the natural approach.

MODELING

When children acquire their native language under natural conditions, their parents, older siblings, and other caregivers serve not only as sources of the comprehensible input considered necessary for acquisition to occur, but also serve as models of the language that the children will eventually speak. It is important to repeat and underscore the fact that language is not consciously taught but automatically picked up from the input provided by models and the context clues that make it comprehensible. Initially, the children's output is reduced, limited, and error-filled. Eventually, however, largely before formal schooling begins, the children have incorporated much of the complexities of the adult language into their budding linguistic competence.

When children begin school, they will still require further language instruction in order to succeed academically and eventually in the adult world. Teachers can fulfill a good part of their responsibility for the continuing language development of their students by modeling the kind of English that is expected in the school environment. The effectiveness of such modeling may not be immediately apparent since language development is often gradual and imperceptible. Teachers may be tempted to correct errors that are developmental in nature and are likely to resist correction until the students progress beyond their present stage of development. Such teachers are best advised, however, to resist such temptation, and patiently trust that their presence as models of standard English is sufficient to insure that the usage they model will eventually emerge in the English of their students. It may not emerge during the term that the students are under their tutelage, but eventually it will. At least that is the outcome predicted by studies of natural language acquisition.

In addition to simply speaking correctly in the presence of students, teachers may model in more conscious and proactive ways. In situations directly following correctable usage by a student, teachers may be prepared to respond in other ways that do not have the potentially demeaning, or anxiety-producing effects of correcting. For instance, if a student says

"Mr. Clark, I brung my homework."

Mr. Clark might, instead of responding in the traditional manner "You *what*? *brung*?" or the like, putting the child on the spot, model the correct form *brought*, in his response, for example

"Oh, that's great. You brought your homework."

Such modeling, in the immediate context following the student's incorrect usage occurs at a time when the student is most likely to see the contrasting form of his usage to that of the teacher. Such modeling appears to be just as likely as a harsher form of traditional correcting to contribute to permanent development of standard usage by the child.

ROLE PLAYING

Recent work in language acquisition from a sociolinguistic perspective (Anderson 1990) indicates that children acquire, at a rather early age, the ability to vary their linguistic output according to the social roles of the participants in the speech event. Children quickly become aware of differences in the speech of persons in various roles such as the doctor, the nurse, the grocery clerk, and the school principal. Such studies suggest that a child's acquisition of standard English might be facilitated by role-playing activities that focus attention upon the stylistic variation in the English spoken by persons in various roles.

As children engage in role playing they can be led to discuss how their English varies according to role differences and learn to apply labels such as standard English, slang, or other labels to different varieties. Certain exotic roles such as sports idol, rap artist, and disc jockey might prove more interesting to children than more conventional roles. The exotic roles can be just as effective as more conventional roles in stimulating useful discussions of language variation. What is most promising about role-playing activities, within a policy of full recognition of AAE, is the opportunities that it opens up for discussing standard and nonstandard English in an objective, neutral, and relatively harmless manner.

IMMERSION AND GROUPING STRATEGIES THAT FACILITATE LANGUAGE ACQUISITION

When language is acquired under natural conditions, a variety of significant persons in addition to teachers serve as models and as sources of comprehensible input for new learners. Krashen (1992) reminds us of the common phenomenon of immigrants and long-term visitors to foreign countries acquiring proficiency in a host language totally through *immersion*, without receiving any formal instruction. Educators planning instructional programs for newcomers and immigrants, as well as citizens who are not native speakers of standard English, should take into account the potential for involving learners in immersion experiences both within and outside of the classroom.

Within the classroom, teachers can promote immersion-like experiences by assigning students to mixed-level groups in which students with lower levels of proficiency may benefit from input provided by peers who model native or near-native proficiency. Teachers who are accustomed to presenting lessons designed for students at the same level, in homogeneous groups, may be uncomfortable with the idea of mixed-level groups. A further obstacle to grouping students of mixed levels of language proficiency may stem from established programs for educating students of Limited English Proficiency (LEP) in separate classrooms. Schools with separate instructional programs for LEP students would have to implement a policy of mainstreaming such students in order to maximize mixed-level grouping practices in mainstream English classes.

Another way in which students are sometimes assigned to homogeneous groups outside of the mainstream school curriculum is through placement in speech therapy and other forms of special education. Such placements are relevant to the present discussion because of evidence that all too often AAE speakers are inappropriately placed in special education because of nonstandard features of their dialect. In later chapters on assessment and school practices we present detailed statistics on the overrepresentation of African American students in special education. Here we only wish to underscore the fact that school practices remove AAE speakers from mainstream classes may have the inadvertent consequence of minimizing opportunities for them to benefit from the immersion-like qualities of mixed-level student groupings.

Outside of the classroom, immigrant students may find some of the richest opportunities to improve their English proficiency through immersion. Such opportunities are minimized, however, to the extent that students isolate themselves to social interaction within ethnic enclaves where mainstream English is rarely heard. The mere fact of their residency in the country, however, guarantees that they will receive considerably more English immersion than students of English as a foreign language in a non-English-speaking country. At a minimum, such students will encounter English when transacting necessary business at shopping centers, schools, and governmental agencies, and passively from the mass media of television and radio. Native-born AAE speakers acquire standard English under conditions of limited opportunity for immersion similar to that of immigrants.

Educators should consider every possibility for supplementing in-class effort to facilitate standard English acquisition by AAE speakers by planning and/or encouraging field experiences that embody opportunities for immersion in a standard English environment. Such field experiences could include activities attended by students from various ethnic backgrounds that include opportunities for cross-cultural interaction, as well as reciprocal visits between members of language minority and mainstream students on a group or individual basis.

Should foreign language teaching methods be used for the teaching of standard English to AAE speakers? Through the years, proposals have been advanced for teaching standard English to speakers of African American English based on the assumption that, for all practical purposes, African American English is a foreign language. There are good and valid reasons for creating techniques for teaching African American children using methods inspired by second language teaching. Educators, however, should be cautious about carrying the analogy too far. One obvious area where the analogy breaks down is that African American children, unlike children for whom English is a second language, begin their schooling with a language that is, strictly speaking, English (Baugh 1995). Furthermore, their language has a high degree of similarity with classroom English, so much so that the children can understand most of what is said to them by teachers. Likewise, teachers can understand most, if not all, of what AAE-speaking children say to them. Whatever barriers to comprehension might exist between standard-English speaking teachers and AAE-speaking children can be bridged as easily by teaching AAE to the teachers as it can by teaching the children standard English.

In the case of children for whom English truly is a second language, it is necessary to make special provisions in the instructional program in order for them to *understand* the language of instruction. There is no corresponding need, however, to instill standard English as a second language into African American children. A child limited to AAE does not have the same kind of barrier to participation in an English-medium science class as would be faced by a child limited to a different native language such as Vietnamese.

Programs to develop standard English proficiency in Black English speakers are often motivated as much by a desire to make the students' language acceptable to teachers and future employers as it is by a genuine need to bridge a communication barrier posed by differences in the standard and vernacular varieties of English. There is great potential for exploiting the general implications of language acquisition theory for classroom teaching. In particular, it has been noted that such practices as modeling and role playing are consistent with the natural approach to language instruction, and that approach has received more attention from foreign language professionals and linguists than from English language arts teachers. Many of the teaching practices associated with sheltered English, such as heavy use of visuals and other kinds of contextual clues to aid comprehension would be beneficial to any student. Some teaching methods traditionally associated with foreign language instruction, such as pattern-practice drills and correcting, are discouraged, however, by advocates of the natural approach to learning a second language. In the following section we discuss a particular claim of language acquisition theory with implications for teaching writing known as the reading hypothesis.

THE READING HYPOTHESIS

Krashen's (1992) claim that language acquisition is facilitated by comprehensible input applies primarily to spoken language. It suggests that learners, given time and sufficient input, will begin to speak without any conscious or deliberate efforts to teach them how and without forcing them to practice. When applied to written rather than spoken language, Krashen's theory implies that if a learner is given sufficient input in the form of comprehensible reading material, the child will become more skilled, not only in reading, but in writing as well. Just as learners will use contextual clues in the speech situation to comprehend speech containing new forms of spoken language and eventually acquire those new forms, they will use contextual clues on the printed page to acquire new words in written form.

In practical terms, the reading hypothesis suggests that teachers should allow time for students to engage in free reading on the assumption that the more they read, the more skilled they will become in all aspects of written language including vocabulary development and spelling. According to this theory, children who read a great deal will expand their vocabulary without necessarily participating in vocabulary-building lesson activities and will become better spellers without consciously attempting to master lists of spelling words. Teachers who want to experiment with this approach only need to set up a reading center in their classroom and set aside times for free reading. According to Krashen, popular reading material such as comic books can be as effective as more serious kinds of material in promoting the acquisition of written language. If some students can only be motivated to read popular literature, it might be prudent for a teacher to include such literature in the reading center on the theory that it is better to read comic books than no books.

As it relates to the policy of leaving AAE alone, the reading hypothesis suggests a way in which teachers can facilitate the development of reading and writing skills for AAE-speaking children without assaulting their linguistic self-esteem. Just as they can refrain from correcting spoken language utilizing harmless approaches such as modeling and role playing activities, they can also refrain from harmful ways of correcting children's written output and concentrate on the goal of making them avid readers, confident that the written language they initially absorb passively through reading will eventually be produced actively as writing.

THE WRITING PROCESS

It was noted above that the policy of leaving AAE alone applies most categorically to children's spoken language, and to a lesser degree to their written language. Recent approaches to writing instruction discourage traditional methods of correcting student writing, such as the use of a red pencil to mark all of the grammatical, mechanical, or stylistic flaws in a student's writing assignment. Such heavy-handed correcting is now generally recognized as ineffective.

Recent approaches to teaching writing rely less on the red pencil than on the students' learning to see writing as a process and to value constructive feedback. Some students are reluctant to engage in writing because of previous experiences in which a teacher has negatively marked or commented on their work. Often such experiences result in students feeling that their language is unacceptable to teachers and likely to elicit humiliating reactions whenever it is written down. In the worst cases, such students have come to see themselves as afflicted with "bad" grammar, perhaps hopelessly so. Teachers can eliminate a great deal of the stress and anxiety that such students are conditioned to expect by teaching writing as a process.

When students are taught writing as a process, they learn that grammar and mechanics are not the only or even the major considerations in the evaluation of written work. They learn that originality and creativity, ingenious development of a main point, and effective use of details are also important components of good writing. By receiving positive feedback on other aspects of their writing, students who feel bad about their grammar may come to feel that they are more capable of achieving success and overcome previous inhibitions.

Students who are reluctant to write because they anticipate negative comments on their grammar may be encouraged by being instructed to produce a rough draft and told that they need not be concerned about grammar at the rough draft stage. After all, they can expect the rough draft to undergo one or more major revisions before it is ready to be edited and proofread. It would be a waste of time to correct the grammar on a sentence or paragraph that may later be totally changed or eliminated. Students should learn to wait until they are sure that their sentences and paragraphs are in final form before they set out to correct any errors of grammar or mechanics.

When students are learning the writing process, they can be told that it is all right to compose their rough draft freely in whatever dialect they speak naturally with the understanding that they will edit it later to the standards of written English. Teachers may decide and communicate to students how much credit they will receive for the rough draft and each subsequent revision of their work, and how much they can expect to be marked down, if at all, for dialectal patterns of their spoken language that appear in their written work. Teachers may set goals, in collaboration with students, for mastery of particular rules of grammar and refrain from grading students negatively for grammar errors in areas that they have not mastered. If instruction is adequately planned, there is no need for the language of AAE speakers or other vernacular speakers to be devalued in the process of their learning to produce standard written English.

Is oral proficiency in standard English a prerequisite to reading and writing? Programs to develop bidialectalism in African American students are sometimes predicated on the assumption that it is necessary for students to learn to speak standard English before they can learn to read and write it. The language that AAE-speaking children bring with them to school is fully adequate, however, for immediate classroom purposes, including learning to read and write standard English. As long as they are capable of speaking standard English by the time they make the transition from school to work, they will be prepared to meet the expectations of employers in job interview situations. Teachers should be clear on their reasons for valuing bidialectalism and be careful not to inappropriately use oral proficiency in standard English as a criterion for academic placement and advancement.

It was noted above that the formal standard that governs written and formal spoken language is different than any spoken dialect. Whenever speakers of American English learn to read and write, they learn to acquire a variety of English that differs in certain respects from their informal spoken language. In general, students learn to read by learning to match the sound-meaning correspondences of their spoken language with a single set of visual symbols consisting of various combination of letters on the printed page.

Learning to read is a complex phenomenon that is taken up in greater depth in later chapters. For present purposes, we shall focus upon the aspect of reading that entails the ability to decode visual symbols corresponding to forms and elements of spoken language. At the elementary level of decoding, Standard Written English (SWE) has a high degree of *dialect neutrality*. Most of the basic vocabulary that appears in beginning reading material is common to all dialects, including AAE. The word *house*, for example, has a variety of dialectal pronunciations, represented by the phonetic transcriptions [haws], [hæws] and [hUws]. The written word is equally accessible to speakers of the various pronunciations, who simply learn to match their particular dialectal pronunciation to a dialectally neutral visual form. Many other basic words such as *mouse, brown, loud*, and *clown* share the dialectal variability of the word house.

Some dialect features affect speakers of some dialects more than others. In certain dialects, pairs of words such as *marry* and *merry* are pronounced differently, whereas in other dialects such pairs are pronounced the same, that is, as homonyms. Learning to spell such pairs of words correctly is clearly an easier task for speakers who pronounce them differently than for those who pronounce them the same. The good news is that such features are distributed among dialects in such a way that all speakers get their fair share of difficult cases.

Speakers of dialects that pronounce words like *marry* and *merry* alike tend to have distinct pronunciations for pairs of words like *horse* and *hoarse*, or *caught* and *cot*. Conversely, many speakers who pronounce the latter words alike, and have difficulty spelling them, pronounce words like *marry* and *merry* differently. In the balance therefore, the dialect neutrality of SWE is not affected by differences in the correspondences between spoken and written forms of particular words.

The neutrality of SWE with respect to differences in spoken language is greatest with dialects that conform to expectation of the informal standard. The kinds of dialect differences in pronunciation discussed in the preceding paragraphs tend to be acceptable to teachers in the dialect areas where the features are common. Speakers of some dialects, for example, do not pronounce the *r* in words like *park*. Such speakers do not have to learn the standard 'r-full' pronunciation of such words before they learn to read and write. As a rule, teachers do not attempt to teach students to pronounce such words differently as a prerequisite for their learning to read them correctly.

Some teachers may be less willing to accept dialectal variation in the pronunciation of words that conform to dialects that they consider nonstandard than they are to accept variation within the range of what they consider standard. Some teachers, for instance, may accept uncritically the widespread attitude that the word *creek* has a correct pronunciation that is violated by speakers who employ the pronunciation [krIk]. Such teachers may go as far as to reject the reading performance of a student who reads a word such as *creek* with what he or she considers incorrect pronunciation. Johnson (1975) points out the inequity of teaching practices that inappropriately classify as reading failure what is better characterized as *dialectal interference*.

An example of dialectal interference in reading by an AAE student involves the possessive pronoun *their*, which in AAE is the same as the subject pronoun they, as illustrated by sentences 1 and 2.

1. *They not ready.* "They're not ready."
2. *They mamma not ready.* "Their mother is not ready."

In Johnson's view, a teacher should accept as correct a sentence such as *their daddy is at home*, read as "they daddy is at home" by an AAE speaker. The difference should not be considered an error but a case of dialectal interference.

Well-meaning programs to instill *standard English proficiency* in AAE-speaking children sometimes make a conscious effort to "standardize" the children's oral language by replacing stigmatized pronunciations, such as [mawf] for *mouth*, with what is considered the standard pronunciation. It should be clear from the preceding discussion, however, that a student who produces the oral form [mawf] in response to the visual stimulus mouth is reading the word correctly. The continuing existence of teachers who might judge it as an instance of reading failure might provide some justification for a program to make students immune to such teachers, but a better and fairer way to address that problem seems to be training teachers to take dialectal interference into account in the assessment of reading success (Dandy 1991).

Each teacher and each school district will ultimately have to decide what goals and priorities they want to set for the acquisition of standard English proficiency by AAE speakers and what special intervention programs, if any, to implement toward that end. The foregoing discussion has examined the extent to which it might be necessary or desirable to modify the oral language of AAE speakers in anticipation of the requirements of Standard English reading material. In the next section we discuss a range of approaches to facilitating reading success for AAE speakers by making written material available in AAE, and on topics drawn from African American culture.

DIALECT READERS AND MULTICULTURAL LITERATURE

The idea of producing initial reading material in AAE derives directly from the recognition of AAE as a language in its own right, and the corresponding right of AAE speakers to be taught in a language that they understand. In bilingual education programs, children who speak languages other than English are taught to read in their native language and have access to initial reading material written in that language. The idea of using *dialect readers* to teach African American children to read was enthusiastically endorsed by a group of linguists who contributed to a volume on the proposal (Baratz & Shuy 1969). One issue discussed by the contributors to Baratz and Shuy is the choice of orthography, that is, the question of how AAE should be represented on the printed page. The general consensus of those linguists is that conventional English spelling would best serve the needs of students whose ultimate goal is to be able to read texts in standard English.

Given the above-mentioned dialect neutrality of written English and the fact that most of the core vocabulary of AAE is the same as that of mainstream English, there is no reason to expect that the written form of individual words should cause any more difficulty for AAE speakers than for speakers of other dialects. The greatest differences between AAE and Standard English are grammatical. The promise of dialect readers for easing the task of teaching AAE speakers to read, therefore, lies in the potential they offer for replacing standard English grammatical constructions with AAE equivalents when there are significant differences. As an illustration of how pervasive such differences may be, consider the following sample text in its Standard English and AAE versions.

SAMPLE TEXT: STANDARD ENGLISH VERSION

Alisha and Tamara are best friends. Alisha is nine years old. Tamara is nine too. Alisha is taller than Tamara. Alisha lives near the school. Tamara lives near the park. Tamara likes to play baseball. Alisha likes to play baseball too. Yesterday Alisha and Tamara were at the park. They were playing baseball. They were having fun.

SAMPLE TEXT: AAE VERSION

Alisha and Tamara best friends. Alisha nine years old. Tamara nine too. Alisha taller than Tamara. Alisha live close to the school. Tamara live close to the park. Tamara like to play baseball. Alisha like to play baseball too. Yesterday Alisha and Tamara was at the park. They was playin' baseball. They was havin' fun.

AAE-speaking children who achieve proficiency in reading material written in AAE, may still have problems reading texts written in standard English, but they would clearly be better prepared for the standard English texts. They would be able to transfer most of their previously learned core vocabulary, and lessons could focus on teaching grammatical patterns that are unfamiliar to AAE speakers.

One problem with the dialect readers proposal stems from the novelty for many Americans of recognizing AAE as a language in its own right. Persons conditioned to mislabel AAE as "bad" English may be confused by texts written in AAE and see them as efforts to teach an inferior form of English to Black children. Such confusion seems to have stymied the earliest efforts to implement the dialect readers proposal. The failure of a pilot series of dialect readers to gain widespread acceptance is often attributed to Black parents' rejection of the concept (Fasold 1990; Rickford & Rickford 1995). In more general terms, however, such rejection seems to be a consequence of the fact that American society does not yet recognize AAE as a medium of classroom instruction.

One particular version of the dialect reader proposal that was implemented with some apparent success in the 1970s is known as the *Bridge* reading program (Simpkins, Holt, & Simpkins 1977). Unlike the earlier programs that focused on initial reading material, the Bridge program was designed for children at the secondary level who were not reading at grade level. The Bridge program consists of a series of narratives incorporating various degrees of African American language in such a way as to facilitate reading development of AAE-speaking students. Experimental field testing of the Bridge program on seventh to twelfth graders, reported in Simpkins and Simpkins (1981) suggest that the Bridge program is more effective than traditional ways of teaching remedial reading. Rickford and Rickford (1995) recently tested a version of the Bridge program in East Palo Alto California and found that many students, especially boys, preferred the AAE reading material.

The apparent success of the Bridge program may be attributed in part to its reliance on *literature-based instruction*. In contrast to traditional approaches to remedial instruction that tend to rely on rote memorization of vocabulary items and grammatical patterns, literature-based approaches depend upon the teachers' ability to focus upon such features as they occur in works of literature. Rather than assign worksheets that drill the use of apostrophes, for example, a teacher might select a fictional piece containing dialogue calls the students' attention to dialectal variation in the use of full, contracted, and zero variants of *is*, *am*, and *are*, and stimulate discussion of how the author uses apostrophes to represent contractions. Ball (1995) presents evidence that a literature-based instructional program is more effective than an "explicit instructional program" for teaching "the various /s/ morphemes" (i.e., plural, possessive, third-person singular, and contracted is) to AAE speakers.

Initial and remedial reading material written in AAE may best serve as one component of a comprehensive curriculum tailored to the particular needs of African American students. In recent years, the potential for literature-based instruction geared specifically to the needs of African American children has expanded with the increased availability of reading material on African-American cultural themes. In addition to the rich body of classical African American literature (e.g., Angelou 1971; Ellison 1952; Hughes 1961; Morrison 1977; Wright 1966), there is a large number of children's books emerging set in African American culture and utilizing African American language, from which teachers could draw (e.g., Baldwin 1976; Clifton 1973).

Labov (1972), discussing the results of his studies of reading failure among ten- to twelve-year-old Black youths in Harlem, attributes "the major cause of reading failure" to "cultural and political conflict in the classroom" (1972, p. 243). As promising as dialect readers may be for easing the transition from AAE to SWE, they are not likely to gain widespread acceptance until educators and the general public are comfortable with the idea that AAE is indeed a language in its own right and also with the corresponding notion of African American bilingualism.

SUMMARY

Advocates of a policy of full recognition of African American English support efforts to teach standard English to AAE speakers, but favor doing it in ways that respect the integrity of the children's home language and culture and do no harm. The policy of full recognition admonishes teachers to leave AAE alone, especially as it applies to the oral language of AAE speakers.

Formal standard English differs from any spoken dialect, and teachers do not, as a rule, attempt to change students' spoken language in preparation for teaching them to read. Some programs for developing bidialectalism in African American children, however, attempt to change the oral language of African American children in preparation for teaching them to read Standard English. Some teachers refuse to accept as correct oral reading by AAE speakers that contains dialectal pronunciations of certain words.

One way of leaving AAE alone is to refrain from correcting the oral language of AAE speakers. Research indicates that the traditional practice of correcting is ineffective. Effective alternatives to correcting, which carry less risk of damage to AAE speakers' self-esteem, include modeling and role playing. On the level of written language, teachers are called upon to seek effective alternatives to the traditional practice of responding to students' writing by marking all errors and requiring students to rewrite it correctly. Suggested alternatives include free reading and teaching writing as a process.

Some of the most promising approaches to the development of African American students' reading and writing skills presuppose acceptance of AAE as a language in its own right. Once such recognition is granted, a variety of approaches currently used in bilingual education merit serious consideration, including the use of dialect readers and programs modeled on Bridge. The increasing availability of multicultural reading material increases opportunities for teachers to implement effective literature-based instructional programs for African American children. Whatever barriers to reading success might be posed by differences between the language of AAE-speaking children and the standard English of teachers and texts can be overcome without heavy-handed attempts to force standard patterns on the children's oral language.

REFERENCES

Anderson, E. (1990). *Speaking with Style: The Sociolinguistic Skills of Children*. London: Routledge.

Angelou, M. (1971). *Just Give Me a Cool Drink of Water 'Fore I Die*. New York: Random House.

Baldwin, J. (1976). *Little Man, Little Man: A Story of Childhood*. London: Michael Joseph Ltd.

Ball, A. F. (1995). Language, learning and linguistic competence of African American children: Torrey revisited. *Linguistics and Education*, 7 (1): 23–46.

Baugh, J. (1995). The law, linguistics and education: Educational reform for African American language minority students. *Linguistics and Education*, 7 (2): 87–105.

Baratz, J. C., & Shuy, R. W. (eds.). (1969). *Teaching Black Children to Read*. Washington D.C: Center for Applied Linguistics.

Clifton, L. (1973). *All Us Come Cross the Water*. New York: Holt, Rinehart and Winston.

Dandy, E. B. (1991). *Black Communications: Breaking Down the Barriers*. Chicago: African American Images.

Ellison, R. (1952). *The Invisible Man*. New York: Random House.

Fasold, R. (1990). *The Sociolinguistics of Language: Introduction to Sociolinguistics*, Volume II. Oxford, UK: Blackwell.

Hughes, L. (1961). *Best of Simple*. New York: Hill & Wang.

Johnson, K. (1975). Black dialect shift in oral reading. *The Reading Teacher*, 28:535–540.

Krashen, S. D. (1992). *Fundamentals of Language Education*. Torrance, CA: Laredo Publishing Co.

Labov, W. (1972). *Language in the Inner City: Studies in the Black English Vernacular*. Philadelphia: University of Pennsylvania Press.

Lennenberg, E. (1967). *Biological Foundations of Language*. New York: Wiley and Sons.

Morrison, T. (1977). *Song of Solomon*. New York: The New American Library.

Rickford, J. R., & Rickford, A. E (1995). Dialect readers revisited. *Linguistics and Education*: An International Research Journal, 7 (2): 107–128.

Sedley, D. (1990). Anatomy of English: *An Introduction to the Structure of Standard American English*. New York: St. Martin's Press.

Simpkins, G. A., Holt, G., & Simpkins, C. (1977). *Bridge: A Cross-Cultural Reading Program*. Boston: Houghton Mifflin.

Simpkins, G. A., & Simpkins C. (1981). Cross cultural approach to curriculum development. In G. Smitherman (ed.), *Black English and the Education of Black Children and Youth: Proceedings of the National Invitational Symposium on the King Decision* (pp. 221–240). Detroit: Center for Black Studies, Wayne State University.

Smitherman, G. (1977). Talkin and Testifyin: The Language of Black America. Boston: Houghton Mifflin.

Stewart, W. A. (1969). On the use of Negro dialect in the teaching of reading. In J. C. Baratz & R. W. Shuy, *Teaching Black Children to Read*. Washington DC: Center for Applied Linguistics.

Wolfram, W. (1991). *Dialects and American English*. Englewood Cliffs, NJ: Prentice-Hall Regents.

Wright, R. (1966). *Black Boy*. New York: Harper and Row.

11

SCHOOL BIASES AND AFRICAN AMERICAN CHILDREN

Chapter Overview

Upon reading this chapter you will gain understanding of

- Some cultural practices of African American children
- The major problem of overrepresentation of African American children in special education classes
- The concept of cultural discontinuity and the implications for African American students
- Cultural biases and the education of African American children
- Cultural clashes between African American and European American culture
- Psychosocial and cultural variables that contribute to educational inequities and prejudicial treatment of African American students by teachers
- Traditional American school practices of cultural discontinuity

Historically, public education was viewed as the primary hope for African Americans to escape poverty in America. Contrary to stereotypical beliefs, African American parents care deeply about their children's education. The majority of these parents sacrifice and struggle to enable their children to get an education. There are many examples of parents working long hours, becoming heavily indebted, and selling prized possessions for the sole purpose of supporting their children through college. Yet, despite their courageous efforts and struggles to ensure that their children have an education and greater opportunities, large percentages of African American students do not make it to high school graduation. Many fall through the cracks before completing elementary school. High rates of school dropout affect not only Black students, but Latino, Native American, Asian, and White students as well.

Although the public schools' major objective is to educate all students so that they may function as literate and socially competent citizens, all students are not benefiting from public education. Traditionally, the blame for academic failure was placed solely on the student. Today, social scientists are researching the impact of traditional American pedagogy, school environments, school administrators, teachers, and schooling to determine educational reform needs and directions. Since cultural matters are at the heart of the socialization function of schools, issues related to culture, diversity, and schooling are the focus of educational reform. Research is also underway that focuses on reasons that contribute to dropout, underachievement, and overrepresentation of African Americans in special education classes (Rossi 1994; van Keulen, Brown, Webster, & Elzey 1997).

Over the last forty years, public schools have initiated and implemented numerous programmatic efforts to improve the educational achievement status of African American students without appreciable success. Despite such efforts however, public schools are basically the same as they were during the early twentieth century in principle and practice. Efforts toward homogenization of the population during earlier periods have remained an inescapable part of the educational process. The melting pot theory of the 1960s and the homogenization goal of American education during that period is still rooted in the public school structure and continues to undermine and suppress practices related to multicultural expressions. School administrators and teachers have implemented and supported practices, structures, and attitudes that are in conflict with students' cultures and educational principles related to multiculturalism. As a result, teachers are identified as the major contributor to students' underachievement, overrepresentation in special education, and dropout rates (Darder 1991; Rossi 1994).

This chapter examines the concept of cultural discontinuity as it relates to teachers and African American students in public schools. The theory of cultural discontinuity focuses on aspects of classroom activity, including the way teachers interact with students and the way students interact with teachers and the school culture (Phelan, Davidson, & Cao 1991). Culturally insensitive public schools and classroom practices and cultural biases of teachers, that create conflict and cultural discontinuity for African American students are the primary focus of this chapter.

Educational inequities, underachievement, and overrepresentation of African American students in special education classes in California and the nation are highlighted as consequences of blaming the victim by teachers who do not recognize, acknowledge, or fully understand the significance of being culturally, ethnically, and racially different in America.

European American cultural values, expectations, and contexts represent the deep structural foundation in the way schooling is done in America. Teachers bring to the classroom their cultural values, experiences, attitudes, and contexts that are often in conflict with African American students' cultural values, attitudes, expectations, and contexts. These cultural differences create problems of cultural discontinuity and cultural conflict between African American students and their teachers.

OVERREPRESENTATION IN SPECIAL EDUCATION CLASSES

Throughout California and the nation African Americans, particularly males, are disproportionally represented in much greater numbers than other students from ethnic and racial groups in special education classes. Although overrepresentation is a problem for Hispanic and Native American students as well, African Americans remain disproportionately higher in special education classrooms.

According to the California Department of Education (1994) report, *California: Facts and Statistics*, African Americans represented 2,208,801 or 7.4 percent of the total California population of 29,760,021 in 1990. In that same year, 55,702 or 11.79 percent of African American students were enrolled in special education classes. The total K-12 public school population was 4,950,474, of which African American students represented 8.6 percent. These statistics illustrate the disproportionality of African American students enrolled in special education in California. These trends of overrepresentation have continued in subsequent years with increases in special education enrollment of 63,457 or 12.17 percent in 1992 and 66,648 or 12.33 percent in 1993, and 68,963 or 12.47 percent in 1994. The cumulative growth since 1990 in special education enrollment is 23.81 percent as compared to Whites at 5.88 percent.

There is a considerable overrepresentation among African Americans in special education; likewise, there is a disproportionately lower percentage of African American special education teachers. In 1990–1991, 5 percent of special education teachers were African American , or 6.79 percent lower than the percentage of African American students in special education in California. A stark contrast to these statistics is the number of White, Non-Hispanic special education teachers in California. In 1990–1991, 87.2 percent of special education teachers were White with a White student special education population of 52.22 percent. These statistical trends, reflective of California, are affected because of its increasing diversity in K-12 schools. California's schools are now 58.6 percent non-White.

On a national basis, in thirty-nine states, according to a U.S. News & World Report analysis of Department of Education data, Black students are overrepresented in special education programs compared with their percentage of the total student population. Significantly, the analysis found that Black students are most likely to be overrepresented in special education classes when they are students in predominately White school districts. In some school districts, neither the number of Black students nor household demographics accounted for the high percentage of Black students. School districts with the highest percentages of Black special education students not accounted for by demographics or Black enrollment are: South County Central, East Patchogue, New York; Fordyee, Arkansas; Compton Unified, California; and Emerson, Arkansas. U.S. News & World Report (1993) reports that these findings support arguments by critics of the special education system who attribute the overrepresentation of African American students in the system to cultural bias in testing and placement procedures, not to any inherently high level of disability. Special education classrooms have become convenient places for general education teachers to send racially and culturally different students they don't want in their classrooms; academics in such cases take a back seat.

The overrepresentation of African American students in special education is also attributed to the fact that criteria used for classifying special education students vary from state to state and are often highly imprecise. Secondly, experts say that socioeconomic factors account for some of the disproportionality, but not all. Table 11-1 provides examples of the extent of disproportionality in some states.

As a nation, we should be very concerned about the continuing increase in numbers of African Americans assigned to special education classes. This is no longer just an issue related to ethics, educational equity, and African

TABLE 11-1   Disproportionality of African American Students in Special Education Classes

	Blacks Among All Students (%)	Blacks in Special Education (%)
Delaware	29	41
South Carolina	42	51
Connecticut	14	22
Louisiana	46	53
North Carolina	33	40
Nevada	12	19

Source: U.S. News & World Report, December, 1993

American students. Instead, if the current practices continue, the entire nation will be at greater risk. It is predicted that America's growing population will increase, with more African American and Hispanic American students than any other diverse group of students. By year 2000, the total number of minority children is projected to increase by more than 25 percent and constitute one-third of all children. The number of White, Non-Hispanic children will increase by only two-tenths of 1 percent. By the year 2030, minority children will increase by more than 52 percent and will constitute 41 percent of our child population and 45 percent by year 2080. There will be 6 million fewer White, Non-Hispanic children in 2030 than today. In the twenty-second century, America may become a majority Non-White nation more closely resembling today's world in which two-thirds are Non-White (Children's Defense Fund, 1989).

By year 2000 all children attending America's schools will need to know how to read, write, compute, and think clearly in order to be productive members of the work force. The jobs will require stronger academic skills than any preceding work force. The jobs will require an education beyond high school with almost one-third requiring four or more years of college. An educated, competent work force is becoming more essential to the nation's economic health and ability to compete internationally.

In view of these future projections for the nation, American schools cannot afford to view special education classes as the solution to a national problem embedded in prejudicial school practices, racism, and ignorance about culturally different people. The existing practices of "getting rid" of African American students by referring them to special education is not the solution and must stop. These practices abuse the intent of special education legislation, programs, and services, as well as the African American students' rights to an appropriate education with peers. The goal of public education must be the same for all students; that is, to help students achieve their fullest potential. Unfortunately, this objective creates many problems for school administrators and teachers; most perceive themselves as being quite competent and committed to the education of all students. Without a doubt many teachers are culturally competent, committed, and sensitive to the educational and social needs of students from diverse cultural and language groups. However, the majority of America's teachers and administrators are European American and have not been prepared through experience or formal education and training how to teach African American students effectively, particularly males.

Many teachers still believe that color and culture make no difference and that all people are the same. European American cultural values, attitudes, perceptions, traditions, and the English language are presumed to be universally applicable, beneficial, and desired by all non-European Americans. It is also assumed by many teachers that the cultures of African Americans and other diverse groups do not meet the cultural expectations of European Americans because of presumed cultural deficiencies. These beliefs are often communicated to students by the way teachers treat and interact with them. Too many teachers equate African American students' academic under-achievement in school to perceived cultural deficiencies and the lack of students' desire to learn. These teachers contribute to the current educational system that works best for students from the select population—White Americans. According to the cultural discontinuity theory, the educational system works best for White students because of the continuity they have between their homes, schools, and communities. Only the most assimilated African American students have this type of continuity between their home and school. When cultural continuity does occur for African American children, it is usually due to the fact that their life experiences are similar to those of White European students. These experiences are usually made possible for African American children when European Americans adopt and rear them in predominately White, upper socioeconomic neighborhoods, or when Blacks become so assimilated into the American mainstream they adopt, internalize, and practice European American cultural values.

Cultural discontinuity between the school and home can affect African American and other culturally and linguistically different students nega-tively. Many students are inappropriately assigned to special education because of cultural discontinuity and not disabilities. Many of these students' futures are ruined because of special education classifications and labels. For the majority of African American males, once labeled and assigned to special education, they are doomed; they do not get out and the placement is usually dead-end and permanent. In the majority of cases, they spend the rest of their school years in special education classes. How can this happen? This happens because too many general education teachers view special education as the place to refer students whose behaviors, language, and learning styles are not congruent with their perceptions and expectations. Students are frequently referred to special education because teachers' behaviors and expectations conflict with their students learned behaviors and expectation in their homes. These cultural clashes are more pronounced in classrooms for some students and teachers than others. In either case, due to cultural discontinuity factors, most teachers expect the students to bend solely to their cultural perspectives, thus making it more difficult for students to concentrate on and learn subject matter taught in school. Special education has become the dumping ground for many culturally different students simply because they have not achieved social competence as bicultural students. This situation is further com-pounded when teachers lack cross-cultural competence to understand the dynamics of cultural discontinuity and the impact of it on students who are bicultural and bilingual.

The majority of reasons for referrals of African American students to special education are attributed to "behavioral problems," which are frequently differences that are in keeping with the perspective of cultural discontinuity. It is interesting to note that many of the students enrolled in special education classes by day are considered "fine and culturally competent" after they leave school. This is not to imply or even suggest that there are no African American students in need of special education services. There are African American students with various types and degrees of diagnosable disabilities. However, the problems related to overrepresentation in special education classes seem not to be directly related to disabilities but rather their teachers' attitudes and lack of understanding of cultural differences and disabilities.

Since the 1970s, numerous psychosocial and cultural variables have been identified as contributing to overrepresentation of African Americans in special education classes, underachievement in school, and underrepresentation in gifted and talented classes. Key cultural perspectives argue that:

1. African Americans have a distinctly different culture with its own language and child-rearing practices through which African American children learn instrumental competencies (McAdoo 1988).
2. America's schools do not recognize or utilize African American students' competencies for teaching, learning, and testing.
3. Overrepresentation of African American students in special education is directly related to cultural discontinuity between students and teachers, home and school environments, curriculum and learning.
4. Assessment instruments and practices used to evaluate African American students determine differences and not deficits.

In view of these cultural perspectives, some current educational practices in America's schools that contribute to cultural discontinuity and educational inequities that frequently result in overrepresentation of African Americans in special education classes, underachievement, and school dropout are discussed.

CULTURAL DISCONTINUITY

Cultural discontinuity refers to the lack of continuation or cohesion between two or more cultures. As mentioned, the theory of cultural discontinuity focuses on teacher and student interactions, school and classroom culture, and the students' home culture. In America, the majority of African American children experience cultural discontinuity because they are born into one culture but have to learn very early how to survive in two—the African American culture and the European American culture. Although the impact of cultural discontinuity is greater for some African American children than others due to socioeconomic differences, neighborhoods in which children are reared, and other factors, they usually do not experience cultural discontinuity until they enter school. At that time, the cultural continuity and cohension experienced in their home, church, and community begin to shift to school experiences that are very different. The school principal, teachers, classroom environments, instructional materials, and activities are so different that the initial experience becomes a source of fluctuating mixed emotions of curiosity and wonderment. It becomes apparent that "school" is not in harmony with their home, language, culture, and existing repertoire of experiences, perceptions, expectations, and lifestyle. Because of these major differences, most Black children begin to experience feelings of isolation, loneliness, curiosity, confusion, and uncertainty (van Keulen et al. 1997).

African American children's first day of school and for subsequent years to follow is similar to visiting a foreign country for the first time where differences are abundant—the people, dress, language, food, music, customs, architecture, attitudes, values, and traditions. The initial feelings commonly associated with such an array of differences are a mixture of excitement, anxiety, and isolation. The excitement is usually associated with the new experience, and the anxiety is usually associated with trying to figure out exactly what to do and how to do it in this foreign country without offending the people. Isolation is felt when familiar surroundings, repertoire of experiences, practices, customs, and language that served you well in European American culture do not fit into the culture or context of your new surroundings. You are experiencing cultural discontinuity—a break in the cohension of your day-to-day experiences back home. African American children do not have to leave the country to experience cultural discontinuity—they experience it in their own country when they leave their homes and communities to interconnect with European Americans in the mainstream and other diverse cultural societies in America. Feelings of discontinuity are even more pronounced for African American students coming from lower socioeconomic and inner city backgrounds (Hale-Benson 1986).

TRADITIONAL AMERICAN SCHOOLS

Traditional American schools perpetuate cultural discontinuity for students from different cultures by promoting only those perspectives, values, beliefs, attitudes, and traditions of European American culture. This practice creates tremendous cultural clashes between African American and other students from different cultural and linguistic diverse backgrounds.

In recent years, pervasive research literature asserts that culture and language affect learning (Banks 1981; Boykin 1982; Hale-Benson 1986; Hilliard 1989; Piestrup 1973; Tharp 1983; Villegas 1991) and most teachers plan instruction and activities with little regard given to the diverse cultural and linguistic backgrounds of the students. Many European American cultural practices which create cultural discontinuity in America's schools for African American and other children who are culturally and/or linguistically different, have been identified by Hamayan and Damico (1991). Cultural clashes occur when school administrators, teachers and other school personnel from the American mainstream culture do not recognize or acknowledge the cultures and languages of their students as valid and legitimate. When this occurs, African American and other students are forced into a dual educational process necessitated primarily by inequality of treatment in the schools and American society. Examples of twelve cultural variables resulting in cultural clashes and discontinuity are as follows:

1. Cooperation versus competition
2. Time
3. Bodily movements
4. Proximity
5. Touching
6. Eye contact
7. Gender
8. Individual versus family orientation
9. Verbal and nonverbal communication norms
10. Fate versus individual responsibility
11. Perceptual style
12. Cognitive style

These variables are discussed for the benefit of teachers who want to become cross-culturally competent in the integration of the African American cultural ethos into the pedagogical process.

1. Cooperation versus Competition. Cultures vary in how value is placed on competition and cooperation among individuals. Our public school culture encourages competition; that is, doing better than others is usually considered proof of mastery and is rewarded. For example, most games played in our schools have a winner and a loser; as a result, it does not take very long for children to learn to compete in order to win. Highly competitive attitudes are pervasive in all areas of mainstream American schools and society. Competition is highly valued and the winners are rewarded. Winning is such a highly valued cultural attribute of European American culture that children, youths, and adults sometimes cheat and steal to win.

In contrast, children reared in cooperative societies, where competition is not generally understood or valued, work together with a mutual goal in mind. For example, children from cultures that value cooperation may be taught by their parents to wait until everyone has finished a cooperative task before they indicate that they have finished first because to do so may embarrass the one that finishes last. Cooperative cultures do not acknowledge or reward individual competition.

Students from cultures that value and reward cooperation instead of competition will be at a serious disadvantage in America's classrooms and testing situations. These students are at a disadvantage until they learn the dual roles required to survive in two cultures—their home culture and the mainstream culture. Until these students have gained cultural competence to function successfully in both cultures, they will likely have difficulties arising from the lack of connectedness between their home culture and the mainstream school culture.

African American children's cultural style is typically one of cooperation and sharing in the home, church, and community. Cooperation is an expected value that is taught in relation to family, relatives, and friends. Black children are reared to help their siblings, parents, relatives, and friends carry out tasks. They hear the words repeatedly as young children through adulthood, "Help your . . ." with whatever tasks there are to be completed. These cooperative expectations and experiences of the home are responded to differently in the school. The highly competitive expectations of the school creates cultural discontinuity for Black children wishing to practice cooperation.

The cooperation versus competition variable affects the educational performance, classroom conduct, and behavior until the Black child learns the expectations of the school culture. If competition is expected at school in order to be successful, then they need to learn it, practice it, and perfect it at school. When they go home, they also have to learn how to switch back to expected home behaviors and practices.

The basic cultural orientation of African Americans is one of cooperation, sharing, collective responsibility, and interdependence. In this regard, cooperative grouping arrangements should be used as a teaching strategy. Although there are many models for cooperative grouping, they all seem to involve some form of heterogeneous pupil grouping (variety of ability or achievement levels, disabled and nondisabled, different races and ethnic groups, males and females) that work together toward a common goal. In comparison with competitive or individualistic arrangements in the classroom, a number of reviews have concluded that cooperative learning techniques can achieve both cognitive and affective goals (Johnson, Maruyama, Johnson, Nelson, & Skon 1981; Sharan 1980; Slavin 1980). Team learning also has a positive effect on motivation (Slavin & Karweit 1984), self-concept of ability (Ames 1981), and race relations (DeVries & Slavin 1976; Slavin & Madden 1979).

African American students tend to be more responsive in classroom environments where teachers use approaches such as open discussions, sharing of ideas, and cooperative learning teams. African American students tend to be least responsive when instruction is teacher-centered, materials and topics lack a multicultural perspective and view of the world, and a passive teaching style is used to discourage interaction and movement among students.

2. Time. Time is another variable that is viewed differently by various cultures. In general, European Americans place a great deal of emphasis and importance on being on time and using time efficiently. Therefore, wasting time and tardiness are frowned upon and viewed negatively. Punctuality is expected and rewarded. The general time rule is to always be at a scheduled appointment at least ten to fifteen minutes early because this makes a favorable impression.

In some cultures time is more expendable; the quality of interpersonal relationships may take priority over punctuality (Hamayan & Damico 1991). African Americans tend to think in terms of approximations of time rather than punctuality. An "in-culture" expression, "C.P.T."—which means "Colored People's Time," is a commonly used expression. When meetings or parties are scheduled, an African American may ask another what time the meeting or party will begin. The response may be, " 7:00 p.m." For further clarity, the next question may be, "C.P. Time?" If the answer is "yes," this means that the meeting or party will begin about twenty or thirty minutes after the appointed time. If the answer is "no, 7:00 p.m." this signals that the meeting or party will begin on schedule and they should be on time.

With respect to time, African American children learn about time expectations based on situations within and outside of the cultural context. For example, the type of social events dictate whether it's appropriate to show up on European American time as scheduled or late on C.P. Time. Showing up on C.P. Time is especially popular among youths because their late appearance captures the moment—all eyes and attention are on them. This is their time and it is referred to as the "grand entrance."

Another interesting cultural aspect related to the concept of time is the student's preference toward a polychronic or monochronic orientation. Polychronic cultures mean that the people of these cultures are, in general, used to handling several interactions and activities at the same time. Whereas, monochronic cultures encourage doing one activity at a time. The saying, "business before pleasure" reflects a monochronic orientation; whereas, polychronic cultures promote business and pleasurable activities as a whole (Hamayan & Damico 1990).

In the United States, mainstream students are usually taught to be monochronic and encouraged to focus on interactions and activities one at a time. These values can be observed in practice in classrooms and homes where children are not permitted to do but one task at a time and without possible distractions, that is, no talking, no friends, no visiting, no music while studying. Teachers with the same cultural orientation usually have monochronic teaching styles, which means they will insist on doing only one activity at a time from start to finish before beginning something else. Students with a polychronic orientation will definitely clash with these teachers' expectations and style.

African American children usually have a polychronic orientation. This means most are accustomed to doing more than one thing at a time. For example, many African American children are accustomed to studying while listening to music, tapping a pencil to the rhythm and beat, or listening to conversations that are within hearing distance. Another interesting observation is a group of three or more African American students socializing and interacting; their interaction style is considerably different from that of European Americans. All appear to be talking at the same time with intermittent listening, laughing, and commenting during the discourse. Teachers who are not familiar with this cultural interaction style may interpret the group's interaction as rude conduct by their standards, or even suggest that they are arguing. In fact, neither of these events is occurring—they are having a good time. They are attending to everything that is said by each speaker, understanding it, and responding appropriately.

In the classroom, teachers can learn from African American students by observing them carefully to see which of the students demonstrate polychronic cultural orientations and which ones demonstrate monochronic orientations and adapt the teaching styles and classroom environments accordingly.

Another important example to consider is the process of assessment with respect to monochronic and polychronic cultural orientations. The assessment process used in schools usually operates from a monochronic orientation. This means that students need to operate meticulously one step at a time within specified time frames if they are likely to succeed. Black students with a polychronic orientation will likely have difficulty adhering to monochronic operating procedures required in the test situation. Plus, their polychronic orientation will likely clash with the required testing process, the test, and the examiner because they represent European American mainstream monochronic orientations.

Cultural differences with respect to monochronic and polychronic orientations can be easily misunderstood by individuals outside of the African American culture. If mainstream America expects a more passive or monochronic style of behavior from students, the Black child's active or polychronic behaviors could be interpreted through the European American teacher's cultural filter as being deviant or disordered. The most common problem reported by teachers in which they need assistance relates to "behavior problems." African American students, as described by many teachers, are always exhibiting active bodily movements by tapping their feet, fingers, or pencil in rhythmic motions. These behaviors are often considered a behavioral problem because, as many teachers so aptly state it, "they just can't sit still" or "they are hyperactive." In view of these behavioral style differences, one may conclude that passive-style students are less apt to be reprimanded by the teacher because of the correspondence of student's behaviors to the teacher's cultural norms and expectations. On the other hand, the active students clash with the teacher's cultural norms and expectations, which means these students are most likely to be reprimanded more often and referred for evaluation for possible special education placement.

If classrooms do not promote reasonable movement and talking among students, then one should ask, "Where does active learning fit into today's educational schema?"

3. Bodily Movements. Bodily movements vary across cultures in type, range and meaning. The way people stand, their arm movements, how they walk and their walking pace, their facial expressions, eye movement, positioning, restrictiveness, and expansiveness of motions are examples of a individual's movement repertoire (Almanza & Mosley 1980). Although movement repertories vary from person to person, some movements are more typical in one culture than another.

Schools do not understand or support the natural energy levels of Black children according to Hale-Benson (1986). Black children are described as entering school with excitement and enthusiasm, only to have the school crush their freedom, creativity, and spirit. They are not permitted to channel their natural energy until given permission to release it. This creates discontinuity for them between their homes and school. This early sign of cultural clash at school begins for some Black children as early as preschool. This is often the beginning of cultural conflict between teachers and Black children, especially Black male children.

Most African American students are accustomed to home environments where there is an abundance of stimulation, intensity, and variation. For example, their home environments may consist of a television playing a significant portion of the time as well as constant music playing. In addition, family members and friends may occupy much of the living space with a variety of activities and talking taking place. These factors contribute to stimulating home environments that produce greater "psychological and behavioral verve in Black children than in White children" according to some of the earlier social scientists (Goldman & Sanders 1969; Maran & Lourie 1967; Wachs, Uzgiris, & Hunt 1971). Exposure to constant high and variable stimulation, leads to a higher level of activity. In view of these findings, it is suggested that classroom environments reduce monotonous academic tasks and seat work in favor of increased variation, stimulation, and movement as a part of the learning process.

4. Proximity. Proximity means nearness to something or someone. Different cultures use, value, and share space differently. In some cultures it is considered appropriate for people to stand close to each other, face-to-face while talking to each other. In another culture, such proximity is considered a major violation of one's personal space. For example, North Americans prefer to have more space between speakers than South Americans. African Americans prefer more space between speakers than European Americans. Persons who come too close when talking are considered invaders of one's personal space. This creates levels of considerable discomfort, causing the African American to move a few steps backward to establish a comfortable distance to communicate.

In school classrooms, hallways, and playgrounds, cultural proximity is observable. It is not uncommon to hear Black students say, "Get out of my face." meaning that you have invaded their personal space. Black students have cultural norms as well as their teachers. The problems arise when the cultural proximity norms clash. This usually occurs when teachers invade the student's personal space, making it uncomfortable to interact.

Just as different cultures have cultural proximity differences for comfortable communication, individuals from those cultures also have other preferences about space. Some cultures prefer close working space whereas others prefer wide-open working space. Proximity also plays an important role when students are assessed and can affect the student's performance. Depending on the nature of the assessment being done, the assessor may require distances during testing that may cause the student to feel stressful and uncomfortable. To avoid cultural proximity clashes, the teacher should observe the student's interactions with others and simply ask the students if they are comfortable when interacting with them.

5. Touching. Different cultures have clearly established rules and expectations about touching. These rules vary from culture to culture. What may be considered acceptable touching in one culture may be highly offensive in another. For example, in some European countries, it is acceptable for men to embrace upon greeting each other; whereas, in American culture, the handshake is the acceptable custom upon greeting another male.

African American children are taught to be physically restrained with strangers. They are taught from an early age not to allow strangers to touch them. They learn through observation and parental permission who to greet and how to greet them. During the early years, Black children observe how their parents greet people to determine their appropriate response. Whether relative, friend, or foe, if African American parents are restrained in their greetings, their children usually act accordingly.

In most instances, young Black children will not greet people by touching initially; instead, they usually extend verbal greetings at the direction of their parents. For example, you may hear a Black parent say, "Give your auntie a hug" or, "It's okay to speak to him, I have known him for years." Again, there are exceptions to these learned practices based on how and where the African American parents were reared. In some instances, their practices may not be in keeping with African American cultural practices.

Although African American children are typically restrained with strangers, they are provided an abundance of physical contact with adults and siblings in the home with family. Touching is reserved for family and very close friends. In some other cultures, parents are less demonstrative and prefer to have a more formal relationship with their children. African American children are reared to view their relationships differently with children and adults. Their relationships with adults are viewed as formal and with children as informal. Adults are to be respected and elders are to be held in high esteem. Black children typically think of their relationship with teachers as formal as well as with other adults. This means that behaviors and language style considered appropriate for their peers are considered inappropriate for adults. These behavioral norms and distinctions have noticeably deteriorated with the decline of African American teachers in our nation's schools.

Touching behaviors and expectations are different across cultures. Therefore, teachers should not assume that touching African American students is acceptable even when touching is intended to convey a form of praise or reward. Teachers are often offended when the student's response is "Don't touch me" in these types of situations. African American students, on the other hand, have been culturally conditioned to respond positively to verbal praise. When teachers' and students' touching rules conflict, discomfort usually arises and interferes with learning.

6. Eye Behavior. Students from different cultures use their eyes for many meaningful purposes beyond seeing. Some students from different cultural groups actively communicate nonverbally by the movement of their eyes and eyebrows. Some students show respect by not looking persons of authority in the eye. This is particularly true of many Latin American and Asian American cultures. European Americans, on the other hand, place different cultural values on the use of eye contact. Most teachers expect direct eye contact with the students when speaking to them. If the student does not look the teacher in the eye when spoken to, the teacher often interprets the response as disrespectful or a sign of inattention. This is another example of cultural discontinuity. The teachers expectations are clashing with the learned expectations of students from different cultures.

African American children usually turn their heads to one side with lips closed and pointed downward to the floor when scolded in the home. This is an ancient pose of "asking forgiveness." This pose is also used to counter accusations when falsely accused. African American children may also turn closed eyes away from a speaker or look upward into space with their eyes open to indicate total rejection of what is being said. Context is very important when interpreting the use of eyes in different situations. African Americans learn and use nonverbal communication styles using their eyes and facial gestures. For example, African American parents can effectively communicate with their children without opening their mouths to say a word. This is particularly noticeable in Black churches where children often sit with their peers in a different section of the church. If the children create a distraction from the service, parents, by the use of their eyes, eyebrows, and facial expressions can communicate messages of disapproval to them at a distance.

"Look me in the eye" expectations of teachers often conflict with cultural values taught in the home. Black children, who are reared in homes that strictly enforce the rule of respect by not looking in the eyes of authority figures when being reprimanded, must be thoroughly confused when teachers insist upon their "looking them in the eye" thus treating them disrespectfully.

7. Gender. Different cultures have different expectations for males and females. According to Hamayan and Damico (1991), in many traditional Colombian and Asian families, young boys are fed, dressed, and pampered. Girls, on the other hand, care for younger siblings, clean, cook, and are given a great deal of responsibility within the home and are usually often restricted in their independence outside the home.

The African American family can best be identified for its adaptability of family roles. Fathers and mothers share the responsibility for child care. Black women and men have historically worked outside the home even though their wages deprived them of economic, social, and political equity. Older children participate in caring for the younger siblings, sharing household chores, and working jobs outside the home to contribute to the support of the family. In general, African Americans are not as concerned about sex role identities as European Americans. Of course, these differences relate to the history of African Americans in this nation. Therefore, they are more concerned with overcoming obstacles based on racial membership than with gender affiliation.

8. Individual versus Family Orientation. Individual achievement does not motivate all students. For example, students from some cultures view their roles as family members as more important than their roles as individuals. In these instances, students may be better motivated to perform in school when told that their family will be proud of them (Gillimore 1981).

With respect to African American children, family praise and recognition are very important. Recognizing the cooperative aspects of African American culture and family orientation, African American children seek to please their families by doing well in school, in sports, and at work. Family and community pride are important attributes of the culture; therefore, they do not want to embarrass or disappoint either.

According to Wilson (1987), it is important to understand that attending school for most African American children is often a difficult process. They are called upon at a young age to alienate themselves abruptly from their home culture and are expected to maintain a precarious psychic balance between the Black and White worlds. This process leads to rebellion against a neurotic process that demands that they become a "not-self" and shed their identity in order to be educated and succeed in school. These conditions do not provide African American students a positive base for motivating them to want to learn, achieve, or be in school. These experiences can be less damaging to the children's overall social and emotional development and well-being if teachers were more aware of and sensitive to how they affect student outcomes.

9. Verbal and Nonverbal Communication Norms. Underlying education in America is the assumption that all students understand the common meanings of verbal and nonverbal communication norms and rules considered acceptable in the classroom. This assumption is incorrect. In the verbal domain, rules for talking vary from culture to culture. Some cultural groups may regard loud talking as rude, whereas another culture may regard it as a natural form of expression and friendliness. Some cultures discourage conversations between children and adults and males and females until such time it is considered appropriate.

African American children are typically verbal and have a considerable repertoire of nonverbal communication skills. They also have a distinctly different linguistic system currently referred to as African American English. Traditionally, references in the literature about African American's English have referred to it as an approximation of mainstream American English or substandard English with negative connotations. Psycholinguists, on the other hand, view and define the language spoken by approximately 80 percent of African Americans as a legitimate linguistic system. It has been established that the same rules and linguistic system requirements of other languages are found in African American English. Therefore, it is important to emphasize again that African American English is a valid linguistic system governed by the same rules as other languages.

Teachers' attitudes and responses to African American children's language create language discontinuity and confusion for the children. After all, the majority of Black children are considered competent communicators in their home and communities when they go to school. They speak the language that is taught, heard, spoken, reinforced, and expected by adults and siblings in the home and peers in the communities. Their language serves them well until they go to school. Upon entering the public school, the language that works quite well for them at home is not sufficient or desired in the school. Why do teachers believe it necessary to get rid of an African American child's primary language in order to teach then a second language—mainstream American English? The practice of eradicating a child's primary language first before teaching mainstream American English is not enforced with children from other countries whose primary language is not mainstream American English. Rejecting the children's language is a rejection of them, their family, friends, and community. Is this really the message teachers intend to convey to African American students?

By respecting the African American child, socially and cross-culturally competent teachers accept the whole child including the language. These teachers understand the child, and foster self-confidence, self-esteem, and psychological well-being by educating the child. Educating means facilitating the acquisition of knowledge and social competence through experiences.

Because most teachers and administrators are unfamiliar with psycholinguistics and sociolinguistics, they judge the students' spoken language by what is known and familiar to them—mainstream American English. When this occurs, they often assume that something is wrong with the language spoken by African American children. When the language of Black children does not fit European American teachers' language expectations for the use of their language, their initial response is to change the students' language to fit their norm. Few teachers stop to investigate whether the language is legitimately different. Instead, many teachers conclude in the early primary grades that speakers of African American English have a speech and language pathology requiring therapeutic intervention, especially when the students return to school speaking the same language that the teacher had worked so hard to change by correcting weeks before.

As mentioned earlier in this text, assumptions are made and acted upon about African American students' language that are inappropriate. This is a prime example of cultural discontinuity between teachers and students that often results in negative and unnecessary consequences for the students. Since parents teach and reinforce African American English every day in the home, it is highly recommended that teachers spend more time in the classroom focusing on teaching and modeling mainstream American English. Since the goal of education is not to eradicate children's home languages in order to teach mainstream American English, teachers should spend less time and energy on the home language and more time on teaching mainstream American English. This is the language they will need to become effective speakers, readers, and writers in mainstream America, and students need this knowledge and skills to switch their language code based on situations and context.

Teachers contribute to the discontinuity that exists between the children's home and school by trying to shape and mold culturally and linguistically different students into "their own image." This means that Black children are not accepted as they are and their culture and language are devalued. This phenomenon causes difficulty for Black children until they have acquired code-switching skills to enable them to switch from the first code (African American English) to the second code (mainstream American English). Until these skills have been developed, the majority of Black students need to decode and translate verbal and written words into their own language. This creates an almost insurmountable obstacle, causing young children in the primary grades to feel baffled in classroom situations. According to the results of research, standard English for the speaker who uses another language exclusively is for all practical purposes a foreign or second language (Baratz 1973).

In this regard, Baratz (1973) indicates that a child's difficulties with standard English are very similar to the difficulties of any non-English speaking immigrant. If the Black child speaks "bad" mainstream American English, then the White child speaks "bad" African American English, and if the Black child does this because he or she is supposed to be disadvantaged or deficient, the White child must also be disadvantaged or deficient.

Schools should reinforce feelings of worth and cultural continuity among students. This can be done by integrating historical facts and contributions of African Americans in the curriculum. The role of the teacher is to make the student's world and the classroom congruent. For example, when teaching American literature, African American writers should be integrated into the curriculum; when teaching music, African American musicians and music should be included in the curriculum. The integration of different cultural perspectives, contributors, and experiences, which reflect the students' lifestyle and history, into the classroom curriculum and activities, will enhance cultural centering in the classroom, as well as benefit all the students.

10. Fate versus Individual Responsibility. Many cultures place a great deal of emphasis on individual rights and responsibilities, whereas some cultures believe that control lies outside of the individual. In other words, external forces are largely responsible for what happens to people. When students from these cultures come to school, they bring with them attitudes and expectations about fate and individual responsibility.

African American children are taught to be responsible to the family and themselves. They also learn about external forces such as racism, which inhibits and suppresses their parents' individual rights. The extent that students believe they have control over their destiny generally corresponds to their motivational levels. If students believe they are in control, they tend to do their best because they believe they can influence the outcome through their own efforts. On the other hand, if students believe that there are prede-termined forces external to themselves that will determine their destiny regardless of their efforts, they will not try as hard to influence outcomes through their own efforts.

The amount of responsibility and persistence an African American stu-dent is willing to assume in school situations is heavily influenced by teacher responses and their cultural views regarding fate and individual responsi-bility. Research shows that when teachers demonstrate to students that they believe they can achieve academically, they do achieve; likewise, when teach-ers demonstrate to students that they believe they cannot achieve academi-cally; they do not achieve.

11. Perceptual Style. A student's cultural background influences what and how they perceive their environment (Luria 1976). If three students from different backgrounds were given a picture of a tall city building, each would perceive it differently based upon his or her environmental experiences and cultural knowledge. A student reared in the inner city may perceive the build-ing as an office building where people busily go in and out during the day. Another student reared in a remote rural area may see the building and con-centrate solely on the elevator because of an elevator ride once in a tall build-ing, and the third student may look at the building and focus primarily on the design of the building since he or she has never seen a building of this mag-nitude. These examples illustrate how different students' exposure, experience, and knowledge affect their perception and interpretation of what they see.

Witkin, Moor, Goodenough, and Cox (1977) suggest that certain cultures cultivate field-independent learners and others cultivate field-dependent learners.

Field independence refers to the ability of an individual to perceive specific details within a complex pattern as discrete entities. A student with a field-independent perceptual style is able to see details apart from the whole. In contrast, field-dependent perceptual style refers to the ability of an individual to perceive details only in relation to the whole. A student with a field-dependent perceptual style will have difficulty making critical discriminations among competing perceptual stimuli. America's schools and formal testing processes tend to favor students with field-independent perceptual styles.

Students from cultures that cultivate field-dependent perceptual styles seem to have more difficulty identifying items in isolation from the total con-text. This does not mean that one perceptual style is better than the other; instead, it means that individuals from different cultures perceive of their environments differently. African American students tend to perceive in terms of the whole picture instead of its parts. Since context is important to perceptions and learning styles, it is critical that teachers take these factors into consideration when introducing new concepts, teaching reading, and administering tests to African American children. Their academic performance will likely improve if contextual teaching strategies are used.

12. Cognitive Style. Cognitive style refers to the way individuals process information. Processing information means taking what is perceived and abstracting, categorizing, and forming concepts about it (Hamayan & Damico 1991). According to Hale-Benson (1986), cognitive styles are greatly influenced by childrearing practices within different cultural groups.

Many classifications are used to describe different cognitive styles: Some students may be classified as having a holistic, global, relational, or intuitive learning style, whereas other students, in contrast, may be characterized as having a reflective, methodical, or analytical cognitive style. These classifications must be viewed on a continuum. Although students have a predominant cognitive style, they can respond with a variety of styles in response to demands and situations.

Students who typically display the analytical cognitive style are academically more successful. These students tend to be methodical and reflective when analyzing information before deriving an answer. For these students, there is continuity with expected academic tasks, test taking skills, and cognitive style.

Students who display holistic cognitive styles tend not to do as well in testing situations because of the discontinuity of test taking cognitive style expectations. Cognitive style clashes may occur in the classroom between the teacher and students. Many teachers assume that all children learn the same way and proceed to teach using their cognitive style without consideration for the different cognitive styles among the students. In these situations, students often experience discontinuity with their teachers' cultural experiences, knowledge, and teaching style. The lack of congruence with students' learning styles is problematic and contributes to poor academic achievement.

Twelve cultural and social variables have been identified and discussed that interfere with African American students' learning and academic success. Chapter 12 identifies strategies that school administrators, teacher preparation programs, and teachers may wish to consider when structuring classrooms and planning instruction for African American students.

SUMMARY

Overrepresentation of African Americans in special education classes is undoubtedly related to cultural and language differences between teachers and students. Many culturally insensitive instructional practices that occur in schools affect African American and other students from diverse backgrounds negatively. These practices are often the result of teachers' lack of cross-cultural competence and pedagogical sophistication to adapt the curriculum and classroom environment to sustain cultural continuity for students from different cultural, racial, and ethnic groups.

In view of the projected demographic trends for the future, the nation's schools cannot continue the practice of placing African American students, particularly males, in special education. Retraining of school administrators and teachers must begin to educate them about children and families whose cultures and lifestyles are different from their own. Students should not be subjected to inappropriate educational placements and practices because teachers lack the necessary knowledge, skills, and experiences to effectively teach them. Many African American students are victimized and denied an equal education because of some teachers. Current practices of overrepresentation also deny students their civil and legal rights. Consideration must be given to the diverse cultural and linguistic backgrounds of all students when planning instruction (Almanza & Mosley 1980; Clark-Johnson 1988; Cummins 1984). The goal of public education must be the same for all students—that is, helping them achieve their full potential.

Effective teachers of African American students create meaningful and successful learning activities that take into consideration their cultural and background experiences. Franklin (1992) found that in examining teacher-student interactions, affective-oriented teachers were more successful than task-oriented teachers in improving African American students' academic achievement. Affective-oriented teachers are described as being kind, optimistic, understanding, adaptable, and warm. They are also group conscious, cooperative, and sociocentric.

Instructional planning should incorporate small groups with peer and cross-age groupings. Heterogeneous ability groups working together on learning tasks and activities are effective with African American students. Since African American students are reared in people-focused families and communities where interaction and stimulus variability are highly valued, cooperative groups are compatible with their cultural characteristics.

Cultural continuity between home, community, and school can be achieved for African American students using instructional strategies that are effective with them. Task variability, culturally competent and sensitive teacher-student interaction, social learning in peer and cross-age groups, and cooperative groups are effective instructional strategies. Although research findings suggest that these instructional strategies are effective, they should not be viewed as rigid prescriptions for success, but as guidance in making instructional decisions.

PRACTICAL APPLICATION

Teachers can help improve problems associated with educational inequities and cultural discontinuity for African American students by utilizing the following practical applications.

1. Become aware of cultural differences and how these differences affect learning by reading and observing these differences in students.
2. Learn more about your own culture and background.
3. Use a multicultural curriculum with a print-rich classroom environment. Choose books and classroom materials that reflect the students' lifestyles, cultures, and heroes.
4. Use culturally significant books as the literature base for instruction.
5. Develop classrooms that represent cultural democracy.
6. Engage students to participate in cooperative learning activities.
7. Empower students through trust, opportunity, praise, and belief in their success.
8. Praise students for genuine effort and achievement.
9. Increase your expectations for Black students.
10. Become aware of special education legislation and the intent of the law.
11. Do not arbitrarily refer African American students to special education classes because of their languages and/or behavioral differences.
12. Engage the students to participate in active learning activities.
13. Participate in cross-cultural curricular activities.
14. Learn and teach about cultural, ethnic, and linguistic differences in a positive and respectful manner.

REFERENCES

Almanza, H. P., & Mosley, W. J. (1980). Curriculum adaptation and modification for culturally diverse handicapped children. *Exceptional Children*, 46:608–614.

Ames, C. (1981). Competitive versus cooperative reward structures: The influences of individual and group performance factors on achievement, attributions and affect. *American Educational Research Journal*, 18:273–287.

Banks, J. A. (1981). *Multiethnic Education: Theory and Practice*. Boston: Allyn & Bacon.

Baratz, J. (1973). Teaching reading in an urban Negro school system. In F. William (ed.), *Language and poverty*. Chicago: Markham.

Boykin, A. W. (1982). Task variability and the performance of Black and White children: Vervistic explorations. *Journal of Black Studies*, 12(4):469–485.

California Department of Education (July, 1994). *California: Facts and Statistics*. Sacramento: California Department of Education, Research, Evaluation and Outcome Unit.

Children's Defense Fund (1989). *A Vision for America's Future.* Washington, DC: CDF Publications.

Clark-Johnson, G. (1988). Special focus: Black children. *Teaching Exceptional Children,* 20(4):46–47.

Cummins, J. (1984). *Bilingual and Special Education: Issues in Assessment and Pedagogy.* San Diego: College-Hill Press.

Darder, A. (1991). *Culture and Power in the Classroom: A Critical Foundation for Bicultural Education.* Westport, CT: Bergin & Garvey.

DeVries, D. L., & Slavin, R. E. (1976). *Teams-Games Tournament: A Final Report on the Research.* Baltimore: Center for Social Organization of Schools, John Hopkins University.

Franklin, M. E. (1992). Culturally sensitive instructional practices for African American learners with disabilities. *Exceptional Children,* 59 (2):115–122.

Gillimore, R. (1981). Affiliation, social contexts, industriousness and achievement. In R. Monroe, & B. Whiting (eds.), *Handbook of Cross-Cultural Human Development.* New York: Garland.

Goldman, R., & Sanders, J. (1969). Cultural factors and hearing. *Exceptional Children,* 35:489–90.

Hale-Benson, J. (1986). *Black Children: Their Roots, Culture and Learning Styles.* Baltimore: The John Hopkins University Press.

Hamayan, E. V., & Damico, J. S. (1991). *Limiting Bias in the Assessment of Bilingual Students.* Austin, TX: Pro-Ed.

Hilliard, A. (1989). Teachers and cultural styles in a pluralistic society. *NEA Today,* 7(6):65–69.

Johnson, D. W., Maruyama, G., Johnson, R., Nelson, D., & Skon, L. (1981). Effects of cooperative, competitive and individualistic goal structures on achievement: A meta-analysis. *Psychological Bulletin,* 89 (1):47–62.

Krashen, S. D. (1992). *Fundamentals of language education.* Newbury Park, CA: Laredo.

Luria, A. R. (1976). *Cognitive Development: Its Cultural and Social Foundation.* Cambridge, MA: Harvard University Press.

Marans, A., & Lourie, R. (1967). Hypotheses regarding the effects of child-rearing patterns on the disadvantaged child. In J. Hellmuth (ed.), *The Disadvantaged Child.* Seattle: Special Child Publications.

McAdoo, H. P. (1988). *Black families.* Newbury Park, CA: Sage.

Piestrup, A. (1973). *Black dialect interference and accommodation of reading instruction in first grade* (monograph no. 4). Berkeley: University of California.

Phelan, P., Davidson, A. L., & Cao, H. T. (1991). Students' multiple worlds: Negotiating and boundaries of family, peer and school cultures. *Anthropology & Education Quarterly,* 22(3):224–250.

Rossi, R. J. (1994). *Schools and Students at Risk.* New York: Teachers College, Columbia University.

Sharan, S. (1980). Cooperative learning in small groups. Recent methods and effects on achievement, attitudes, and ethnic relations. *Review of Educational Research,* 50(2):241–271.

Slavin, R. E. (1980). Cooperative learning. *Review of Educational Research,* 50(2):315–342.

Slavin, R. E., & Karweit, N. L. (1984). Mastery learning and student teams: A factorial experiment in urban general mathematics classes. *American Educational Research Journal*, 21(4):725–736.

Slavin, R. E., & Madden, N. A. (1979). School practices that improve race relations. *American Educational Research Journal*, 16:169–180.

Tharp, R. G. (1983). Psychocultural variables and constants: Effects on teaching and learning in schools. *American Psychologist*, 44(2): 349–359.

U.S. News and World Report. (December 13, 1993). Separate and unequal: U.S. News Investigative Report. *U.S News & World Report*, 12:48–60.

van Keulen, J., Brown, B., Webster, J., & Elzey, F. (1997). *Why Is There an Overrepresentation of African American Males in Special Education?* San Francisco State University, Department of Special Education. A Three Year Research Study Funded by the California Department of Education, Specialized Services Branch, Sacramento, California. Contract Number 2043.

Villegas, A. (1991). Culturally responsive pedagogy for the 1990s and beyond. Trends and Issues paper, No. 6.

Wachs, T., Uzgiris, I., & Hunt, J. M. (1971). Cognitive development in infants of different age levels and from different environmental backgrounds: An explanatory investigation. *Merrill Palmer Quarterly*, 17:283–316.

Wilson, A. N. (1987). *The Developmental Psychology of the Black Child.* New York: Africana Research Publications.

Witkin, H. A., Moore, C. A., Goodenough, D. R., & Cox, P. W. (1977). Field independent cognitive styles and their educational implications. *Review of Educational Research*, 47:1–64.

12

IMPORTANCE OF SPOKEN LANGUAGE TO READING SKILLS

Chapter Overview

Upon reading this chapter, you will gain an understanding of:

- African American children's language and literacy in the home and school
- Culture and language variations of African American children
- Reading and writing in multicultural classrooms
- Three types of schemas used in reading
- Differences between two instructional models
- Literacy and cooperative language arts
- A framework that elaborates a critical literacy approach to educating culturally diverse students

In order for children to learn how to read, they must learn the "specialized" variety of language used in books. Book language is considerably different from any variety of American English and the language which the majority of Black children speak. Although there are differences in written English and the spoken language of Black children, the differences are not enough to interfere with their learning how to read or their understanding of what they read.

This chapter covers language and literacy in the home and school. Teacher attitudes and practices toward Black children and their language patterns are also examined in relation to teaching reading. Specific linguistic functional and structural differences of African American English are discussed and contrasted with mainstream American English to illustrate how these differences can interfere with some Black children's ability to acquire reading skills. Suggestions are provided for teachers in their selection of reading materials and the development of multicultural lessons to integrate into the language arts curriculum.

The process by which children begin to learn to read begins in the home. It is crucial that schools recognize the role played by the home in developing reading programs for young children. Like most children, Black children begin figuring out reading when they first notice written language. At some point during the toddler years they begin to understand that there is meaning connected to the "squiggles" called print. When toddlers have the opportunity to observe readers getting messages from written language, they begin to model what they see and "read" by making up messages and saying them in a "reading" voice with inflections differing from normal speech (Lay-Dopyera & Dopyera 1993). Young children also notice examples of written language that appear to have particular utility. For example, a three-year-old child may look at the word configuration of the word "McDonald's" on a sign along with the golden arches and say, "That says, that's where to eat."

Young children also imitate reading behaviors observed in the home. They will observe their parents' and siblings' behaviors when reading and will often imitate their behaviors by picking up their books, magazines, and newspapers to "read." It is not at all unusual to find a three-year-old sitting in the parent's favorite chair holding a book or newspaper upside down "reading" with gestures identical to the parent or sibling. When asked, "What are you doing?" you will likely be told, "Reading."

According to Gibson and Levin (1975) and Lavine (1977), most children acquire information about writing as toddlers. By seeing print frequently, they learn about the visual features of written language—letters and words. Their awareness of letters and words is often shown in their scribbles, which include forms and features that resemble letters even though they are not precisely the letter symbols of the alphabet.

According to Lay-Dopyera and Dopyera (1993), early writing, which to the causal observer may appear to be only scribbling, often has configurations matching the orthography of the child's culture. At age four, children in Saudi Arabia scribble differently from children in the United States. Harste, Woodward, and Burke (1984) point out how the American four-year-old places wavy lines from left to right and creates a whole page of such lines starting at the top of the page and finishing at the bottom. In contrast, a four-year-old in Saudi Arabia uses a series of very intricate curlicue formations with lots of dots over the script, and an Israeli child makes shapes that look mostly like Hebrew characters and moves from right to left. They also point out that young children who have not yet had any formal instruction in reading and writing format their "writing" on the page in the traditional manner of their cultural orthography, whether it is a letter, list, story, or map. Children try to make their writing conform more and more closely to the print they observe about them; as they do so, children in this culture make a series of discoveries that may include the following:

1. Writing uses the same shapes again and again.
2. Writing consists of a limited number of letters used over and over in different combinations.
3. The same letters can be written in different ways—manuscript, print, cursive writing, and type style variations. (Harste et al. 1984, p. 303)

Children's knowledge that supports literacy grows and changes over a span of years. Contrary to what some believe, literacy does not begin at the time of reading instruction at school. Instead, literacy emerges and becomes increasingly functional and elaborated across preschool and primary years. By the time most children enter first grade, they have figured out that there is a one-to-one correspondence between spoken words and written words. Learning that written words they see, when read, will be heard as a separate spoken word is a major milestone. To facilitate prereading experiences, children need to have many experiences of seeing print, seeing it read, and seeing spoken words transformed by a writer into print (Harste et al. 1984).

Since literacy begins at home, young children need models and materials that can enhance their literacy. Ideally, support from adults and other children in a "print-rich" environment will greatly enhance children's reading and writing skills. Current theories of literacy development hypothesize that we develop literacy by means of "comprehensible" input (Krashen 1992), which means that more reading results in better literacy development. This means that children who are exposed to print-rich environments, and are read to or read more, perform better on reading tests, comprehension, vocabulary, writing, and grammar.

In view of Krashen's theory of literacy development, adults working in preschools and elementary grades should provide many opportunities for young children to see print, hear stories, and engage in scribbling and writing of letters and words. These are forms of comprehensible input that will enhance their abilities and understanding about written words, spoken words, and better vocabulary.

Black children who come from print-rich environments where the parents model and reinforce emerging literacy skills will likely enter first grade equal to their White counterparts having had the same or similar experiences. The primary differences will most likely be in the language spoken by Black children and the written language in print. This means that Black children may bring different assumptions about the world to the printed page, so teachers must be aware that Black children's interactions with text may be different from White mainstream American English speaking children. These differences are often caused by not having written word–spoken word correspondence, and these differences are what most teachers do not understand. Typically, Black children's spoken home language is not represented in conventional storybooks or textbooks. Therefore, learning to read for some Black children involves making meaning of the letters, words, and sentence structure, as well as the identification of words. On the other hand, White children typically have congruence in the language they speak at home with the written words found in conventional print. This lack of congruence for African American children is where culture and language variation makes a difference in language, speech, and learning. These are also areas where teachers need knowledge and understanding of cultural differences to prevent the promotion of misconceptions about Black children as individuals and false perceptions about their abilities to learn.

It is also interesting to note that according to Krashen (1992), there are documented cases in the research literature of children learning to read and write without instruction and before entering school. This phenomena supports the comprehensible input hypothesis mentioned earlier.

However, too frequently teachers make erroneous assumptions about Black children's abilities to learn; they often perceive their cultural, language, and racial differences as deficits. In some instances, Black children may need a little more time, a smaller instructional group or a sensitive teacher acting as a coach who rewards success and can address specific literacy needs; this need is not exclusive to Black children. On occasion, children from other cultural groups may need the same type of assistance and support with their literacy needs.

LANGUAGE AND LITERACY: THE BLACK CHILD

According to Wells (1973) and Halliday (1973 & 1974), children's language learning develops for functional reasons. This means that language is acquired in response to the learner's need to interact with the environment and to gain control of his or her environment. These functional language experiences begin to emerge as young Black children have relevant and meaningful experiences. These experiences are essential for them to learn to discriminate sounds, words, and sentence patterns required by various functions and to be able to relate oral language to print. These functional experiences are not unique to Black children; they occur in all languages and cultures.

Black children will acquire mainstream American English reading and writing skills, as well as enhanced speaking and listening skills, when their learning environments promote comprehensible input through meaningful language and literacy functional experiences. In the home, Black children are expected to talk and learn how to read and write. They model their speech, reading, and writing behaviors based on models within their environment and positive responses. Their family members usually focus on the content of their message when they speak and not the form. In this same regard, when they read, write, or scribble, they often receive positive responses to their reading and writing skills based on their intended message and not their language code. The responses to emerging literacy in the home are often positive; however, when these same behaviors are transferred to school, they often receive oral feedback from teachers that contradicts familiar at-home language practices and behaviors. In time, these contradictions create feelings of low self-worth and confusion since each child's language represents the norm of his family and community.

According to Crawford (1993) reading and writing will begin to emerge [for Black Children] in a multicultural classroom when the following conditions are met:

1. Students engage in reading and writing experiences in a literate environment where literacy is modeled and demonstrated, literacy is embedded into the content across the curricula, meaningful print surrounds the learners, learners have stimulating and motivating access to books and tools for writing, and learning activities are based on rich content that stimulates learning.
2. Teachers assume learners are capable and competent, and they provide challenging and intellectually rigorous learning experiences.
3. Daily literate experiences are relevant, meaningful, and functional, and they integrate multiple language processes.
4. Teachers and students collaborate in developing experiences that are meaningful for learners, and they have ample opportunities to interact and respond in cooperative learning activities.
5. Students have interactive participation with teachers who are literacy demonstrators as well as literacy models.
6. Students take responsibility for their own learning through options, self-selections, goal-setting, and supportive assistance of others.
7. Students have opportunities to acquire literacy in sociocultural contexts in which they interpret reading and writing as an important function in real life for enjoying learning.
8. Students are reinforced and facilitated as they take risks in developing ownership for appropriate graphophonic understandings.
9. Parents and community group members are collaborative in developing school programs and curricula. (pp. 50–51)

According to Crawford (1993), reading and writing, like oral language, are not learned just because students are taught skills. Young children's cognitive view of the world, developed in their primary language acquisition, becomes the basis for the cognitive sociocultural blueprint or framework schema used for interacting and responding in language and literacy. As the cognitive structures are developed and refined from experiences, a network of interrelations develop among the schemas through active listening, participating, and experimenting with input from the environment. According to laboratory and informal evidence, cognitive development is not a result of deliberate conscious attempt to absorb new ideas through study; instead, cognitive development occurs incidentally and subconsciously while attempting to solve problems of interest and while engaged in critical thinking situations.

Knowledge is viewed as a by-product of experience (Krashen 1992; Smith 1988, 1990).

Three types of schemas used in reading have been identified:

1. Domain-knowledge of topics, concepts, and processes for reading a specific topic or type of material.
2. General world knowledge—understanding situation-specific social relations, causes, and activities.
3. Knowledge of rhetorical structures—conventions for organizing and signaling the organization of texts. (p. 53)

In order to achieve mainstream American English proficiency and literacy, two dimensions must be realized: Language proficiency has two levels—a less demanding level of speaking used for basic communication and a more demanding level of language required for academic purposes. The second level requires relatively complex, elaborate language and is crucial for academic success in language and literacy because of cognitive-level requirements (Cummins 1981; Genesee 1986).

Black children, like most children, can expect to have some difficulty learning how to read and write. After all, these are new skills requiring coordination and integration of mental processes, perceptual and motor skills. Black children's cognitive sociocultural blueprint and environmental experiences may conflict with the mainstream cognitive schemas—values, attitudes, beliefs, and traditions that are necessary for understanding reading (Steffensen 1987), especially when content, themes, and experiences are alien to their cultural contexts. Black children will learn to read with less difficulty and gain an increased understanding of materials when books represent their cognitive schemas and cultural contexts.

Schema theory contends that comprehension results when "input" is matched with preexisting background knowledge. When incoming data is found by the brain to be contradictory, one of two things happens. Either the schema is amended by the new information or the information is rejected in favor of the existing schema (James 1987).

In view of the schema theory, prior experiences of Black children cannot be ignored; their prior experiences with language and literacy are important to acquiring reading and writing proficiency. Literacy and learning at school should be built on the foundation that is already in place when the child first comes to school; to do otherwise will hinder the process. Lipson (1984) suggests that even able readers might run into difficulties when the text either contradicts their factual knowledge or is contrary to their deeply held world perceptions.

Cultural differences also affect comprehension. Black children can be literally excluded from *understanding* when they read materials, themes, and topics that do not provide appropriate clues to activate their schemas, or when they do not possess schemas in their cognitive sociocultural blueprint to understand. This is another example of incompatibility between the reader (Black children) and writers of school texts. The writers usually anticipate that all readers can extract meaning from what is written without knowing what the readers can really do.

To illustrate this point, Anderson and Barnitz (1984) reported the effects of cultural differences on reading comprehension between urban, working-class African American students and European American students from an agricultural area. They discovered that

> Both groups of students read a letter sent from one African American male friend to another, who had moved away, describing an episode in the school cafeteria. The letter quoted a verbal exchange among students such as "You so ugly that when the doctor delivered you he slapped you in the face." The European American students interpreted the passage as involving physical aggression while the African American students generally interpreted the passage in relation to the verbal style common to their community. . . .(p. 105)

This is an example of how students fail to comprehend and misinterpret meaning when they lack formal schemas to match the text's cultural information. In the example above, the European American students demonstrated the lack of schemas to understand unfamiliar cultural information that caused incorrect perceptions based on their cognitive sociocultural blueprint (James 1987). This is an excellent example of such a mismatch. When Black students have a match with the text's cultural information or story structures, they find the text or materials easier to read, understand, and comprehend no matter how complex it is syntactically and rhetorically. In this regard, care needs to be exercised in selecting textbooks because irrelevant information results in fewer connections and greater ambiguity for Black students (Pritchard 1990).

To emphasize the importance of schemas to matching the text's cultural information, Lipson (1984) in another study, chose an equal number of children from a private Hebrew day school and a Catholic school to read a culturally neutral passage about divers in Japan, and, in counterbalanced order, passages entitled "Bar Mitzvah" and "First Communion." Children from both groups performed better on the completely unfamiliar neutral passage on Japan than when reading partially familiar passages from the other religious group that contained analogous information. Their religious content schema acted as a barrier rather than a bridge to understanding the other religious events.

With regard to Black children's language and literacy, proficiency in mainstream American English should be seen as a *goal* and not a prerequisite to becoming literate. Increasing their command of mainstream American English *will not*, in and of itself, improve Black children's ability to think critically, since their own language can serve just as well for verbal expression and reasoning (Au 1993). Most Black children have emerging literacy when they arrive at school; however, today's hurdles confronting young Black children upon arrival often interfere with their language, literacy, and learning skills. Many find it extremely difficult to concentrate on literacy, learning, and language in school because of the numerous ambiguities and incongruences found within the school's learning environment. It is unimaginable by most mainstream Americans what *school* and *education* experiences are like for most Black students. Meeting racial, ethnic, cultural and linguistic conflict, isolation, resentment, ridicule, negative attitudes, and low expectations by many White teachers, administrators, and counselors is a major burden for students to bear for twelve to sixteen or more years. These burdens can make literacy and learning more difficult for Black children than their White counterparts because they have to learn how to *cope* in addition to reading, writing, and speaking mainstream American English.

TEACHER ATTITUDES AND BLACK STUDENTS' LANGUAGE

Some teachers have negative attitudes toward Black students' home language and culture; this causes many students to feel alienated and resentful and therefore refuse to participate in school literacy activities (Fairchild & Edwards-Evans 1990). Au (1993) cited an example taken from Piestrup (1973), of a group of first grade students reading sentences printed on long strips of cardboard. When it is Lionel's (C1's) turn to read, the teacher spends the time correcting his pronunciation. The text being read aloud is in italics:

Teacher This one, Lionel. This way, Lionel. Come on, you're right here. Hurry up.

C1 Dey, —

Teacher Get your finger out of your mouth.

C1 Call —

Teacher Start again.

C1 Dey call, "What i' it? What is it?"

Teacher What's this word?

C2 Dey.

C1 Dat.

Teacher What is it?

C2 Dat.

C3 Dey.

C4 (Laughs.)

C1 Dey.

Teacher Look at my tongue. They.

C1 They.

Teacher They. Look at my tongue. (Between her teeth.)

C1 They

Teacher That's right. Say it again.

C1 They.

Teacher *They.* OK. Pretty good. OK, Jimmy. (Au 1993, p. 131)

Piestrup (1973) points out how the teacher, in the example, actually disrupts the continuity of the reading lesson by focusing on surface features of Lionel's speech. She is unaware of the fact that Lionel's pronunciation is correct in African American English and indicates that he understands that the word is *they*. In African American English the regular pronunciation rules for the sound represented by *th* are quite different from mainstream American English. The particular sounds that *th* represent are mainly dependent on the context in which *th* occurs. At the beginning of a word the *th* is frequently pronounced as a *d* in African American language, so that words such as "the," "that," and "they" are pronounced as "de," "dat," and "dey" (Adler 1993, p. 57).

In this and other examples, teachers' behaviors and responses can alienate Black children from learning by subtly or blatantly ridiculing them and rejecting their speech and language. Teachers can discourage children by constantly "correcting" their speech and implying through words, gestures, and even silence that they know very little.

In these instances, Black children may exhibit their resistance to the teachers' negative attitudes by engaging in verbal play with peers or withdrawing into a sad or angry silence. These coping strategies give Black students momentary relief in troublesome situations, but the process of coping in school also cuts them off from opportunities to learn to read in school. This creates a double bind for the student—rejection when they do participate and alienation when they do not. Black students need to be taught through meaningful communication and input from the environment. How can teachers use Black students' existing language abilities to promote school literacy? Models of instruction that appear effective in promoting school literacy for Black students are based on the assumption that literacy learning begins in the home, *not the school*, and that instruction should build on the child's literacy foundation established in the home.

Taylor (1983), suggests that knowledge for the functions of literacy used to maintain social relationships precedes knowledge in the forms of literacy needed for the names of letters of the alphabet. Young Black children have experiences with literacy in their homes that can serve as the basis for further growth in reading and writing. Teachers should not assume that Black children enter school *without* emerging literacy skills and experiences. The difference may lie solely in the *amount* of early exposure and opportunities of some Black children to draw pictures, scribble, and interact with books and magazines to enhance early "input" experiences with literacy.

Teale (1987) referred to the terms *emergent literacy* as the early signs of reading and writing shown by children before they begin to read and write in ways recognized by most adults. The terms *emergent* or *emerging* means that children are always in the process of becoming literate.

Several in-depth studies have looked at home literacy events experienced by children of diverse backgrounds before they entered school. One such study was conducted by Taylor and Dorsey-Gaines (1988) of four African American families living in an inner-city neighborhood. The children living in each family were perceived by their parents to read and write. The adults of these families used literacy in many different ways. For example, one adult discussed his favorite poems and shared lists of books he had read and intended to buy. Another adult received and replied to letters from family and friends almost daily and saved poems and articles clipped from the newspaper. All four families made extensive use of literacy in their dealings with public agencies, reading and filling in forms, and providing documentation. The researchers' observations left no doubt that the children in these families were growing up in literate homes (Au 1993).

According to Teale (1987), young children appear to grow into literacy in much the same way as they learn to speak, without formal instruction. Current theory in language acquisition stipulates that "language acquisition is a subconscious process; while it is happening, we are not aware of it happening. In addition, once we have acquired something, we are not usually aware we possess any new knowledge" (Krashen 1992).

Children learn to speak by engaging in meaningful acts of communication with people around them and by constructing their own ideas about the principles of language (Wells 1986). Children provide evidence that they can construct their own ideas about language, rather than merely imitate the speech of adults, in their construction and use of words. For example, a young child just learning speech and language may say "foots," "goed," and other forms of speech that adults do not use. However, in these instances the children are showing an understanding of the rules of the English language, such as the use of -ed to indicate past tense and -s to indicate the plural form.

In these examples, Holdaway (1979) described this process of learning to speak as one of *successive approximation* whereby children engage in the full process of speaking and gradually perfect their efforts over time. When babies are learning to speak, adults do not criticize them for failing to pronounce words such as *bottle (ba-ba)*, *mother (ma-ma)*, and *daddy (da-da)* correctly. Instead, the parents usually provide positive feedback in the form of a smile or hug and say something like this, "Bottle, do you want your bottle?" Just as babies are not criticized in their efforts to learn to speak, Holdaway (1979) argues that the process of learning to read and write should be viewed in the same way. Children's efforts to read and write should be seen as acts of successive approximation in which they gradually move from emergent literacy toward conventional literacy, and then toward increased understanding and sophistication. Research on good writing style indicate that it is due to reading, not writing, and writing makes profound contributions to cognitive development (Krashen 1992).

Children should not be belittled for making errors; instead, they should be shown the necessary skills expected to advance them beyond errors. Teachers should remember that for *all* students, literacy learning is a process of successive approximation and comprehensible input (Au 1993; Krashen 1992). When students are learning to read and write, they should engage in the full processes of reading and writing during meaningful acts of communication. For example, teachers should give Black students the opportunity to correct reading errors and to answer questions by increasing the wait-time. In other words, teachers should not intervene so quickly with the correct responses; instead, they should give the students a chance to do their own thinking and reasoning. When Black students are denied the opportunity and time to think through ideas on their own, the chance to expand their understanding and knowledge of literacy is denied. Furthermore, they will never develop high levels of literacy if instruction is rote memorization, drills on skills in isolation, short wait-times, interruptions, overcorrections, and ridicule. In the opinion of the author, these teaching strategies contribute to low levels of literacy and self-esteem among Black students in our schools and high levels of psychological stress and school dropout rates.

Black students need to be involved in meaningful, motivating communication experiences for literacy learning. School activities and functions related to literacy should be relevant and should inspire students to read books about African American culture and other cultures; as well as write plays, fiction, poetry, songs, letters to family members, relatives, classmates, autobiographies; keep journals, eye witness reports, stories, book reviews, and so on.

Black students need teacher support—that is, knowing when to give the necessary guidance for growth in literacy and knowing when to give support by allowing time and space for them to construct their own understanding of reading and writing. A proper balance between the two types of support should be established by all teachers (Au 1993).

Instruction, utilizing the constructivist model concepts, may be more suitable for most Black children. First, instruction is defined as: "helping the student to become interested and involved in a meaningful activity, then providing the student with the support needed to complete the activity successfully" (Au 1993, p. 40).

Au (1993) indicates that this definition grows out of the school of thought known as *social constructivism*. Models of literacy instruction consistent with this definition are known as constructivist, process, or transactional models. For example, the whole language philosophy is an educational application of social constructivist thought that has become quite influential in schools.

The constructivist models of instruction is the notion that learners must actively construct their own understandings. In contrast to the constructivist model are the transmission models of instruction, which assume that skills and knowledge can be transmitted or passively absorbed (Weaver 1990). Transmission models are also called "skills" or "mastery models" of instruction and are based largely on theories of Carroll (1963) and Bloom (1976). The differences between constructivist models and transmission models are found in Table 12-1.

Teachers are encouraged to base the classroom literacy program on the concepts of the constructivist model. Reading instruction should be based on relevant, high-quality children's literature and writing should be conducted through purposeful forms of writing. When teachers interact with students, they should do so for the purposes of exchanging ideas and not for the purpose of correcting pronunciation and grammar. Can you imagine how frustrating it might be, if you were in the process of conveying an important message and the listener abruptly interrupted you after every word to correct your pronunciation by saying the word, then on occasion, to demonstrate how to say the word with their teeth, tongue, and mouth movements? These types of responses to language differences turn students off to literacy learning. Instead of using these teaching tactics, teachers should focus more on ideas being conveyed by the students and modeling the use of mainstream American English, including pronunciation, grammar, and vocabulary through

TABLE 12-1   Differences Between Instructional Models

Constructivist Models	Transmission Models
1. Learners actively construct their own understandings.	1. Skills and knowledge can be transmitted or passively absorbed.
2. Teaching proceeds from the whole to the part.	2. Teaching proceeds from the part to the whole.
3. Literacy is embedded in social contexts.	3. Literacy is taught as skills in the abstract, without regard for social context.
4. Students are encouraged to explore the functions of literacy.	4. Little or no emphasis is placed on the functions of literacy or the relationship of skills to these functions.
5. Instruction is student-centered; individual differences are taken into account.	5. Instruction is skills-driven; little emphasis is given to individual or group differences.
6. Instruction emphasizes the processes of thinking; recognizing the place of students' life experiences and cultural schemata.	6. Instruction focuses on product; little recognition given to students' life experiences and cultural schemata.
7. Instruction allows for cultural diversity	7. Instruction may reflect the values of the mainstream, to the exclusion of the other cultures.

Au, K.H. *Literacy Instruction in Multicultural Settings.* Texas: Harcourt Brace Jovanovich, 1993, p. 48.

meaningful reading and writing activities and conversations. Opportunities for contrasting the mainstream culture and the culturally different languages and communication styles should also be integrated into the curriculum so all children may benefit from this knowledge. This will permit students to hear the differences and to discuss the differences in writing styles, grammar, and pronunciation without placing value on different languages as "good" or "bad." It should be emphasized here that the authors recognize the need for African American children to learn how to read, write, and speak mainstream American English with maximum efficiency in order to function as literate, socially competent, productive adult citizens within the mainstream of American society; however, the issues and concerns relate to process—how teaching these skills should add to the students' educational growth and not to lowering their self-esteem and interest in literacy and learning.

Banks and McGee-Banks (1989) have focused considerable attention in their writings about ethnic minorities and educational equality and the role of teacher attitudes, expectations, and competencies in perpetuating educational inequality for ethnic minorities. They raise an important question worthy of consideration—"How can teachers who have grown up in ethnically isolated communities and in a racist society teach ethnic minorities as well as they can Anglos?" Furthermore, Banks and McGee-Banks (1993) find this question crucial in equations of educational equality, especially when most teachers are racially White, culturally Eurocentric, middle-class and trained in White, Eurocentric colleges and universities to teach White, Eurocentric students.

These facts cannot be ignored in view of the growing numbers of Black students and other ethnic minorities attending America's schools. Banks and McGee-Banks (1989) contributes school failure and academic underachievement of students from ethnic minority populations to some factors which are teacher specific. They include the following:

1. Most teachers know little about students from different ethnic groups' life-styles or learning habits and preferences.
2. They tend to be insecure and uncertain about working with African American, Hispanic, Asian, and Native American students and to have low expectations of achievement for these students.
3. Too many teachers still believe that minority students either are culturally deprived and should be remediated by using middle-class Whites as the appropriate norm or do not have the capacity to learn as well as Anglos. Teachers form expectations about ethnic minority children based directly upon race and social class, . . . pupil test scores, appearance, language style, speed of task performance, and behavior characteristics, which are themselves culturally defined.
4. Teacher's expectations are more influenced by negative information about pupil characteristics than positive data.
5. Teachers transmit these attitudes and expectations in everything they say and do in the classroom. Black and other ethnic minority students' responses to these expectations become self-fulfilling prophesies. They come to believe that they are destined to fail, and they act accordingly; whereas Anglo students internalize the high expectations teachers have for them and accordingly believe they are destined to succeed (p.184)

SELECTING READING MATERIALS AND ACTIVITIES

In selecting reading materials and activities, teachers need to think about the importance of student outcomes in literacy, social-cultural identity, cognitive consequences, linguistic skills (mainstream American English and African American English), and academic achievement.

When teachers do not respect Black students' cultural values and expectations, they threaten their sense of cultural identity and self-esteem as mentioned earlier in the text. However, when teachers accept Black students' home language and use books, other materials, and activities that incorporate their culture, teachers signal their recognition of Black students' values and concern for their self-esteem. Self-esteem and confidence are very important to academic success because students with high self-esteem will have the confidence to take on new challenges in reading, writing, and other academic tasks.

With respect to cognitive consequences, teachers need to be aware that most research on the learning styles of African Americans conclude that from all indications their knowledge is gained most effectively through kinetic and tactile senses, through the keen observation of the human scene, and through verbal description. This difference in perception manifests itself not only in world view, but also in modality preference, cue selection, and pictorial perception (Banks & McGee-Banks 1989).

Research on linguistic skills show that language and literacy instruction in the first (home) language gives students certain advantages that can help them to become literate in mainstream American English. These advantages come in the form of skills that can be transferred from one language to another (Au 1993).

In the area of academic achievement, African American students will learn best in schools where the schools' cultures are accepting and not oppressive; where teachers and administrators have high expectations about their learning, a curricular emphasis on sociocultural integration, and the use of assessment, evaluation tools, and procedures that are appropriate and respectful of individual, cultural, and language differences.

Tiedt and Tiedt (1990) provided a summary of studies of the language arts curriculum and instruction that gives a knowledge base from which teachers can begin planning the development of a multiculturally based language arts program. The following basic assumptions should guide them in their development of multicultural lessons to infuse into the language arts curriculum:

1. A strong thinking-language base is necessary for success in reading and writing. Thinking and language permeate all learning.
2. Reading and writing cannot be taught in isolation. Integrating language arts reinforces learning efficiently and effectively, especially when reading is relevant to students' interests.
3. Beginning readers need to learn basic phonics; this information provides them tools they can use to decode words and reinforce their learning through reading and writing whole language. Decoding (unlocking meaning from words presented in the English code) and encoding (spelling/writing words according to the English code system) should be

presented as complementary processes during meaningful reading and writing activities.

4. Students learn to read, write, and think by being in print-rich environments and by receiving comprehensible input. "We learn to read by reading, and good writing is the result of reading" (Krashen 1992).
5. Literature should be an integral part of instruction across the curriculum at all levels. It should be presented as something to be read and also as an example of good writing by real people who are sharing their thinking.
6. Both reading and writing entail a transaction between author and audience as they work together to construct meaning. The work of both reader and writer are influenced by prior knowledge—what each brings to the task of making meaning. All learners come to school with a store of prior knowledge, which includes their cultural backgrounds. (Tiedt & Tiedt 1990, p.186)

Devillar, Faltis, and Cummins (1994) describe another literacy framework conceptualized by Ada (1988) that elaborates an approach to the education of culturally diverse students. Ada's framework outlines how zones of proximal development can be created that encourage culturally diverse students to share and amplify their experiences within a collaborative process of critical inquiry. Four phases are distinguished in what is termed "the creative reading act." Each phase is characterized by an interactional process either between the teacher and students or among peers. The "text" that is the focus of the interaction can derive from any curricular areas or current event.

The four phases are considered equally applicable at any grade level in a creative reading act and may happen concurrently and be interwoven. The four phases are called: (1) descriptive phase, (2) personal interpretive phase, (3) critical analysis phase, and (4) creative action phase. A brief description follows for each of the four phases.

1. Descriptive Phase. In this phase, the focus of interaction is on the information contained in the text. Typical questions at this level might be: "Where, when, how did it happen?" "Who did it?" "Why?"

2. Personal Interpretive Phase. After the basic information in the text has been discussed, students are encouraged to relate it to their own experiences and feelings. Questions that might be asked by the teacher at this phase are: "Have you ever seen (felt, experienced) something like this?" "How did what you read make you feel?" "Did it make you happy?" "Frighten you?" "What about your family?" Ada (1988) points out that this process helps develop students' self-esteem by showing that their experiences and feelings are valued by the teacher and classmates. It also helps students learn that true learning occurs only when the information received is analyzed in the context of one's own life experiences and emotions.

3. Critical Analysis Phase. After the students have compared and contrasted what is presented in the text with their personal experiences, they are ready to engage in a more abstract process of critically analyzing the issues or problems that are raised in the text. This process involves drawing inferences and exploring what generalizations can be made. Appropriate questions during this phase might be: "Is it valid?" "Always?" "When?" "Does it benefit everyone alike?" "Are there any alternatives to this situation?" "Would people of different cultures (classes, genders) have acted differently?" "How?" "Why?" This phase further extends students' comprehension of the text and issues analyzed by encouraging them to examine both the internal logical coherence of the information or propositions and their consistency with other knowledge and prospective.

4. Creative Action Phase. This phase consists of translating the results of the previous phases into concrete actions. The dialogue is oriented toward discovering what changes individuals can make to improve their lives or resolve the problems presented. For example, after relating a school problem or the issue to their own experiences and critically analyzing causes and effects, they might decide to take creative actions to address the problem, for example, writing to elected officials to express concern or highlighting the issues in the school's newsletter. This phase can be seen as extending the process of comprehension insofar as when one acts to transform aspects of his or her social realities to gain a deeper understanding of those realities (pp. 384-385).

SUMMARY

The process by which Black children learn to read and write begins in the home. Home culture, language, and experiences are the foundation for school literacy learning and the acquisition of mainstream American English. Contrary to what some believe, literacy does not begin at the time of reading instruction at school. Instead, literacy emerges and becomes increasingly more functional and elaborate during the preschool and primary years. Support from adults and print-rich environments will greatly enhance children's reading and writing skills. Likewise, children's language learning develops for functional reasons. These functional language experiences begin to emerge as young Black children have relevant and meaningful experiences. When certain classroom conditions are met, Black children's language and literacy thrive. These conditions take into consideration that young Black children's cognitive view of the world, developed in their primary language acquisition, becomes the basis for their cognitive sociocultural blueprint or framework schema used for interacting and responding in language and literacy. Teachers' attitudes and practices can sustain old patterns of schools' failure to recognize Black children's culture, language, and early home expe-riences, or they can build on the home language, culture, and emerging liter-acy experience for greater school and academic success. Current theories and research of literacy development advance the theories that children learn to read by reading, develop good writing by reading, that cognitive develop-ment occurs incidentally and subconsciously, and knowledge is a by-product of experience.

PRACTICAL APPLICATION

1. Provide students with a print-rich classroom environment. Introduce a variety of books about different cultures, histories, and heroes. Books should be at different levels to accommodate and encourage successful reading experiences.
2. Do not practice correction of written and spoken language of African American students; instead, practice teaching and modeling of main-stream American English speaking and written forms.
3. Accept and respect the children; they represent their family's culture, race, ethnicity, language, and expectations.
4. Do not make assumptions about African American students' literacy based on their race, culture, ethnicity, or language.

REFERENCES

Ada, W. F. (1988). Creative reading: A relevant methodology for language minority children. In L. M. Malave (ed.), *NABE '87. Theory, Research and Application: Selected Papers*. Buffalo: State University of New York Press.

Adler, S. (1993). *Multicultural Communication Skills in the Classroom*. Boston: Allyn & Bacon.

Anderson, B. V., & Barnitz, J. G. (1984). Cross-cultural schemata and reading com-prehension instruction. *Journal of Reading*, 28 (2):102–108.

Au, K. H. (1993). *Literacy Instruction in Multicultural Settings*. Fort Worth, TX: Harcourt Brace Jovanovich.

Banks, J. A., & McGee-Banks, C. A. (1989). *Multicultural Education: Issues and Perspec-tives*. Boston: Allyn & Bacon.

Banks, J. A., & McGee-Banks, C. (1993). *Multicultural Education: Issues and Perspectives* (2nd ed.). Boston: Allyn & Bacon.

Bloom, B. S. (1976). *Human Characteristics and School Learning*. New York: McGraw-Hill.

Carroll, J. (1963). A model for school learning. *Teachers College Record*, 64:723–733.

Crawford, L. W. (1993). *Language and Literacy Learning in Multicultural Classrooms*. Boston: Allyn & Bacon.

Cummins, J. (1981). The role of primary language development in promoting educa-tional success for language minority students. In California State Department of

Education, Office of Bilingual Bicultural Education, *Schooling and Language Minority Students: A Theoretical Framework* (pp. 3–49). Los Angeles: California Evaluation, Dissemination, and Assessment Center.

Devillar, Faltis, & Cummins. (1994). *Cultural Diversity in Schools: From Rhetoric to Practice.* Albany: State University of New York Press.

Fairchild, H. H., & Edwards-Evans, S. (1990). African American dialects and schooling: A review. In A. M Padilla, H. H. Fairchild, & C. M. Valadez (Eds.), *Bilingual Education: Issues and Strategies* (pp. 75–86). Newbury Park, CA: Sage.

Genesee, F. (1986). The baby and the bath water or what immersion has to say about bilingual education. *NABA Journal*, 10:227–254.

Gibson, E. J., & Levin, H. (1975). *The Psychology of Reading.* Cambridge, MA: MIT Press.

Halliday, M. K. (1973/1974). *Exploration in the Functions of Language.* New York: Elsevier North-Holland.

Harste, J. C., Woodward, V. A., & Burke, C. L. (1984). *Language Stories and Literacy Lessons.* Portsmouth, NH: Heinemann.

Holdaway, D. (1979). *Foundations of Literacy.* New York: Ashton Scholastic.

James, M. O. (1987). ESL reading pedagogy: Implications of schema-theoretical research. In J. Devine, P. L. Carrell, & D. E. Eskey (eds.), *Research in Reading in English as a Second Language* (pp. 175–188). Washington, DC: Teachers of English to Speakers of Other Languages.

Krashen, S. D. (1992) *Fundamentals of Language Education.* Ontario, CA: Laredo.

Lavine, L. O. (1977). Differentiation of letter-like forms in prereading children. *Developmental Psychology*, 13:89–94.

Lay-Dopyera, M. & Dopyera, J. (1993). *Becoming a Teacher of Young Children.* New York: McGraw-Hill.

Lipson, M. Y. (1984). Some unexpected issues in prior knowledge and comprehension. *The Reading Teacher*, 37, (8):760–765.

Piestrup, A. M. (1973). Black dialect interference and accommodation of reading instruction in first grade. Monographs of the language-behavior research laboratory, No. 4. Berkeley, CA: University of California.

Pritchard, R. (1990). The effects of cultural schemata on reading processing strategies. *Reading Research Quarterly*, 25 (4):273–295.

Ruddell, M. R. (1993). *Teaching Content Reading and Writing.* Boston: Allyn & Bacon.

Smith, F. (1988). *Understanding Reading* (4th ed.). Hillsdale, NJ: Lawrence Erlbaum.

Smith, F. (1990) *To Think.* New York: Teachers College Press.

Steffensen, M. A. (1987). The effect of context and culture on children's L2 reading: A review. In J. Devine, P. L. Carrell, & D. E. Eskey (eds.), *Research in Reading in English as a Second Language* (pp. 41–57. Washington, DC: Teachers of English to Speakers of Other Languages.

Taylor, D. (1983). Family Literacy: *Young Children Learning to Read and Write.* Portsmouth, NH: Heinemann.

Taylor, D., & Dorsey-Gaines, C.(1988). *Growing Up Literate: Learning from Inner-City Families.* Portsmouth, NH: Heinemann.

Teale, W. H. (1987). Emergent literacy: Reading and writing development in early childhood. In J. E. Readence & R. S. Balwin (eds.), *Research in Literacy: Merging Perspectives* (pp. 45–74). Thirty-sixth Yearbook of the National Reading Conference. Rochester, NY: National Reading Conference.

Tiedt, P. L., & Tiedt, I. M. (1990). *Multicultural Teaching: A Handbook of Activities, Information, and Resources.* Boston: Allyn & Bacon.

Weaver, C. (1990). *Understanding Whole Language: Principles and Practices.* Portsmouth, NH: Heinemann.

Wells, G. (1973). *Coding Manual of the Description of Child Speech.* Bristol, UK: School of Education, University of Bristol.

Wells, G. (1986). *The Meaning Makers: Children Learning and Using Language to Learn.* London: Heinemann.

13

EMPOWERING AFRICAN AMERICAN CHILDREN

Chapter Overview

Upon reading this chapter, you will have a better understanding of:

- Teachers' influence on empowerment of African American students
- Institutional characteristics of schools that empower or disable African American students
- Ways parents and teachers can enhance pride and empowerment in African American children
- Ways to develop positive self-images and self-esteem in African American children
- Parents' influence on self-esteem, self-discipline and empowerment

This chapter focuses on the importance of having Black children *centered* in the classroom and strategies for enhancing their academic achievement and motivation for schoolwork. Parent and teacher roles are discussed with respect to the causal analysis of *why* and *how* Black students experience school failure and *what* can be done about it. A theoretical framework for intervention, developed by Cummins (1989), is examined in relation to helping Black students learn how to handle stress related to school experiences. Empowerment is identified and discussed as a *major* variable of strength for Black children and the importance of their feeling empowered. Several strategies that can be used to enhance empowerment by teachers, parents, and community are presented with particular attention given to building self-respect and developing positive self-images and self-esteem.

TEACHERS' INFLUENCE ON EMPOWERMENT

The role of the teacher is to make a student's world in the classroom congruent with his or her world at home and community. For African American children, this means that the classroom language, environment, curriculum, experiences, books, materials, strategies, and so forth should incorporate their students' culture, language, and experiences that occurs outside the classroom. It means helping Black students to become *centered* in the classroom.

Centering means treating Black students with respect, ensuring that they learn about self, other cultures, and the world. Centering also means developing positive self-images, self-esteem, and self-confidence among Black students through interacting with other students from different ethnic, cultural, and linguistic backgrounds. Black students who are centered in the classroom tend to feel self-confident, calmer, and ready to learn. These inner feelings are critical to achievement in school and the society. Through centering, Black students will be able to discover freedom and strength from within.

This is made possible because the classroom experiences are centered in cultural ways that make learning interesting and intimate. Students receive reinforcement in their own historical experiences. It has been found through observations, inquiry, and discussions that "children who are centered in their own cultural information are better students, more disciplined, and have greater motivation for schoolwork" (Asante 1992, p. 29–30). Asante further indicates that as "ridiculously corny" as it may seem, "many Black children have never been touched at their psychological centers, never been reached in their cultural homes. They see school as a foreign place because schools do foreign things. Of course, many Black students master the 'alien' cultural information, but others have great difficulty getting beyond the margin in which they have been placed" (Asante 1992, p. 30). Black students who are centered in the classroom are able to engage in genuine dialogue with the teacher comfortably without fear of negative feedback; they are able to receive guidance and facilitation in learning rather than control; they are encouraged to engage in student-to-student talk within a collaborative learning context; they are encouraged to use meaningful language to communicate rather than suffer from "overcorrecting" of surface forms; there is a conscious integration of language use and development in all curricular content; the teacher focuses on developing higher level cognitive skills rather than factual recall; and, the learning tasks generate intrinsic rather than extrinsic motivation (Cummins 1988).

Teachers who are genuinely committed to Black student equity and excellence in education make a commitment to the *educator's ethical responsibility* to empower students and become informed as to the causes of Black students' academic difficulties. These teachers also have strategies for helping Black children overcome these difficulties (Cummins 1988). They will advocate for the *curriculum* that provides for the inclusion of Black student's culture; not the death of it in order to learn White cultural information. School administrators and teachers need to look at how they have encouraged Black students to primarily concentrate on learning about the White culture—an exclusionary approach to education. Even though Black students may learn about White culture, when they do so at the exclusion of their own, they are left without *cultural grounding*, they have their sense of *cultural place* destroyed. This is usually an unquestioned experience of Black students, especially when they are quite young, naive, and impressionable. They are trusting and believe that school is in their best interest. They are usually unaware of what is happening to them at the time, and the realization does not come until years later. For many Black students this causes emotional stress and confusion about what is being taught and expected at school versus what is being taught and expected at home. Because of this confusion, some Black students will "abandon, in their minds, their own cultures in order to become like Whites culturally, hoping this will bring them closer to the White norms" (Asante 1992, p. 30). In this respect, it seems quite apparent that many Black children learn how to *culture-switch* as well as code-switch in order to survive in America's schools and society. They learn how to use the characteristics of the mainstream culture when in school and switch back to their own culture's characteristics once they return to their community and home. They are expected to learn two cultures, socially share two cultures, and learn two linguistic systems in addition to the subjects taught at school. This is the result of living in and being socialized in two societies. However, the mainstream society only reinforces one in the schools. The fact that teachers can teach American literature and not refer to one African-American writer is doing a disservice to students of all cultural backgrounds. Likewise, teachers who teach American history and do not refer to one African American who contributed to the history and building of this nation do a disservice, as well as the teacher who teaches music and does not mention one composition by an African American. This is "de-centering African American students and miseducating the rest of the children" (Asante 1992, p. 30). Teachers who work for student empowerment become empowered, and when "the best teachers soar like eagles, their students soar with them" (Asante 1992). Once centered in the classroom, Black students will be able to channel their personal energy to learning instead of using it to ward off emotional stress and abuse. These inner feelings are critical to achievement in school and the society.

Empowerment of Black students in schools is dependent on the extent to which teachers are willing to redefine their roles individually and collectively with respect to Black students, their families, and community. The first step in the redefinition process is to acknowledge that Black students are failing academically, not primarily because of language differences, but because they are disempowered as a result of particular kinds of interactions with well-intentioned teachers. Disempowerment results in shame and the loss of power to control their own lives in situations where they interact with members of the mainstream, for example, in classrooms. Consequently, Black students perform in school the way most teachers expect them to perform—poorly. The poor performance in turn reinforces the teachers' perceptions of them as deficient. The numerous incongruences that exist among the two cultural and linguistic groups (African American and mainstream America) create a vicious cycle for Black children in their efforts to receive an education that is supposedly beneficial for them. They are caught between two worlds and all the problems inherent in both. In order "for real change to occur toward correcting this unfair and psychologically unhealthy situation, educational interventions must be oriented towards empowerment—toward allowing Black students to feel a sense of efficacy and control over what they are committed to doing in the classroom and in their lives outside the school. In other words, real change must challenge the power structure (i.e. the institutionalized racism) that disables Black children." The process of role definition involves a commitment to *empower* Black students both personally and academically (Cummins 1989).

A theoretical framework for intervention has been developed by Cummins (1989) that examines the causal analysis of *why* and *how* students experience school failure. The central hypothesis of this framework is that Black students are disempowered educationally in very much the same way that their communities are disempowered by interactions with societal institutions. The converse of this is minority students will succeed educationally to the extent that the patterns of interaction in school reverse those that prevail in the society at large. In short, Black students are "empowered" or "disabled" as a direct result of their interactions with teachers in the schools. These interactions are mediated by the implicit or explicit role differences that teachers assume in relation to four institutional characteristics of schools. These characteristics reflect the extent to which: (1) Black students' language and culture are incorporated into the school program, (2) Black community participation is encouraged as an integral component of Black children's education, (3) the pedagogy promotes intrinsic motivation on the part of Black students to use language actively in order to generate their own knowledge, and (4) professionals involved in assessment become advocates for Black students by focusing primarily on the ways in which Black students' academic difficulty is a function of interactions within the school context rather than legitimizing the location of the "problem" within Black students (Cummins 1989, p. 58).

Each dimension can be analyzed along a continuum with one end reflecting an *intercultural* or *anti-racist orientation* and the other end reflecting the more traditional *Eurocentric-conformity (assimilationist) orientation*. The overall prediction is that the latter orientation will tend to result in *personal and/or academic disabling* of Black students whereas the anti-racist orientation will result in Black student *empowerment*, which implies the development of the ability, confidence, and motivation to succeed academically (Cummins 1989).

There are four institutional characteristics of schools that can contribute to the empowerment of Black students:

1. **Cultural and Linguistic Incorporation.** Research data suggest that for minority groups who experience disproportionate levels of academic failure, the extent to which students' language and culture are incorporated in the school program constitutes a significant predictor of academic success. With respect to Black students and the natural incorporation of their language and culture, the teacher's role definitions can be characterized along an "additive-subtractive" dimension. Teachers who see their role as adding a second language and cultural affiliation to Black students' repertoire are likely to empower students, whereas teachers who see their role as replacing or subtracting Black students' primary language and culture in the process of assimilating them to the mainstream culture are more likely to disable them.

2. **Community Participation.** It has been argued that Black students will be empowered in the school context to the extent that the communities are empowered through their interactions with the school. This means that when teachers involve Black parents as partners in their children's education, they seem to develop a sense of efficacy that is communicated to their children with positive academic consequences. The teacher's role definitions associated with community participation can be characterized along a *collaborative-exclusionary* dimension. This means that teachers operating at the collaborative end of the continuum actively encourage Black parents to participate in promoting their children's academic progress in the home and through involvement in classroom activities. The collaborative orientation may require a willingness on the part of the teacher to work closely with teachers or aides who can speak African American English in order to communicate effectively and in a non-condescending way with Black parents. This also means that Black parents will genuinely participate in school decisions, be accepted, respected, and valued by teachers and school administrators.

At the other end of the continuum are teachers with an exclusionary orientation. These teachers tend to regard teaching solely as their job and are likely to view collaboration with Black parents as either irrelevant or actually detrimental to their children's progress. They often view parents as part of the problem since they use African American English to interact with their children at home. Many Black parents do not participate in schools after the first attempt because they encounter teachers with the exclusionary orientation and are left feeling unwelcome, powerless, manipulated, and intimidated;

other parents just hear about these negative experiences from their relatives and friends and decide at that moment never to participate in their childrens school.

Dramatic changes in Black students' school achievement can be realized when teachers take the initiative to change their exclusionary orientation to one of collaboration. Of course, some teachers do better than others in relating to Black parents and in forming true parent-teacher partnerships. In either case, teacher attitudes define their roles and relationships with Black parents. Most have accepted rather than challenged the power structure in which education of Black students take place. These attitudes are communicated subtly to Black students and contribute directly to the disabling of Black students.

3. Pedagogy. Two major orientations are identified with respect to pedagogy. These differ in the extent to which the teacher retains exclusive control over classroom interaction versus sharing some of this control with students. The dominant instructional model in most western societies has been termed a *transmission* or *banking* model; and the other an *interactive/experiential* model. In implementing the transmission model, the teacher's role is to impart knowledge and skills that he or she possesses to students who do not yet have these skills. The teacher initiates and controls the interaction, constantly orienting it towards the achievement of instructional objectives. Transmission model teachers, unfortunately, may be responsible for inducing learning difficulties in Black students in that Black students designated "at risk" frequently receive intensive instruction that confines them to a passive role and induces a form of "learned helplessness." Instruction that empowers students aims to liberate them from dependence and encourages them to become active generators of their own knowledge. The transmission model of teaching is said to contravene central principles of language and literacy acquisition because it does not allow for reciprocal interaction between the teachers and students.

The interactive/experiential model incorporates proposals about the relation between language and learning by a variety of investigators (Barnes 1976; Lindfors 1980; Wells 1986). The promotion of literacy conforms closely to the approaches to reading as discussed by (Goodman & Goodman 1978; Smith 1979) and on encouraging expressive writing in the early grades (Chomsky 1981; Graves 1983).

An important aspect of the interactive/experiential model is that "talking and writing are means of learning." The major characteristics in comparison to a transmission model are as follows:

1. Genuine dialogue between student and teacher in both oral and written modalities

2. Guidance and facilitation rather than control of student learning by the teacher; encouragement of student-student talk in a collaborative learning context
3. Encouragement of meaningful language use by students rather than correctness of surface forms
4. Conscious integration of language use and development with all curricular content rather than teaching language and other content as isolated subjects
5. A focus on developing higher level cognitive skills rather than factual recall, and task presentation that generates intrinsic rather than extrinsic motivation. (Cummins 1989, p. 64)

In essence, pedagogical approaches that empower students encourage them to assume greater control over setting their own learning goals and collaborate actively with each other in achieving these goals. They are actively involved in expressing, sharing, and amplifying their experiences within the classroom.

4. Assessment. As mentioned in Chapter 11, assessment has served to legitimize educational disabling of many Black students. This has been accomplished by locating academic problems of the school system within the students. Recognizing the nature of most school structures—exclusionary orientation toward Blacks; transmission models of teaching that suppress Black students' language and experiences and inhibits active participation in learning—the assessment process is bound to discover academic difficulties in Black students that are attributed to psychological dysfunctions. What do psychologists expect when they use psychological tests that are inappropriate, unfair, and work against Black students?

The alternative role definition that is required to reverse the "legitimizing" function of assessment is an "advocacy" orientation. This means that psychologists, special educators, and regular classroom teachers must end the traditional function of psychological assessment with Black students. They need to become advocates for Black students in critically scrutinizing the social and educational context within which a child has developed. Assessment needs to be broadened so that it goes beyond psychoeducational considerations and takes into account the child's entire learning environment. To end the disabling of Black students and their overrepresentation in special education classes, assessment must focus on the extent to which Black children's language and culture are incorporated within the school program, the extent to which teachers collaborate with Black parents in a shared enterprise, and the extent to which Black children are encouraged to use their language in the classroom to amplify their experiences when interacting with other children and adults.

It should be remembered that racism in the assessment process is structural, the actual discriminatory assessment itself is carried out by well-intentioned individuals who, rather than challenge the social and educational system, have accepted an educational structure that makes discriminatory assessment virtually inevitable (Cummins 1989, pp. 57–67).

BUILDING SELF-RESPECT

Self-respect means taking pride in oneself. Parents and teachers can contribute in many important ways to helping Black children take pride in themselves. One way of helping them develop pride is to help them build feelings of empowerment within by promoting their higher order thinking capabilities. When parents and teachers behave respectfully with Black children, they feel respected and this strengthens the very core of their being. Respectful behaviors with Black children allow them to develop that aspect of self that is important to their overall psychological growth. With self-respect well developed, Black children are empowered; without it, they are demeaned.

Teachers begin building self-respect early in a child's development by showing respect and valuing him or her. Teachers show respect when giving recognition to them for who they are and what they do. Respect is shown to Black children when they are allowed to exercise options of choice and when their choices are acknowledged. Respect is shown to them when they are allowed to verbally express their thoughts and opinions, which are valued. Respect is shown to them when they are allowed to make decisions that affect their lives and when their decisions are valued. Respect is shown to children when they are allowed to be free and soar like eagles. When Black children receive recognition and respect for all that represents them individually and collectively, this type of recognition and respect make them feel esteemed. They come to view themselves as persons of worth. This does not mean that children should have choices about *everything* they do; instead, it means that many opportunities should be allowed for Black children to make choices. Decision making is an essential condition of growth and personal power.

Respect is not shown for children by deferential treatment, by rejection, by insincere praise, and by deception. Respect is shown Black children through interactions when teachers thoughtfully "hear" what they have to say. Respect is shown to Black children by listening to their messages and understanding what is being said and felt. Respect is shown through genuine treatment, compassion, and understanding.

Teachers can play an important role in building Black children's respect for themselves. These teachers are ones who develop trusting relationships with Black children. They are respected by Black children for their consistency, honesty, diplomacy, nurturing, and caring. They model self-respect and give respect. These teachers are able to empower Black children through accepting their differences and praising their worth. They shape the lives of Black children through genuine praise and recognition, and these teachers are remembered by Black children when they become adults. These teachers are powerful forces in shaping Black children into adults, and they are remembered for empowering them and respecting them as children. These teachers are also remembered for understanding how they felt, and how they were appreciated for who they were and what they did. These teachers asked Black students for their ideas and listened with interest; they valued their choices and opinions and used them in making important classroom decisions. When respect is shown for Black children, self-respect grows. Through self-respect, Black children are empowered.

In contrast to being respectful and building self-respect in Black children is being disrespectful to them and diminishing their will. Some teachers take advantage of Black children simply because they have the power and are physically larger. Other teachers believe that children are "to be told , to be shown, to be directed, to be controlled" in such a way that children are not allowed to express their opinions and share ideas; cannot explore and discover; cannot make choices; and cannot be free to grow. These teachers tend to believe this is the way to organize a classroom for learning and believe they have the right to do so because they are the *adult and teacher*. These teachers manipulate Black children and shape their behaviors so that they can do only what the teacher says they can do. These teachers exercise their power over them and by doing so disempower the children. These teachers are also powerful role models and they demonstrate to Black children how to behave with power over others (Wassermann 1987).

DEVELOPING POSITIVE SELF-IMAGES AND SELF-ESTEEM

By the age of three, if development has gone well, children have a sense of assurance about who they are and what they can do. They are old enough to have developed personalities and some ideas about things in their environment. Their sense of self will serve as an influence on their future development. Typical three-year-olds have also developed many stable views that will influence their involvement, their reactions to various stimuli, and their expectations of others. The child at age three may have already formed a sense of himself or herself as being attractive or ugly, good or bad, weak or strong. These self-views develop out of the interactions of the prior three years and, while they persist, they will strongly influence future interactions. The three-year-old child's sense of identity is quite pliable and susceptible to adult and peer influences during this period of development; therefore, his or her current self-concept can be reinforced and strengthened, or extended to include additional perspectives during preschool and early elementary school years (Lay-Dopyera & Dopyera 1993).

Self-concept as described by Kunjufu (1984) means the individual's understanding of the expectations of society and his peers and the kinds of behavior that the individual selects as a style of life. People discover who they are and what they are from the ways in which they have been treated by those who surround them in the process of growing up. In this regard, every person tries to be the kind of person that he or she thinks is expected by his or her environment. For example, when children are told and shown by their parents and teachers that they are *bright*, they try to meet this expectation and tend to achieve academically. In contrast, when parents and teachers indicate to children that they have very low expectations of them by their remarks and attitudes, the children perform at levels in keeping with the adult's estimates of their ability regardless of their true ability.

Many studies have been conducted that demonstrate the effects of teachers' expectations on the children in their classrooms (Clark 1965; Glasgow 1980; Rist 1977; Rosenthal & Jacobson 1968). These findings indicated that, where children are perceived as bright, articulate, and motivated, the children fulfill the prophecy of success. Where children are perceived as slow, dull, and unmotivated, they reproduce the behavior and attitudes that support negative teacher expectations.

Darder (1991) stated that in assessing the impact of teacher expectations on Black students, it is important to understand what Caroline H. Persell (1977) calls the "genesis of teacher expectations." The genesis of teacher expectations involves a number of essential factors.

> First, it includes the social context, which incorporates the prevailing social attitudes associated with race, class structure, and the social, political, and economic ideology.
>
> Second, teacher expectations are influenced by the specific pedagogical theories and conceptual frameworks, as well as educational structures and practices, instilled by teacher training programs. This category reflects the climate of expectations surrounding testing, tracking, and record-keeping.
>
> Third, crucial in the development of teacher expectations are the teacher's personal experiences related to race, education, and peer socialization.
>
> And fourth, teacher expectations are found to be significantly influenced by student characteristics such as race, class, appearance, behavior, and test performance. (p. 18)

According to Darder (1991), teachers' expectations function primarily as an unconscious mechanism that helps to explain their hegemonic function and their resistance to change. In view of this type of power and authority over students, teacher expectations related to poor and Black students can result in any of the following consequences:

- Teachers are more likely to hold negative expectations for poor and Black children than for middle-class White children.
- Teacher expectations are affected by testing and tracking procedures that are themselves biased against poor and Black children.
- It is precisely such negative information that suggests it is more potent in its consequences than positive expectations.
- Expectations are related to teacher behaviors and to student cognitive changes even when IQ and achievement are controlled.
- Given the less powerful position of poor and Black children in society, they appear to be more influenced by teacher expectations. (p.18)

In view of the power of teacher expectations, Rosenbaum (1976) places a strong emphasis on the question of how teachers' expectations affect the manner in which they allocate attention in the classroom. He says that the most important teacher bias is related to the distribution of attention.

> Ryan (1981) argues that teachers' expectations and attention that students receive or fail to receive greatly influences their level of achievement in the classroom. According to Darder (1991), recent studies of Ryan (1976, p. 134) have shown that, even when there is little substantial difference in the quantity of interaction between high-expectancy and low-expectancy groups, the qualitative differences are great. With students of whom they hold high expectations, teachers more often praise correct answers or "sustain" the interaction if the answer is incorrect—that is, they repeat or rephrase the question, give a clue, and in general try to get the student to continue to work toward a correct response. With pupils of whom they expect little, teachers are more inclined to accept correct answers with minimal praise and criticize incorrect answers. In addition, the teacher is much more likely to limit her or his interactions with these students to matters of class organization and discipline. (Ryan 1976, pp. 18–19)

With respect to socioeconomic influences on teachers' expectations, Persell (1977) observed that students who are at the bottom rungs of the social ladder are more likely to be influenced by teacher expectations than those from the upper and middle classes. As a result of these observations, it appears that Black students are much more likely to have their achievement negatively affected by negative teacher expectations. This type of structural dominance and negative expectations function together to depress the academic achievement of the majority of Black students while supporting the educational success of students from the dominant culture.

Teachers must recognize their damaging effects on students' self-esteem and change the manner in which they work with Black students in the classroom. Their pedagogy and negative experiences disempowers and erodes Black students' positive self-esteem. Cultural democracy is missing in classrooms, teachers' discourse, and practice.

The development of self-esteem begins to emerge from the very first contact the child has with his or her family. These early experiences during infancy and toddlerhood gradually develop an awareness of self, just as environmental experiences and maturation will shape the child's self-concept and self-esteem. The goal of parents and teachers should be that of enhancing the development of positive self-images and self-esteem in Black children by providing them positive experiences and positive Black role models.

The terms *self-esteem* and *self-image* are often used interchangeably. However, in this text, self-esteem is defined as *the opinion of oneself*; whereas self-image is defined as *a likeness symbol—a mental picture of oneself.* These concepts are closely related and one does affect the other. For example, the child with a highly favorable opinion of himself or herself will most likely have a positive mental picture of himself or herself. Self-image is thought to be more of a process or catalyst that affects self-esteem. In this chapter, the focus is on the relationship of self-esteem and self-image to Black students' performances in school.

Children are extremely sensitive to messages that are given to them directly and indirectly and verbally and nonverbally by teachers. They start learning and sensing how people really feel about them by the silent messages they receive. Children can feel rejection just like they can feel acceptance. They can feel negative racial attitudes that affect their self-image. A child's self-image is learned by looking at him- or herself through the "mirror" of society. As society looks back at the child, the child senses, feels, sees, and assigns meaning to whatever is positive and negative in his or her life.

The self-image of Black children has been historically unstable and volatile. This was evidenced in research conducted by Clark and Clark (1950) on negative and confused racial attitudes frequently expressed by Black children. The Black children who participated in the studies usually expressed a preference for White dolls and they rejected Black dolls. Clark concluded that by age five, Black children are aware of the fact that to be Black in contemporary American society is a mark of inferior status. Follow-up research studies by Goodman (1952) and Moreland (1962) confirmed Clark's findings.

In 1974, Poussaint reported that Black children had developed a greater self-esteem than reported in previous research findings. Research reported on self-image and self-esteem of Black children in the early 1970s showed that

Black youngsters in these studies preferred people of their own color to Whites. These results are encouraging and are probably a tribute to the "Black and Proud" movement by Blacks during the late 1960s and early 1970s. Self-esteem among Blacks reached an incredible high in America. Blacks felt empowered and defined themselves in positive terms—Black, beautiful, and proud. Standards of beauty were redefined by African Americans for African Americans based on their heritage and roots. Blacks saw themselves in the mirror and many liked what they saw and fully accepted what they saw for the first time.

This movement enlightened many Black parents about the importance of enhancing their children's self-esteem, self-image, and sense of empowerment. Most Black children were quite confused about their identity and double-consciousness. They were discovering their roots with pride while being mindful of satisfying the expectations of two cultures. DuBois (1969) described Black self-esteem, which is reflective of the dual socialization of Black children in America:

> This double-consciousness, this sense of always looking at one's self through the eye of others, of measuring one's soul by the tape of a world that looks on in amused contempt and pity. One ever feels his twoness—an American, a Negro; two souls, two thoughts, two unreconciled strivings, two warring ideals in one dark body, whose dogged strength alone keeps it from being torn asunder. (p. 45)

Self-esteem is one of the most important possessions a person can have. Self-esteem makes it possible for children to feel good about themselves, to believe in themselves, and to be proud of themselves. Self-esteem is courage, power, assertiveness, strength, and self-acceptance. Parents affect their childrens self-esteem by enhancing it or lowering it in what they say and how they say it to their children. For example, when parents say, *"You are a bad boy,"* the child has been criticized rather than the behavior. Many parents will say, *"You did a bad job"* or *"You are ugly when you act like that"* or *" Why can't you be a good boy?"* when talking to their children. These words can be devastating to the development of self-esteem in children. In many cases, long after the parents have forgotten what they said, children cling to the memories and feelings associated with those demeaning experiences. They remember as adults how terrible and worthless their parents made them feel and how, in some instances, they wished they could become invisible as children to avoid the pain.

Parents must take responsibility for developing positive self-esteem and self-images in their children. This can be done through nurturance. Nurturing means to love, take care of, develop, discipline, and support. Nurturing also means providing predictability and stability for children in the home. Just as parents feel they are deserving of respect, children should also be respected and valued. Just because children are physically smaller than adults does not mean that they are inferior human beings.

Unfortunately, some well-intentioned parents abuse their children emotionally and spiritually. These are parents who do not listen to or respect their children. These are parents who are typically too strict, quick to call names, lack expressions of love and affection, and criticize their children unmercifully. These parents are found in all cultural, racial, ethnic, and language groups. Their children's spirits are broken at a very young age and they seem delayed in social and emotional growth by the time they reach preschool.

Self-esteem is also influenced by the school. Performance in school is a by-product of self-esteem and high expectations. As mentioned throughout this book, teachers bring to school their own attitudes, beliefs, values, and biases. As a result, each classroom will likely reflect the cultural characteristics of the teacher and his or her style for interacting with students; thus, no two classrooms should be identical. However, most classrooms in America are very similar because the majority of teachers are White and reflect Eurocentric values and attitudes. In this respect, some teachers will enhance their students' self-esteem through positive interactions, respect, praise, and acceptance of each student for his or her uniqueness. These teachers can stimulate Black students to higher levels.

In contrast, there are teachers who are disrespectful, rude, and obnoxious toward Black students as described in Chapter 12. Some teachers actually appear to derive pleasure from making students feel uncomfortable, unsure, and devalued. These teachers are typically those who are quick to punish (not discipline) Black students, especially the boys, and the punishment usually exceeds the "crime." These teachers have a negative effect on the overall development of Black children—their psychological, intellectual, social, and emotional growth. These repeated negative experiences can cause students to feel angry toward and resistant to any authority. Although Black children are typically very resilient and can respond to a variety of "tough" situations and circumstances, some break emotionally when continuously taunted by teachers. In this respect, there are teachers who literally push Black students out of school and onto the streets. Then, the very same teachers wonder why some Black youths behave the way they do.

As we have witnessed throughout history, for most Black children, it takes only one person to genuinely care about them in order for their performance to improve. Many Black students have responded to a coach, teacher, teacher aide, or librarian who has shown them respect and believed in them. These role models adopted by the students often become their surrogate parents. The surrogate parents give emotional support, encouragement, praise, and respect. These Black students have someone who has high expectations for them and they work harder to achieve what is expected.

Historically, the Black church influenced Black children's self-esteem and social behavior. It is often said that both the church and the family can be credited for the survival of Black people during slavery (Kunjufu 1984). However, between 1950 and 1980 there was a declining influence. The University of Michigan conducted a survey in 1950 and again in 1980 in an attempt to try to determine the major influences on children. The findings are listed below.

1950	*1980*
(1) home	(1) home
(2) school	(2) peers
(3) church	(3) television
(4) peers	(4) school
(5) television	(5) church
(Kunjufu 1984, p. 17)	

These findings represent the declining influences of the church. What happened to the church? Why are children losing interest in the church? The answers to these questions vary, but people's responses to these questions are usually based on their own experiences. In general, the most frequent answers you are likely to hear from Blacks are: (1) The church is too passive; (2) the church keeps you on your knees praying instead of on your feet fighting; (3) Black people should not be worshipping and glorifying a "White man" meaning pictures and images of Jesus Christ; and (4) too many hypocrites occupy the church pews; they say one thing and do another. These are just a few reasons why some Black adults have chosen not to attend or send their children to church. Historically, the Black church has been the religious institution where religious, social, and educational activities occur for Blacks. It has been the *backbone* that held the Black community together through preaching, teaching, praising, and praying. For many Blacks, the church is their spiritual sustenance; it gives them courage, patience, and incredible inner strength.

The Black church has influenced and continues to influence the lives of many Black families. Black children who are actively involved in the church from childhood are affected by what they see, hear, and learn at church. Attending church is a way of life for many Black children; they internalize the values, images, and memories of positive church experiences and most remember them for life. These positive church experiences thus influence the decisions and choices they make during adolescence and adulthood. When church experiences are positive for young Black children, most will continue to view the Black church as an important part of their lives and will continue to attend church even after leaving home for college or careers. The Black church remains a positive institution for many Blacks. In most instances, Black children and adults can celebrate something positive that the church did for them, for example, building character, setting standards for behavior and/or developing self-confidence.

At the present time in our history, many Black children do not attend church because of many competing forces. For example, advanced technology has brought to Blacks entertainment devices such as electronic games, televisions, radios, videos, cassettes, computers, cars, and other devices so that many Black children prefer to be entertained than attend and participate in church activities. They typically find these electronic devices more interesting and stimulating than church services and Sunday school. Therefore, many may opt to stay home to be stimulated and entertained by turning a knob or switch. Television is not only a competitor with the church, it is a competitor with the family life of Black children. This should be of major concern to Black parents because television's images can have a positive or negative effect on Black children's' self-esteem and self-image. Unfortunately, the majority of images portrayed of Blacks on television are negative. For many Black children the impact of this "age of advanced technology" is contributing to their deteriorating interest in self, home, church, and school. This is a growing national problem affecting too many children and youth.

Black church attendance will likely continue to be on the decline until some strategies have been identified that will interest and attract Black children. It is worth the investment of time and energy of Black churches and community leaders to seek ways to actively involve Black children in meaningful activities and experiences that will benefit them, the church, and the community. If this challenge is not perceived as a priority for action in Black communities, more Black children will be lost.

PARENTS' INFLUENCE ON SELF-ESTEEM, SELF-DISCIPLINE, AND EMPOWERMENT

Parents are the first educators of their children, and the family is the primary agent of child socialization. This means that children are influenced in their individual and social development by a variety of factors. The family, peer relations, school, church, media, broader community, and society play an integral part in shaping children's personalities and equipping them with the skills necessary for social survival. Of these factors, the family is the most important influence through the socialization process. The socialization process begins when the child is born. The parents begin the process with the physical and emotional care and protection of their child. During this period, the parents' involvement and family experiences will shape the way their children will see themselves, the larger world, and their place in it. Culture is also transmitted to the child during the socialization process.

Family experiences and status's have a tremendous influence on the formation of the child's self-esteem and self-image. From birth forward, parents need to provide their children with consistent emotional support, love, affection, and encouragement in order to help them develop positive self-images and the confidence needed to deal effectively with the challenges and adversities of life (Sermones 1990). For young children, the family is the first social group of which they become members, and parents represent their first teachers, guides, and role models.

Many parents do not think of themselves as teachers. Most envision a teacher as being one who is formally trained and credentialed to teach in a classroom. Black parents are no exception to this perceived notion. Many Black parents do not realize how much they teach their child and influence their behaviors, literacy, and learning prior to their going to preschool and/or kindergarten. Likewise, many Black parents do not realize how much learning is taking place in the course of their day-to-day interactions with their children. Many parents are unaware of how these early years are critical in determining what the children will be like as adults.

PARENTAL INFLUENCE ON BLACK CHILD DEVELOPMENT

In this section, particular attention will focus on the importance of love, parenting challenges, interaction, praise, encouragement, predictability, consistency and discipline to empowerment of children. Parents can influence their child's overall development, empowerment, and school achievement by the type of early experiences children encounter prior to going to school.

Love

Children need unconditional love. Through the love of parents and family members the child learns how to love. Love is demonstrated through nurturing care and providing for the child's basic needs. Love is giving and advocating for the child's maximum growth potential—physically, emotionally, socially, and intellectually. Love is teaching the child about family beliefs, norms, values, symbols, artifacts, and means of communication that are significant to the family's identity and culture. Love is socializing the child to know what patterns of behavior are expected and those that are unacceptable. Love is teaching the child rules that will help guide, protect, and make him or her feel secure. Love is interacting with the child affectionately and listening to what he or she has to say. Love is enriching the child's language and cultural experiences to enable him or her to participate fully in meaningful ways in the home, community, and broader society. Love is modeling behaviors that parents expect of the child and praising him or her when attempts are made to imitate those behaviors. Love is strength, courage, and endurance. Love for the child should be always and everlasting.

Parenting Challenges

These are particularly sensitive times for Black parents in America—economically and emotionally. The portrayal of so many negatives by the media about Black children and families, as related to inappropriate conduct and crime, is probably as disturbing as the national unemployment and underemployment of Blacks. The media has been quite successful recently in giving the general public very negative impressions about Black adults and Black children—particularly Black males—as being primarily involved in unlawful conduct. These media images are very disturbing to most Black parents and the Black community because they know that the majority of Black children are *not* engaged in inappropriate or unlawful conduct. Such negativism reinforces negative perceptions and images of Black children by the American mainstream and corrupts the positive images and perceptions of other groups about Blacks. These unfair representations of Blacks by the media are just another example of racist practices that make it more difficult for Black parents to rear their children in a way that they will receive fair treatment and respect in America's schools and society.

Black parents are faced with major challenges. Most want to be outstanding parents and strive to be the best parents possible. Of course, no parents are perfect. However, even the outstanding Black parents have additional burdens placed upon them in their child-rearing practices that mainstream American White parents do not have to contend. They have to socialize their children to know how to live and survive in two cultures and two societies. They have to teach their children how to contain their aggression around Whites, while freely expressing it among Blacks. Although some people call this a survival technique, it is thought to contribute to Black-on-Black violence (Comer & Poussaint 1992).

Of all professions, parenting brings with it major responsibilities, joys, challenges, successes, and failures. For Black parents, raising healthy children in such an emotionally unhealthy society is becoming increasingly more difficult. The majority of Black parents know that positive parenting is essential to the development of physically, socially, and emotionally healthy children, and also understand the importance of providing their children with as many diversified experiences as possible to discover talents and interests. They also know that parenting is a full-time responsibility and involves double-duty child rearing to influence and shape the behaviors and lives of their children. This is a very demanding profession for which most "parent practitioners" have not been trained.

Most Black parents (as well as others) learn parenting skills by trial and error with their first-born. Unfortunately, parenting and child development classes are not offered in schools prior to students' high school graduation. Parenting is a very important "profession" in which most students have an interest and most pursue at some time in their lives. In spite of the fact that parenting is learned by doing, research indicates that first-born children tend to receive more attention, affection, and discipline than children born later. These first-borns also tend to become higher achievers than their siblings who tend to be more relaxed and sociable (Dunn & Kendrick 1983; Forer 1976). For example, first-born children tend to earn better grades in school, score higher on IQ tests, and appear more likely to go to college. In this regard, Black parents are encouraged to repeat the love and care given to the first-born to all the later-born siblings. They should also try to practice parenting skills that show love for their child. Some of these parenting characteristics are:

- Try to remain calm and in control.
- Be kind and loving to your children.
- Exercise discipline not punishment.
- Do not be too busy for your children.
- Be positive, optimistic, and realistic with your children.
- Respond to your children positively verbally and nonverbally.

Interaction

Interaction means communication. Black parents do communicate with their children. However, their communication style is different from that of the White mainstream. Black families socialize their children so they will learn the forms and functions of language that will help them achieve some degree of self-identity as a group member and also to meet the needs of everyday interactions. Anthropologists, social historians, and folklorists have detailed the long-standing rich verbal forms of African American rhymes, stories, music, sermons, and joking (Folb 1980; Hannerz 1969; Levine 1977; Smitherman 1970; Whitten & Szwed 1970). Black parents wishing to enhance their children's opportunities for greater academic success need to add to their current practices many opportunities for the children to tell what they know and not just show what they know. Although parents traditionally interact with their children through storytelling, it is just as important for them to read to the children as it is to tell stories. Introduce books and other materials with print and encourage their reading by listening to them and modeling reading behaviors. Encourage the child to scribble and draw pictures about stories and other events. Talk to and listen to the child. Parent-child communication will increase the child's understanding of language and how it works, as well as increase the children's vocabulary and comprehension. Ask children questions that are open-ended that will encourage language elaboration instead of "yes" and "no" responses. These type of ongoing parent-child interactions will enhance the child's language development and emerging literacy, build self-esteem, and improve chances for school success.

Praise

Praise means to congratulate, approve, adore, build up, dignify, honor, compliment. Black children need to be acknowledged in their efforts to grow as independent, healthy individuals, while at the same time they need to comply with parents', relatives', and peer expectations about standards of behavior. This is quite a challenge for most children because they want to please everyone. It is very important from birth through adulthood to give praise. Parents' verbal praise and demonstrations of affection provide direction for the child and enhances self-esteem. The child should be praised for his or her sincere efforts as well as his or her accomplishments. Children need to hear and see their parents' pride in them through verbal praise, for example, "You did a great job, I am so proud of you" and/or physical expressions such as a hug, kiss on the cheek, or pat on the back. Praise inspires and encourages children just as it does adults. For many Black parents, praise means buying or giving the child something materialistic. This practice is highly discouraged because social praise that is internalized by the child will have much longer lasting effects. In addition, children should not be reared to expect something each time they behave in ways considered appropriate and expected by their parents and society. Praise represents words from the heart that are likely to have lasting effects on the souls and psyches of Black children through adulthood. Praise is an essential ingredient in rearing healthy, happy, and empowered children.

Encouragement

To encourage children means to stimulate, help, support and promote them. Black children need a great deal of encouragement from parents, relatives, friends, and teachers. They need to know that there are people who strongly believe in them and believe that they can achieve. They need encouragement in their efforts to succeed in everything they do from infancy through adulthood. Encouragement energizes the spirit and mind even when the body is tired. Black children need to hear that they *can* achieve in this society. They need encouragement to help them sustain their efforts in performing tasks at home and at school. Black parents need to be there to support their children and help promote their personal and professional goals and aspirations. Black parents need to advocate strongly for their children and their children's education. Black parents who are visible and vocal in the schools as advocates for their children *do* make a difference. School principals and teachers usually respond favorably to Black parents who are assertive and make it clear what they want for their children. Parents, who are owners of the public schools, cannot afford to forfeit their powers and rights to teachers and administrators. Black parents must get involved in their children's education. Parental involvement makes a strong statement of encouragement and genuine caring for children, as well as a statement to schools about the need and importance of involving parents from the community in reforming schools.

Predictability and Consistency

Predictability means to be able to anticipate, foresee, or express an outcome in advance; consistency means constancy and regularity. Many Black children do not have predictability or consistency in their lives. From the time a child is born, it is dependent upon the environment (parents) for its care. Soon after birth, the child begins to experience routines in the hospital and at home. Schedules evolve for feedings, sleeping, bathing, changing, and interacting with the family. Most babies adapt to these schedules, which usually become fairly routine. As an infant, the internal clock also seems to adapt to the schedule. This is noticeable when you hear parents say, "My baby is really on schedule, he wakes up on schedule for feedings and changing." These routines of basic care and nurturing by the parents become predictable events in the infant's daily life. If the baby cries, someone will usually respond; the baby is picked up, fed, changed and/or interacted with. This predictability provides the child with a deep sense of security. This type of predictability is important to rearing healthy children. Many young children who are abandoned by their parents or primary caregivers do not thrive. Young children who seriously lack predictability in their lives or are abandoned tend to suffer tremendous emotional pain and usually find it difficult to feel secure or trust people even as adults. In this regard, Black children need predictability in their lives. They need to know what the household schedules are for home—mealtimes, study time, bath time, bed time, play time, and so on. Being able to anticipate the order of events brings order to the child's life. This is not to suggest that children should be reared on a rigid schedule; instead, children should be reared to know what comes next. Daily routines provide direction, internal control, and security for children.

Discipline

The term discipline comes from the word *disciple (believer, follower)*. This can be translated to mean that the parents are the leaders and their children are the believers and followers. In this event, discipline can be thought of as the ways in which the leaders (parents) are able to motivate and teach the followers (children) rules and regulations for desired behaviors. In this process of teaching the followers, the parents should always remember that children need to be disciplined with love and sincerity. They need to have clearly defined limits and rules for their own security, safety, and well-being. The limits and rules should be reinforced so that the child and parents can feel safe and secure. Children are in danger if they are not taught limits and rules that they are expected to follow.

Discipline is an area of child rearing where many parents have difficulty. Most parents make mistakes trying to handle discipline problems. Of the various discipline techniques used by parents, the ten worst discipline techniques have been identified by Windell (1991), a psychotherapist specializing in family problems. All are ineffective and frequently lead to emotional and behavioral problems in young people. Parents using these techniques are encouraged to stop these "bad" parenting habits and to use alternative discipline techniques that will work for them and their children. The ten worst techniques are:

- Physical Abuse—beating, hitting, slapping, punching, and otherwise physically attacking children.
- Coercion—forcing a child to do something when a child does not comply with the parent's wishes or demands.
- Yelling—yelling does not work, yet so many parents do it. The only way yelling might work is if children dislike hearing their parents raise their voices.
- Demanding Immediate Compliance—this techniques is very closely associated with yelling. Children, like adults, resent being ordered around; therefore, to keep their feelings of self-respect intact, they do not comply immediately when ordered around.
- Nagging—this technique is one of the most ineffective discipline techniques. This technique usually leads to yelling and force. Parents who nag usually do not know how else to get their children to do what they want them to do.
- Lecturing and Advice Giving—giving lectures and sermons to children as a means of discipline is usually a "turn off" for most of them, especially teenagers. They prefer to have parents listen to them and try to understand what they are experiencing.
- Taking Anger out on Children—this technique involves giving an extra dose of anger, criticism, or punishment due to the parent's pressures,

frustrations, disappointments, or difficulties not necessarily related to the child. In these instances, parents will likely say or do things out of proportion to the child's offense.

- Shaming and Belittling—making children feel inadequate, less intelligent, and insecure by putting them down. Shaming them with statements like, "Why are you acting like a baby?" Or, making them feel less intelligent with such statements as, "That's one of the dumbest things you have ever done," or "You are really stupid." Creating anxiety and insecurity by threatening to leave the child with this type of statement, "If you don't stop now, I will leave and never come back," or, "I've had it with you, when you wake up tomorrow morning, I will not be here." These discipline techniques destroy children and should not be used. Instead of making the child strong, these techniques make them emotionally weak and insecure.

- Setting traps—this is a popular technique used by autocratic parents with high expectations. These parents set traps for their children; that is, when they know the child has failed to live up to a certain requirement or rule, they will ask the child if he or she followed the rule or met the requirement. They wait for the child to lie or try to wiggle out of the situation. These parents cause children to become rebellious liars and learn to mistrust any questions asked of them by others. This causes serious communication and relationship problems for these children.

- Imposing Excessive Guilt—by making children feel responsible for the parents' well-being. For example, making the child feel guilty because a parent is an alcohol or drug-abusing parent. In situations like this, a child can be made to feel guilty about marital problems, parents' stress, hard work, and so on. In other words, "If it were not for you, I would not drink" or, "You drive your father to drink" or, " You caused your mother to leave us." Imposing excessive guilt on children for adult (parent) problems is unfair, unhealthy and will likely result in emotional problems for the child later. (pp. 15–26)

Most parents want their children to be happy, productive, and well-adjusted children and adults. In order to have a child who is productive and happy, the child needs to have a positive sense of self-worth. In order for children to have self-confidence and motivation, they must like themselves. Parents can contribute to their childrens self-worth and self-esteem by being good, competent disciplinarians—giving guidance and being positive at the same time. This requires that discipline begins at birth and be related to love and nurturing, and that parents have a healthy respect for their children and their needs at all developmental levels (Windell 1991).

Windell (1991) describes parents who use excessive discipline and bad parenting practices with children as qualifying for the Hall of Shame. Alternative practices can be used to foster self-control, enhance self-concept, encourage desired behaviors, and prevent early and later problems in children.

To begin, parenting is a very challenging profession for which most parents have never received formal training in how to be a parent or how to discipline children effectively. Therefore, most parents use discipline techniques that were used with them by their parents, or they come up with discipline techniques on the spot when needed. In either case, parents often worry about what constitutes appropriate discipline and how to cope with discipline challenges.

Parents can begin practicing effective discipline techniques by setting limits and teaching rules to their children between the first and second year. Rules protect children, give a sense of security, ensure a sense of order, and play an important part in discipline. Rules should start very early and be few, simple, clear, understandable, and age-appropriate.

Parents should be very clear about their reason for rules and use appropriate consequences to enforce rules. The consequences should be reasonable and fair. Consequences for infractions should not result in overreactions by parents to relatively minor offenses. Instead, parents should acknowledge that consequences are not always needed. Sometimes children forget the rule and simply need to be reminded.

Rules are usually established by parents to encourage desired behaviors and safety. In this regard, children are more likely to cooperate with rules if they understand the reasons given for them. However, if there are too many rules governing every aspect of their life, children will likely give up on all the rules.

Desired behaviors in children are often achieved by parents when they use the following techniques:

- Give praise and attention to children. Find time each day to focus on your child's behavior; give praise and positive attention to acknowledge the behaviors that are desired. Do not focus only on negative behaviors; instead, accentuate the positives. Say something positive about behaviors you like; this lets children know what behaviors are desired. Parents should make an effort to notice and acknowledge desired and appropriate behaviors each day. To make sure praise works, parents should watch for desired behaviors; then, shower the children with sincere praise. Tell your children how proud you are of them and for completing desired tasks without being told.
- Express appreciation for their help. Say "thank you, for your help, you did a great job."
- Model ethical behaviors and language. Parents are models for their children. Children carefully observe their parents behaviors, for instance, how they walk, talk, interact with others, and use language. Therefore,

parents should model the type of behaviors they expect from their children. When parents use physical abuse (beating, hitting, slapping) in an effort to curb undesired behaviors, they are telling their children that the use of physical abuse is an acceptable way to obtain compliance. Contradictions of this type in parent behaviors and expected child behaviors often cause confusion and breed contempt in children. In addition to physical abuse, children should not be emotionally abused by parents who resort to yelling profanities and coercing them to comply with their demands just because they "said so." Children respond best to positive, friendly, and encouraging words.

- Parents should not take their anger out on their children. Due to demands and pressures related to parenting and basic day-to-day survival, many parents take out their anger and frustrations on their children. In these instances, children often believe they are the cause of their parent's anger or frustration. Parents should not make children feel responsible or guilty about their well-being. Instead, parents should take responsibility for themselves and their behaviors. When they are angry or frustrated because of something totally unrelated to their children, they should divert their time and attention away from the children onto something else for a while, preferably something relaxing and fun. Interaction with the children should begin when the parents can clearly and calmly focus on their children in an attentive manner.
- Imposed guilt on children is unfair and unhealthy. If it is not controlled, the child may suffer from emotional problems later.

Black children, when reared with love, respect, support, encouragement, praise, appropriate discipline, and role models by parents will have the basic foundation to achieve in school, their community, and society. They know who they are and what they can do. They are centered, self-assured, self-disciplined, and socially competent. They are Black, they are proud, and they are empowered.

SUMMARY

Parents and teachers have a major impact on the development of self-esteem, self-image and self-discipline in Black children. Parents can enhance their child's sense of empowerment through love, support, praise, encouragement and modeling appropriate behaviors while enabling the child to make choices about his or her life.

Teachers can enhance self-esteem in Black children by respecting them as individuals, which means respecting their culture and their language. Teachers who are genuinely concerned about education equity and excellence for

Black children will ensure that their classroom incorporates their language and cultural experiences in the curriculum. Teachers will also ensure that Black children are centered in the classroom through curricular experiences to enhance their pride and discover inner strength and sense of freedom. The goal of parents and teachers should be that of enhancing the development of positive self-images and self-esteem by providing encouragement, praise, support, and respect.

Black students who are loved and respected at home, and respected and centered in the classroom in their own cultural information, will likely result in students who are self-disciplined, perform better academically, and are more motivated for school work. These students will have self-respect and feelings of empowerment. They will be proud of themselves and their heritage.

It is critical to the educational and social-emotional outcome of African American children that parents and teachers begin to collaborate and work together. They are responsible for enhancing or impeding the development of ability, confidence, desire of knowledge, respect and honor of differences. The home-school teaching and learning conflicts must be resolved in a genuine spirit of solidarity and within the context of a multicultural society.

Some strategies that can assist in building or strengthening parent-teacher relationships and the empowerment of African American children are listed below.

PRACTICAL APPLICATIONS

1. Teachers can consciously work toward developing culturally democratic classrooms that will allow *all* students to participate freely with others as they learn.
2. Teachers need to become more aware of and sensitive to how they use their power to control and influence children's behaviors and self-image.
3. Teachers should be prepared to teach in culturally diverse schools. Traditional teacher preparation and training programs are not prepared to deal with the changing education and schooling needs of Black and other diverse students. (Read DeVillar, Faltis, and Cummins 1994, pp. 109–110)
4. Teachers need to recognize that parents, regardless of race, language, and income, are the primary influence on their children's growth and development. Work with parents to achieve a balance between personalism and professionalism in order to minimize cultural dissonance.
5. Teachers need to be sensitive and understanding of African American parents' wants for their children; most want them to achieve education, economic, and social success, but they do not want them to have to learn to act White to do so.

6. Teachers need to know how to use the students' cultures to help them achieve academic success and promote cooperative and collaborative learning opportunities among students. Discuss strategies for accomplishing this task with other teachers.
7. Teachers should consciously become aware of how they demonstrate and verbalize belief in their students.
8. Teachers should remember that teaching context is very important to pedagogy and student success. What may work in a suburban middle-class school may fail miserably in an urban, predominately Black school, or vice versa.
9. African American parents need to be supportive of their children and advocate strongly for their educational rights, aspirations, and goals.
10. African American parents need to become more actively involved in their children's education by initiating contact with teachers, expressing their thoughts and concerns, making teachers aware of their educational issues and priorities.

REFERENCES

Asante, M. K. (December 1991/January 1992). Afrocentric curriculum. *Educational Leadership December*, 49(4):28–31.

Barnes, D. (1976). *From communication to curriculum*. Harmondsworth, Middlesex: Penguin.

Chomsky, C. (1981). Write now, read late. In C. Cazden (ed.), *Language in early childhood education* (2nd ed). Washington, DC: National Association for the Education of Young Children.

Clark, K. (1965). *Dark Ghetto: Dilemmas of Social Power*. New York: Harper & Row.

Clark, K., & Clark, M. (Summer 1950). Emotional factors in racial identification and reference in Negro children. *Journal of Negro Education*, 19(3):341–350.

Comer, J. P., & Poussaint, A. F. (1992). *Raising Black Children*. New York: Penguin Group.

Cummins, J. (1988). From multicultural to anti-racist education. In *Empowering Minority Students*. Sacramento California Association for Bilingual Education.

Cummins, J. (1989). *Empowering minority students*. Sacramento: California Association for Bilingual Education.

Cummins, J. (1986). Empowering minority students: A framework for intervention. *Harvard Educational Review*, 58:18:36.

Darder, A. (1991). *Culture and power in the classroom*. Westport: Bergin & Garvey.

DeVillar, R., Faltis, C., & Cummins, J. (1994). *Cultural Diversity in Schools: From Rhetoric to Practice*. Albany: State University of New York Press.

DuBois, W. E. B. (1969). *The Soul of Black Folks*. New York: New American Library.

Dunn, J., & Kendrick, C. (January 1983). Sibling quarrels and maternal responses. *Developmental Psychology*, 19 (1):62–70.

Folb, E. A. (1980). *Runnin' down Some Lines: The Language and Culture of Black Teenagers.* Cambridge, MA: Harvard University Press.

Forer, L. (1976). *The Birth Order Factor: How Your Personality Is Influenced by Your Place in the Family.* New York: D. McKay.

Glasgow, D. (1980). *The Black Underclass.* New York: Random House.

Goodman, K. S., & Goodman, Y. M. (1978). Learning about psycholinguistic processes by analyzing oral reading. *Harvard Educational Review,* 47:317–333.

Goodman, M. (1952). *Race Awareness in Young Children.* Cambridge, MA: Addison-Wesley.

Graves, D. (1983). *Writing: Children and Teachers at Work.* Exeter, NH: Heinemann.

Hannerz, U. (1969). *Soulside: Inquiries into Ghetto Culture and Community.* New York: Columbia University Press.

Kunjufu, J. (1984). *Developing Positive Self-Images & Discipline in Black Children.* Chicago, IL: African American Images.

Lay-Dopyera, M., & Dopyera, J. (1993). *Becoming a Teacher of Young Children.* New York: McGraw-Hill.

Levine, L. W. (1977). *Black Culture and Black Consciousness: Afro-American Folk Thought from Slavery to Freedom.* New York: Oxford University Press.

Lindfors, J. W. (1980). *Children's Language and Learning.* Englewood Cliffs, NJ: Prentice Hall.

Moreland, K. (1962). Racial acceptance and preference of nursery school children in a southern city *Merrill-Palmer Quarterly of Behavior and Development,* 8:279.

Persell, C. H. (1977). *Education and Inequality.* New York: Free Press.

Poussaint, A. F. (August, 1994). Building a strong self-image in the Black child. *Ebony Magazine,* 29.

Rist, R. (1977). *The Urban School: A Factory of Failure.* Boston: MIT Press.

Rosenbaum, J. (1976). *Making Inequality.* New York: Wiley Interscience.

Rosenthal, R., & Jacobson, L. (1968). *Pygmalion in the Classroom.* New York: Holt, Rinehart & Winston.

Ryan, W. (1976). *Blaming the Victim.* New York: Vintage Books.

Ryan, W. (1981). *Equality.* New York: Pantheon Books.

Sermones, J. K. (1990). *Sociology: A Core Text.* Fort Worth, TX: Holt, Rinehart and Winston.

Smith, F. (1979). *Understanding Reading* (2nd Ed). New York: Holt, Rinehart and Winston.

Smitherman, G. (1977). *Talkin' and Testifyin': The Language of Black America.* Boston: Houghton Mifflin.

Wassermann, S. (April 1987). Enabling children to develop personal power through building self-respect. *Childhood Education,* 63(4):293–294.

Wells, G. (1986). *The Meaning Makers: Children Learning Language and Using Language to Learn.* Portsmouth, NH: Heinemann.

Whitten, N. E., Jr., & Szwed, J. F. (1970). *Afro-American Anthropology: Contemporary Perspectives.* New York: Free Press.

Windell, J. (1991). *Discipline: A Sourcebook of 50 Failsafe Techniques for Parents.* New York: Macmillan.

INDEX